Brain Injury and Pediatric Cardiac Surgery

Brain Injury and Pediatric Cardiac Surgery

Richard A. Jonas, M.D.

William E. Ladd Professor of Surgery, Harvard Medical School;
Cardiovascular Surgeon in Chief, Department of Cardiac Surgery,
Children's Hospital, Boston

Jane W. Newburger, M.D., M.P.H.

Associate Professor of Pediatrics, Harvard Medical School; Senior Associate
in Cardiology, Department of Cardiology, Children's Hospital, Boston

Joseph J. Volpe, M.D.

Bronson Crothers Professor of Neurology, Harvard Medical School;
Neurologist-in-Chief, Department of Neurology, Children's Hospital,
Boston

Foreword by
John W. Kirklin, M.D.
Professor of Surgery, University of Alabama at Birmingham

Butterworth–Heinemann

Boston • Oxford • Melbourne • Singapore • Toronto • Munich • New Delhi • Tokyo

Every effort has been made to ensure that the drug dosage
schedules within this text are accurate and conform to standards
accepted at time of publication. However, as treatment recommendations vary in the light of continuing research and clinical
experience, the reader is advised to verify drug dosage schedules
herein with information found on product information sheets.
This is especially true in cases of new or infrequently used drugs.

∞ Recognizing the importance of preserving what has been written,
Butterworth–Heinemann prints its books on acid-free paper
whenever possible.

Library of Congress Cataloging-in-Publication Data

Brain injury and pediatric cardiac surgery / [edited by] Richard A.
    Jonas, Jane W. Newburger, Joseph J. Volpe ; foreword by John W.
    Kirklin.
      p.   cm.
    Includes bibliographical references and index.
    ISBN 0–7506–9567–6 (alk. paper)
    1. Congenital heart disease in children—Surgery—Complications.
2. Brain damage. 3. Infants—Surgery. I. Jonas, Richard A.
II. Newburger, Jane W. III. Volpe, Joseph J.
[DNLM: 1. Brain Injuries—in infancy & childhood. 2. Brain-
–surgery. 3. Heart Surgery—in infancy & childhood. WS 340 B8138
1995]
RD598.B6928   1995
617.4′12′0083—dc20
DNLM/DLC
for Library of Congress   95–40257
                                                 CIP

British Library Cataloguing-in-Publication Data

A catalogue record for this book is available from the British
Library.

The publisher offers discounts on bulk orders of this book.
For information, please write:

Manager of Special Sales
Butterworth–Heinemann
313 Washington Street
Newton, MA 02158-1626

10 9 8 7 6 5 4 3 2 1

Printed in the United States of America

Contents

Contributing Authors

Mitsuru Aoki, M.D.
Assistant in Pediatric Cardiovascular Surgery, Tokyo Women's Medical College; Associate in Pediatric Cardiovascular Surgery, Department of Pediatric Cardiovascular Surgery, Heart Institute of Japan, Tokyo Women's Medical College, Tokyo

David Bellinger, Ph.D., M.Sc.
Associate Professor of Neurology, Harvard Medical School; Research Associate, Department of Neurology, Children's Hospital, Boston

David A. Benaron, M.D.
Director, Biomedical Optics Group and Assistant Professor of Pediatric/Neonatal Optics Group, Department of Pediatrics and Hansen Experimental Physics Laboratory, Stanford University School of Medicine; Attending Neonatologist, Lucile Salter Packard Children's Hospital, Neonatal Intensive Care, Palo Alto, CA

Frederick A. Burrows, M.D., FRCP(C)
Associate Professor of Anaesthesia, Harvard Medical School; Co-Director of Cardiac Anesthesia Service, Department of Anesthesia, Children's Hospital, Boston

Adre J. du Plessis, M.D., M.P.H.
Assistant Professor of Neurology, Harvard Medical School; Assistant in Neurology, Department of Neurology, Children's Hospital, Boston

William J. Greeley, M.D.
Associate Professor of Anesthesiology and Pediatrics and Division Chief, Division of Pediatric Cardiac Anesthesia and Critical Care Medicine, Duke University Medical Center, Durham, NC

Sandra L. Helmers, M.D.
Assistant Professor of Neurology, Harvard Medical School; Assistant in Neurology, Department of Neurology, Children's Hospital, Boston

Paul R. Hickey, M.D.
Associate Professor of Anaesthesia, Harvard Medical School; Anesthesiologist-in-Chief, Department of Anesthesia, Children's Hospital, Boston

Gregory L. Holmes, M.D.
Associate Professor of Neurology, Harvard Medical School; Director, Division of Clinical Neurophysiology and Epilepsy, Department of Neurology, Children's Hospital, Boston

David Holtzman, M.D.
Associate Professor of Neurology, Children's Hospital and Harvard Medical School, Boston

H. Robert Horvitz, Ph.D.
Professor of Biology, Massachusetts Institute of Technology; Investigator, Department of Biology, Howard Hughes Medical Institute, Cambridge; Neurobiologist, Department of Neurology, and Geneticist, Department of Medicine, Massachusetts General Hospital, Boston

Frances E. Jensen, M.D.
Assistant Professor of Neurology, Harvard Medical School; Attending in Neurology, Department of Neurology, Children's Hospital, Boston

Michael V. Johnston, M.D.
Professor of Neurology and Pediatrics, Johns Hopkins University School of Medicine; Attending Physician, Departments of Neurology and Pediatrics, Johns Hopkins Hospital and Kennedy Krieger Children's Hospital, Baltimore

Richard A. Jonas, M.D.
William E. Ladd Professor of Surgery, Harvard Medical School; Cardiovascular Surgeon in Chief, Department of Cardiac Surgery, Children's Hospital, Boston

Karl C. K. Kuban, M.D., S.M., Epi
Assistant Professor of Neurology, Harvard Medical School and Children's Hospital, Boston

Stuart A. Lipton, M.D., Ph.D.
Associate Professor Neurology (Neuroscience), Harvard Medical School; Director, Laboratory of Cellular and Molecular Neuroscience, Children's Hospital; Senior Associate in Neurology, Beth Israel Hospital; Associate in

Neurology, Children's Hospital and Brigham and Women's Hospital; Clinical Associate in Neurology, Massachusetts General Hospital, Boston

Jane W. Newburger, M.D., M.P.H.
Associate Professor of Pediatrics, Harvard Medical School; Senior Associate in Cardiology, Department of Cardiology, Children's Hospital, Boston

Leonard A. Rappaport, M.D.
Assistant Professor of Pediatrics, Harvard Medical School; Associate Chief, General Pediatrics, Department of Medicine, Children's Hospital, Boston

Julie A. Swain, M.D.
Chief, Division of Cardiovascular Surgery, University of Nevada School of Medicine, Las Vegas

S. Ted Treves, M.D.
Professor of Radiology, Harvard Medical School; Chief, Division of Nuclear Medicine, Department of Radiology, Children's Hospital, Boston

Miles Tsuji, M.D.
Instructor in Pediatrics, Joint Program in Neonatology, Harvard Medical School; Attending Neonatologist, Department of Newborn Medicine, Brigham and Women's Hospital, Boston

Robert C. Vannucci, M.D.
Professor of Pediatrics, The Pennsylvania State University of Medicine; Chief of Pediatric Neurology, The M.S. Hershey Medical Center, Hershey

Joseph J. Volpe, M.D.
Bronson Crothers Professor of Neurology, Harvard Medical School; Neurologist-in-Chief, Department of Neurology, Children's Hospital, Boston

David L. Wessel, M.D.
Associate Professor of Pediatric Anaesthesia, Harvard Medical School; Director of Cardiac Intensive Care, Department of Cardiac Intensive Care, Children's Hospital, Boston

David Wypij, Ph.D.
Assistant Professor of Biostatistics, Harvard School of Public Health, Boston

Foreword

Since Bigelow's pioneering work with hypothermia and Charles Drew's use of it in 1959 to ameliorate the potentially damaging effects of total circulatory arrest, arguments have raged as to whether circulatory arrest associated with cardiopulmonary bypass does or does not produce brain damage. Although intuitions indicated that if long enough it surely would, some groups attempted to discount this possibility when the circulatory arrest was associated with profound hypothermia. In my opinion, it was this specific continuing controversy that led to the epochal randomized trial begun at the Boston Children's Hospital in 1988. Again, in my opinion, it was this trial and the world-wide circumstances related to the controversy that generated the broader subject of brain injury and pediatric cardiac surgery.

The editors of this authoritative book, Richard Jonas, Jane Newburger, and Joseph Volpe, were primary movers in both the remarkable randomized trial and in all of the interest and information that appears to have followed it. The editors, in addition to contributing important chapters themselves, have stimulated other experts to write important chapters. Together, the authors have made monumental contributions to a field that has for too long been little explored by true experts in multiple disciplines. Clearly, careful reading of the text will be rewarding for both clinicians and basic scientists.

John W. Kirklin

Preface

Undoubtedly the greatest tragedy for the pediatric cardiac surgical team is to conduct what appears to be a technically flawless procedure only to find that their young patient has suffered profound brain injury. Society has agreed with the extent of this tragedy by awarding some of the largest financial awards seen in medical malpractice courts to the families of brain injured children. Perhaps what should be of equal or even greater concern to those of us working in this field is the possibility that current-day methods of brain protection used routinely during cardiac surgery are inflicting subtle degrees of brain injury on all our patients. Until recently these issues were over-shadowed by the challenge of achieving survival for children with many of the congenital cardiac anomalies. With the advent of modern cardiopul-monary bypass methods, new surgical techniques, and the introduction of prostaglandin E1, most of the survival challenge has been met. Undoubtedly fear of malpractice liability has inhibited many of us from opening this potential Pandora's box. But now the time has come when this area must be systematically investigated.

This book is an attempt to focus upon the issues that seem to us to be most relevant to the problem of brain injury as it relates to children undergoing cardiac surgery. It is in part based upon a conference held at Children's Hospital, Boston, in October 1993, in which investigators from a number of different fields were invited to present their perspective on the problem. It also has allowed us to bring together in a single format the background, methods, results, and inferences derived from our own ran-domized clinical study comparing deep hypothermic circulatory arrest and low-flow continuous cardiopulmonary bypass. The study, like this book and the conference at Children's, reinforces the overriding importance of interdisciplinary collaboration if the problem of brain damage related to cardiac surgery in children is to be both understood and prevented.

We would like to thank the many people who have contributed their time and effort to this book. We thank our many outstanding contributors, including many colleagues at Children's, who were willing to take time away from their numerous other academic responsibilities to prepare their chapters. At Butterworth-Heinemann, Susan Pioli provided essential initial support while continuing editorial guidance has been provided by Cynthia Carlson and Michelle St. Jean-Richards. Laura Young worked tirelessly in assembling and unifying many varied text formats. Most especially, we thank our EEG technicians, lab technicians, nursing staff, perfusionists, respiratory therapists, research and clinical fellows, and residents, who have been a constant source of ideas and inspiration through their curiosity and questioning of accepted dogma.

Richard A. Jonas
Jane W. Newburger
Joseph J. Volpe

CHAPTER 1

Brain Injury and Infant Cardiac Surgery: Overview

Joseph J. Volpe

Introduction

Brain injury and the neurological morbidity related to such injury are important phenomena observed in infants who have undergone cardiac surgery. The modern era of cardiac surgery has been characterized by correction of serious cardiac defects earlier and earlier in infancy; correction in the neonatal period is now common. Despite the application of such complex surgery to small, sick, labile infants, mortality rates have been strikingly low. Thus, the absolute number of surviving infants with brain injury and subsequent neurological morbidity in this setting can be expected to increase. Prevention of this brain injury will require understanding of its basic nature, pathogenesis, and timing.

This introduction will focus on the magnitude of the problem, the neuropathology and the neurology in the human infant, and the pathogenesis. Rational formulations for prevention of this brain injury will follow.

Magnitude of the Problem

The magnitude of this problem relates directly to the large number of affected infants. Thus, approximately 10,000 infants are born every year in the United States with congenital heart disease that is serious enough to require surgery early in life. Although the estimates of brain injury observed following such surgery vary considerably from study to study and according to the outcome measure, incidences are approximately 10% to 30%.[1-11] Thus, there are very large absolute numbers of affected infants yearly.

TABLE 1–1
Neurological Sequelae in Infants after Cardiac Surgery

- Cognitive deficits
- Seizures (acute > chronic)
- Choreoathetosis
- Spastic quadriparesis
- Bilateral motor deficits
  Spastic diplegia
  Spastic quadriparesis
- Hemiparesis

Neurological Features

Although our understanding of the neurology of brain injury associated with infant cardiac surgery is incomplete, the major neurological deficits observed have been cognitive deficits, seizures, choreoathetosis, bilateral motor deficits, and hemiparesis (Table 1–1). Cognitive deficits of various types are most common. Seizures are relatively common, primarily as an acute event. Choreoathetosis, which is somewhat less common, is also principally an acute event. Bilateral motor deficits, however, are more commonly chronic sequelae. The two major types to be recognized are spastic diplegia, in which lower extremities are affected more than upper extremities, and spastic quadriparesis, in which the extremities are affected approximately equally, perhaps upper more than lower. Finally, a substantial minority of affected infants have unilateral motor deficits, particularly spastic hemiparesis. Overall, of the long-term sequelae, the principal neurological features are cognitive deficits, bilateral motor deficits, and hemiparesis.

Neuropathological Features

The neuropathological substrates for the neurological features just described are understood only incompletely.[12–17] Based on the experience at Children's Hospital, Boston, and also as reported elsewhere, the most common neuropathological lesion is periventricular leukomalacia. Selective neuronal necrosis is probably the next most common lesion. Focal and multifocal ischemic brain necrosis, i.e., stroke-like pathology, and parasagittal cerebral injury are somewhat less common.

Pathogenesis

The central theme in pathogenesis appears to be ischemia (Figure 1–1). This pathogenetic theme includes also reperfusion injury following ischemia.

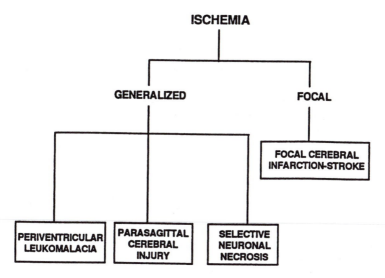

FIGURE 1–1.   Relation of generalized and focal ischemia to the major neuropathology observed in infants following cardiac surgery.

Focal ischemia, i.e., impairment of blood flow within the distribution of a single cerebral vessel, results in the focal cerebral necrosis, i.e., infarction, the stroke-like pathology noted earlier. When multiple vessels are affected, multifocal brain infarction results. Generalized ischemia, however, appears to underlie the other three cerebral lesions: periventricular leukomalacia, parasagittal cerebral injury, and selective neuronal necrosis. Each of these latter three lesions will be discussed in terms of the neuropathology, the identification of that pathology in the living infant, and the specific pathogenetic features.

Periventricular Leukomalacia

Periventricular leukomalacia, the most common of the lesions observed in affected infants on follow-up study, is characterized neuropathologically after a few months by multiple small cystic areas of necrosis, dorsal and lateral to the external angle of the lateral ventricle.[18,19] After many months to a year or more, the cysts may disappear as they are obliterated by an astroglial scar. However, most striking is a marked deficiency of cerebral white matter with a resulting large lateral ventricle. This deficiency of myelination results not only because of the focal periventricular necrosis but also because the acute lesion involves, in addition, more diffuse injury to the differentiating oligodendroglia in the white matter of these infants. The result is an impairment of myelination, because the oligodendroglia are necessary for subsequent myelination of the cerebral white matter.

Periventricular leukomalacia can be identified in the living infant in the acute period by cranial ultrasonography performed through the open anterior fontanelle.[18,19] The acute lesion appears as bilateral, generally symmetric echodensities in periventricular white matter dorsal and lateral to the external angle of the lateral ventricle. It is usually most marked in the white matter around the trigone of the lateral ventricle. After approximately one to three weeks, the echodense lesions are interrupted by small echolucent lesions, which are the ultrasonographic correlate of the cysts observed pathologically. The cysts are visualized best on parasagittal ultrasonographic views, particularly in the peritrigonal regions. After many months, cranial ultrasonograms may no longer show the echolucent cysts because the cysts collapse at the site of the glial scar. However, the lateral ventricular dilation is identified readily at this time and reflects the deficiency of cerebral myelin discussed earlier.

The neurological features of this lesion, i.e., particularly spastic diplegia, relate to the topography of the injury.[18,19] Thus, in spastic diplegia, the lower extremity is involved more than the upper extremity. Because of the focal necrosis in the periventricular white matter, the motor fibers emanating from the cerebral cortex and subserving lower extremity function are preferentially affected. Fibers subserving the function of upper extremities course more laterally and thus are less likely to be injured or are injured less. However, because there is also more diffuse injury to cerebral white matter, association fibers are affected, and this involvement may account for at least some of the cognitive deficits that one sees on follow-up in affected infants.

Why does generalized ischemia result in this topographically very specific lesion? There are two interacting pathogenetic factors involved (Table 1-2).[18,19] The first is the presence of periventricular vascular end zones and border zones. These zones relate to the terminal fields of the long penetrating arteries that originate from the major cerebral arteries in the subarachnoid space. Elaboration of an interconnected terminal capillary bed as well as of anastomotic connections between the penetrators is deficient. These vascular end zones and border zones are present in the human brain in the third trimester. These distal fields are most vulnerable to diminution in cerebral blood flow. Presumably, this vascular anatomic factor is the most important determinant for the occurrence of the focal periventricular infarctions of periventricular leukomalacia.

A second factor or series of factors also must be operative in the pathogenesis of periventricular leukomalacia (see Table 1-2). Thus, as noted earlier, there is clearly more diffuse injury to oligodendroglia, apparently outside the vascular end zones and border zones. Thus, factors relating to the intrinsic vulnerability of early differentiating oligodendroglial cells remain to be elucidated. Leading candidates for the mediators of cell death in this context are glutamate, free radicals, cytokines, etc.[19]

TABLE 1–2
Periventricular Leukomalacia Pathogenesis

- Cerebral ischemia
- Periventricular vascular border zones/end zones
- Intrinsic vulnerability of cerebral white matter

Parasagittal Cerebral Injury

Parasagittal cerebral injury, a second topographically restricted lesion related to generalized ischemia, is characterized neuropathologically by injury to superomedial aspects of the cerebral cortex and subcortical white matter and is bilateral and generally symmetric.[19] The acute lesion is demonstrated best in the living infant by MRI (see Figure 1–2). Functional imaging techniques, particularly those providing measurements of regional cerebral blood flow (e.g., PET, SPECT), are particularly sensitive for detection of parasagittal cerebral injury. In the days following the insult, the areas of injury are manifested by parasagittal regions of decreased cerebral blood flow.

The neurological features of this lesion, i.e., particularly spastic quadriparesis, relate to the topography of the injury.[18,19] Thus, in spastic diplegia, the lower extremity is involved more than the upper extremity. Because of the focal necrosis in the periventricular white matter, the motor fibers emanating from the cerebral cortex and subserving lower extremity function are preferentially affected. Fibers subserving upper extremity function course more laterally and thus are less likely to be injured or are injured less. However, because there is also more diffuse injury to cerebral white matter, associated fibers are affected, and this involvement may account for at least some of the cognitive deficits that one sees on follow-up study in affected infants.

Why does generalized ischemia result in this topographically specific injury? Again, the major pathogenetic factor is the presence of parasagittal vascular border zones and end zones (Table 1–3).[19] The border zones are between the end fields of supply of the middle, anterior, and posterior cerebral arteries. In the anterior cerebrum, the principal border zone is between the middle and anterior cerebral arteries, and in the posterior cerebrum, it is between the middle, anterior, and posterior cerebral arteries. These distal fields are most vulnerable to a decrease in cerebral blood flow. The lesions are most marked posteriorly because all three major cerebral arteries are involved in the posterior parieto-occipital border zone.

Selective Neuronal Necrosis

Selective neuronal necrosis, which is a very important and common type of injury in these infants, is characterized neuropathologically by neuronal

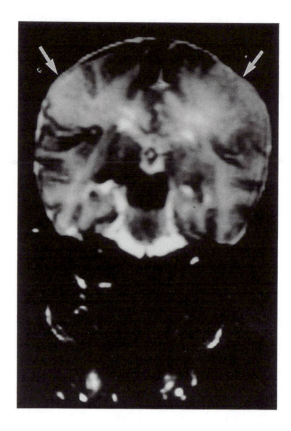

FIGURE 1–2. Parasagittal cerebral injury, MRI scan. T2-weighted, coronal MRI scan obtained four days after a generalized ischemic insult in a newborn shows striking bilateral and symmetric areas of loss of demarcation of gray and white matter in parasagittal cerebral regions, indicative of parasagittal cerebral injury.

injury that is both regionally and cellularly selective.[19] Thus, the neurons of specific regions, such as the CA1 region of the hippocampus or the neocortex, are especially likely to be injured. Moreover, neurons are more vulnerable than are glia.

TABLE 1–3
Parasagittal Cerebral Injury Pathogenesis

- Cerebral ischemia
- Parasagittal vascular border zones/end zones

TABLE 1–4
Selective Neuronal Necrosis Pathogenesis

- Cerebral ischemia
- Regional distribution of excitatory amino acids
- Regional circulatory factors
- Regional metabolic factors

Selective neuronal injury undoubtedly plays some role in the genesis of the cognitive deficits and the seizure disorders that follow infant heart surgery. Moreover, injury to basal ganglia, which exhibits a transient, maturation-dependent, rich expression of excitatory amino acid receptors in the perinatal human brain, may underlie the choreoathetosis that develops in some infants. These clinico-pathological correlations remain to be established conclusively.

Why does generalized ischemia lead to neuronal injury with such striking selectivity? The major pathogenetic determinant for the regional selectivity is the regional distribution of excitatory amino acids and amino acid receptors (Table 1–4).[19] Calcium-mediated events appear to be most important. The mechanisms by which excitatory amino acids lead to this type of neuronal death will be discussed in detail by others. The topographic distribution of excitatory amino acid receptors parallels closely the topographic distribution of ischemic selective neuronal injury. A role for regional circulatory factors also may be contributory because selective neuronal injury occurs particularly in depths of sulci and in parasagittal areas. However, although circulatory factors probably play some role, this role is not as important as that of the regional distribution of excitatory amino acids. Regional metabolic factors relating to glucose and energy metabolism, calcium homeostasis, and free radical scavenging capabilities may also contribute to the selectivity. More data are needed on these issues.

Focal Cerebral Infarction

Focal cerebral infarction or stroke, the result of obstruction to a single vessel, is characterized neuropathologically by destruction of all cellular elements within the distribution of the affected vessel.[19] The bases for the vascular obstruction remain to be proven conclusively. Possibilities include air emboli or other thrombo-embolic phenomena related to bypass circuits or endothelial and white blood cell activation with vascular injury.

Focal cerebral infarction presumably is the basis for the spastic hemiparesis that subsequently is evident in some infants.[19] Because the infarction most often is in the distribution of the middle cerebral artery, the hemiparesis is characterized usually by greater involvement of upper than lower extremity, with prominent affection of the face.

Conclusion

This cursory overview indicates that brain injury in the infant undergoing cardiac surgery is an important problem and is related primarily to ischemia, especially generalized ischemia. The occurrence of topographically restricted injury in the face of generalized insult relates primarily to the interaction of vascular anatomic factors and the intrinsic vulnerability of cerebral oligodendroglia and neurons in the developing human brain. Attempts at prevention must address both aspects of this pathogenesis. Prevention of ischemia will differ in part according to the clinical circumstances because the amount of diminished cerebral blood flow that constitutes dangerous ischemia will depend on such factors as body temperature, concomitant use of drugs that alter cerebral metabolism, or both. Prevention of neuronal injury may include the use of agents that block excitatory amino acid receptors, calcium channels, or attack by free radicals. Prevention of oligodendroglial cell death remains a mystery, although free radical scavengers may prove especially useful. The duration of value for interventions, following termination of the insult, remains to be established in this clinical setting. This information will be crucial in the design of future clinical trials. However, the possibility of pretreatment to prevent ischemic cell death is probably more of a reality in the infant undergoing cardiac surgery than in other areas of medicine. Future research will be of great interest and importance.

References

1. Blackwood MJA, Haka-Ikse K, Steward J. Developmental outcome in children undergoing surgery with profound hypothermia. *Anesthesiology* 1986;65: 437–440.
2. Ehyai A, Fenichel GM, Bender HW. Incidence and prognosis of seizures in infants after cardiac surgery with profound hypothermia and circulatory arrest. *JAMA* 1984;252:3165–3167.
3. Mendoza JC, Wilkerson SA, Reese AH. Follow-up of patients who underwent arterial switch repair for transposition for the great arteries. *AJDC* 1991; 145:40–43.
4. McConnell JR, Fleming WH, Chu WK, et al. Magnetic resonance imaging of the brain in infants and children before and after cardiac surgery. *AJDC* 1990; 144:374–378.
5. Ferry PC. Neurologic sequelae of open-heart surgery in children. *AJDC* 1990; 144:369–373.
6. Furlan AJ, Sila CA, Chimowitz MI, et al. Neurologic complications related to cardiac surgery. *Cerebral Ischemia* 1992;10:145–166.
7. Park SC, Neches WH. The neurologic complications of congenital heart disease. *Neurocardiology* 1993;11:441–463.
8. Newburger JW. Personal communication, 1994.

9. Newburger JW, Jonas RA, Wernovsky G, et al. A comparison of the perioperative neurologic effects of hypothermic circulatory arrest versus low-flow cardiopulmonary bypass in infant heart surgery. *N Engl J Med* 1993;329: 1057–1064.
10. Bellinger DC, Wernovsky G, Rappaport LA, et al. Cognitive development of children following early repair of transposition of the great arteries using deep hypothermic circulatory arrest. *Pediatrics* 1991;87:701–707.
11. Miller G, Rodichok LD, Baylen BG, et al. EEG changes during open heart surgery on infants aged 6 months or less: Relationship to early neurologic morbidity. *Pediatr Neurol* 1991;10:124–130.
12. Bozoky B, Bara D, Kertesz E. Autopsy study of cerebral complications of congenital heart disease and cardiac surgery. *Neurology* 1984;251:155–161.
13. Bjork VO, Hultquist G. Brain damage in children after deep hypothermia for open-heart surgery. *Thorax* 1960;5:284–291.
14. Terplan KL. Patterns of brain damage in infants and children with congenital heart disease. *Am J Dis Child* 1973;125:175–185.
15. Terplan KL. Brain changes in newborns, infants and children with congenital heart disease in association with cardiac surgery. Additional observations. *J Neurol* 1976;212:225–236.
16. Glauser TA, Rorke LB, Weinberg PM, et al. Acquired neuropathologic lesions associated with the hypoplastic left heart syndrome. *Pediatrics* 1990;85: 991–1000.
17. Kinney HC. Personal communication, 1994.
18. Volpe JJ. Current concepts of brain injury in the premature infant. *AJR* 1989; 153:243–251.
19. Volpe JJ. *Neurology of the newborn.* Philadelphia: Saunders, 1994.

PART I

Development of the Central Nervous System

CHAPTER 2

Brain Development and Its Relationship to Patterns of Injury

Michael V. Johnston

When we consider the patterns of injury that may result from insults occurring during infancy, it is worthwhile to consider that the postnatal brain is undergoing a transformation in its organization, especially with respect to synaptic connections among neurons. This chapter outlines the major trends in brain development, especially as they relate to excitatory amino acid neurotransmitter systems.

The very immature fetal brain contains a basically flat or lissencephalic cortex. The task ahead for the brain is to develop a gyrencephalic cortex, where the sheet of cortical neurons expands. To fit inside the skull, the sheet of neurons also forms sulci and gyri. Two structures are especially important targets for brain injury: the hippocampus and basal ganglia.[1,2] The part of the basal ganglia called the caudate/putamen is important in the causation of motor disturbances that are seen after various injuries, including cardiac surgery.[3]

The panorama of brain development follows complicated developmental programs. Figure 2–1 illustrates patterns of brain development showing the relationship between neurogenesis, gliogenesis, synaptogenesis, and development of white matter.[4] Much of the neurogenesis in the brain has been completed by the time of full-term birth in the human (Figure 2–1). Major anomalies in the primitive neural tube, such as spina bifida, occur well before birth at approximately 30 days gestation. During the period of infancy from birth through the first year, when cardiac surgery is frequently undertaken, the major developmental events include completion of neuronal migration into areas such as the cerebellum and glial multiplication. Some of these glia are the oligodendroglia, which form myelin to cover transcortical tracts in the brain itself. Myelination is initiated in the brain stem and

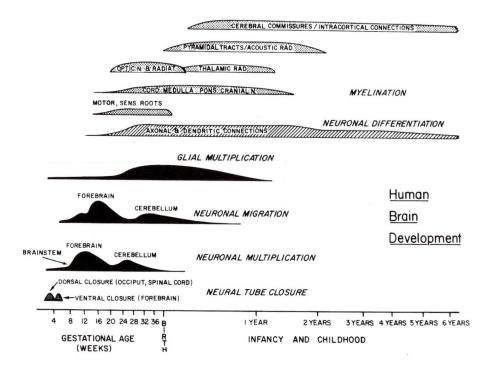

FIGURE 2–1.   Schematic plot of the temporal relationship between major developmental events in the human brain. (Reproduced with permission from Kandt RS, Johnston MV, Goldstein GW. The central nervous system: Basic concepts. In Gregory GA (ed.), *Pediatric anesthesia.* New York: Churchill Livingstone, 1989, pp. 161–162.)

continues beyond 20 years of age in the commissures in the cerebral hemispheres and deep frontal lobe white matter. Developing myelin is very vulnerable to ischemic injury, especially before 32 weeks gestation.[5]

Axons and Dendrites

The elaboration of axons and dendrites forming synaptic connections between neurons accounts for a large fraction of brain expansion during the first year of life. Based on these developmental timetables, injury during the first postnatal year is more likely to disrupt axonodendritic connections and synapses than neuronal multiplication, migration, and white matter formation. Rather than simply developing increased synaptic connections during postnatal development, it is thought that neurons go through a process of overproduction and pruning. This concept was first observed by a Harvard neurobiologist named Conel in a study of human cerebral cortical cytoarchitecture during development. Conel found that there appears to be a more dense matrix of axonodendritic arborization during the first years of postnatal life than there is later in the adult.[6] This turned out to be very important. Synaptic number was quantified by a pediatric neurologist at the University of Chicago, Peter Huttenlocher, who studied in great detail both frontal lobe cortex and visual cortex in the occipital lobe.[7] In a series of studies, Huttenlocher examined the synaptic density per cubic millimeter of brain tissue in human visual cortex and found that a newborn full-term baby has about the same synaptic density as a mature adult, but that from about two months to about two years of age, there is a rapid proliferation of synapses between neurons. From two years of age until adulthood, one of the major developmental events is pruning or elimination of nearly half the synapses in the developing cerebral cortex.

These observations imply that the postnatal period can be divided into two parts as far as synaptogenesis is concerned. From the newborn period onward there is very rapid proliferation of synapses, but from two years of age onward the brain is selecting among populations of synapses, half of which will be lost. There clearly must be processes to stabilize some synapses and to eliminate others.

A composite synapse for excitatory amino acids is illustrated in Figure 2–2.[8] The presynaptic nerve terminal abuts against a dendrite on a postsynaptic neuron. Neurotransmitter is packaged and released into the synaptic cleft. It then comes in contact with a receptor, which either opens an ion channel or stimulates production of a second messenger (or sometimes reduces the production of a second messenger), thereby influencing the chemical and electrical activity of the postsynaptic neuron. The synapse provides a mechanism for modulating neuronal activity, by converting electricity into a chemical signal.

Neurotransmitters

Neuronal activity in the brain is carefully modulated by a balance between glutamate—similar to the flavor enhancer, monosodium glutamate, used in oriental restaurants—and gamma-aminobutyric acid (GABA). Glutamate is the major excitatory neurotransmitter in the brain while GABA is the major inhibitory transmitter. They are released by distinct populations of neurons that are arranged in interactive networks. GABAergic neurons usually are activated shortly after activation of glutamate neurons to prevent overstimulation of postsynaptic neurons.[9] On the other hand, too much unopposed GABA is usually not allowed to reach postsynaptic neurons because this will produce suppressed activity or coma. The balance between sleep and wakefulness is modulated by this balance between these two amino acids, GABA and glutamate, as well as other neurotransmitters. GABA influences

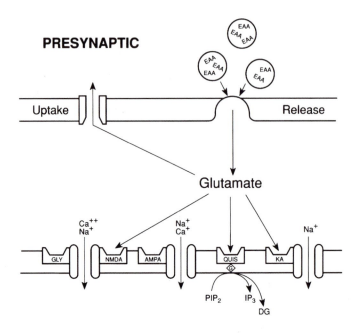

FIGURE 2–2. Composite schematic drawing of glutamate synapses. Glutamate is released from presynaptic nerve terminals and interacts with a variety of receptor subtypes. Some of the receptors operate ion channels (ionotropic), while others stimulate production of a second messenger such as inositol triphosphate (IP₃). Abbreviations: EAA: excitatory amino acid; Gly: glycine; NMDA: N-methyl-D-aspartate; AMPA: a-amino-3-hydroxy-5-methyl-4 isoxazole-propionate, antagonist of glutamate; QUIS: quisqualic acid; PIP₂: phosphatidylinositol 4,5-bisphosphate; IP₃: inositol 1,4,5 triphosphate; DG: diacylglycerol; KA: kainic acid.

neuronal activity by increasing the conductance of chloride, so it tends to hyperpolarize the neuron. Glutamate, through its various receptors, depolarizes the neuron. Following glutamate release, there is usually a very discrete spike with a strong signal-to-noise ratio, quickly followed by an inhibitory postsynaptic potential, mediated by GABA. But if GABA's effect is inhibited and one adds an agonist analogue of glutamate, so-called N-methyl-D-aspartate (NMDA), then repetitive spiking is produced and the balance is disrupted.[10]

There has been a lot of interest in neurotransmitters over the past few years. For example, dopamine is important in control of movement and the neuropeptides that modulate pain perceptions. However these neurotransmitters pale in significance beside the small amino acids, i.e., glycine, aspartic acid, glutamic acid, and GABA, which carry the majority of messages in the brain. Glutamic acid, as the major excitatory neurotransmitter, conducts most of the excitatory electrical activity in the brain. Most of the input into the reader's visual cortex from this page is being mediated by the release of glutamate.[11] In addition, important glutamatergic pathways include the intracortical association pathways, the cortico-spinal pathways, connections in the hippocampus that are important for learning and memory, and corticostriatal pathways.

GABA, on the other hand, is the major inhibitory transmitter. It is noteworthy that GABA differs from glutamate by only a single carboxyl group. Thus, a single carboxyl group, together with the enzyme glutamate decarboxylase that produces GABA from glutamate, determines whether one is in a coma or in status epilepticus.

Aspartic acid is another excitatory transmitter which is used in some pathways. Glycine has turned out to be quite interesting because it can have both inhibitory and excitatory actions. There is an inhibitory glycine receptor site in the spinal cord and brain stem which is antagonized by strychnine. Strychnine can produce seizures by blocking this inhibitory receptor. Recently it was discovered that glycine also plays a major excitatory role. In the forebrain, glycine is a coagonist with glutamic acid, allowing the NMDA-type glutamate channel to be opened.[12] These systems appear to be especially important in the pathogenesis of hypoxic-ischemic brain injury because hypoxia can trigger excessive excitement and "excitotoxicity."[13–16]

Receptors

The complexity and selectivity of the actions of these relatively nonspecific amino acid neurotransmitters are imparted by a variety of specific receptors.[17] When glutamate is released from a presynaptic terminal, its two carboxyl groups can rotate around the central axis, and can create a variety of conformations (see Figure 2–2). Figure 2–3 illustrates a receptor that most comfortably fits the conformation of glutamate in the so-called N-methyl-D-aspartate (NMDA) conformation, and therefore, was named the NMDA receptor. It is linked to a channel which fluxes calcium and sodium.

There are also so-called AMPA or QUIS-type glutamate receptors, which accept glutamate in the conformation of these rigid analogues. The unusual names are derived from the fact that these were rigid analogue compounds that have the highest affinity for physiologically identified receptor subtypes. These receptors flux mainly sodium but sometimes calcium. Another rigid analogue of glutamate, kainic acid, is connected with similar non-NMDA channels. In addition, there are several receptors linked to polyphosphoinositide turnover that produce important intracellular messengers. Therefore glutamate released at presynaptic nerve terminals can have a variety of postsynaptic actions depending on the distributions of

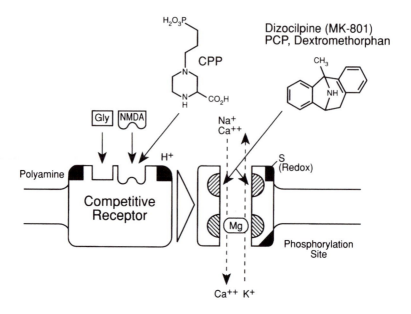

FIGURE 2–3. Schematic drawing of the NMDA receptor channel complex. The amino acids glycine and glutamate must interact with the competitive receptor for the channel to open. Sites for inhibition by polyamines and hydrogen ions are shown. The channel is usually blocked by magnesium. Redox and phosphorylation sites are shown where channel modulation may take place. A site that can interact with Zn^{++} to inhibit the channel is also present on the channel. The compounds CPP (3-(2-carboxypiperazin-4-yl)propyl-1-phosphoric acid), a competitive antagonist, and dizocilpine, a noncompetitive antagonist, are neuroprotective.

glutamate receptor subtypes, their molecular characteristics, and their developmental stage.[6]

Role of Receptors

A major role of excitatory amino acid receptors appears to be to manage the very dangerous trophic molecule, calcium. Normally, there is a 10,000:1 concentration gradient for calcium from outside to inside neurons. One of the major roles for these receptors is to control the gates, or the ion channels, that allow calcium to enter the cell.[18] Perhaps a useful analogy is that the cell membrane is like a dike along the Mississippi River. When the dike is breached, then water, like calcium, can overwhelm the intracellular machinery of plants, killing crops along the river. Plants require water to live but can be killed by too much. Just as a plant needs water, the neuron's cellular machinery needs calcium to thrive. Calcium has important trophic effects, but it is a very dangerous ion that needs to be carefully gated through the neuronal membrane.

The excitatory amino acid receptors have recently been cloned in several laboratories.[19,20] All of the subtypes contain regions of similarity with four transmembrane segments. The second transmembrane segment seems to be very important in determining how much calcium these channels can flux.[21] A single amino acid change can control this feature. The developing brain is endowed with channels that flux more calcium than the adult brain. This is consistent with the stimulating trophic role that calcium plays in immature neurons.[22]

The NMDA Receptor Channel Complex

The NMDA receptor channel complex (Figure 2–3) is one of the more important channels in physiologic and pathophysiologic processes in the developing brain.[6] Glutamate stimulates the so-called competitive site that is linked to the ion channel. Competitive interaction at both the glutamate and glycine sites are necessary to open the channel. The channel allows Na^+ and Ca^{2+} to enter and K^+ to leave. Numerous antagonist drugs for sites within the channel, so-called noncompetitive sites, have been characterized.[16] The best known noncompetitive antagonist is dizocilpine (MK-801), a potent neuroprotective drug against hypoxia and ischemia. Ketamine, the anesthetic, and phencyclidine, the drug of abuse, also block the NMDA channel at this site.

Another important molecular feature of the NMDA receptor/channel complex is that normally it is blocked by magnesium.[23] Neuronal depolarization is required along with stimulation of the competitive receptor to expel magnesium and open the channel. Magnesium at high doses also serves as a noncompetitive glutamate antagonist.

Voltage-Sensitive Calcium Channels

It is important to distinguish between the NMDA-activated calcium channels and the voltage-sensitive calcium channels familiar to clinicians who treat hypertension and cardiac arrhythmias (Figure 2–4). Voltage-sensitive calcium channels, in contrast to the glutamate-stimulated channels, are blocked by drugs such as verapamil. Voltage-sensitive calcium channels differ from the others in that they require only passive depolarization of the membrane instead of neurotransmitter agonist to open the channel. As glutamate is depolarizing neuronal membranes in the nervous system, the voltage-sensitive calcium channels open passively.[24] These channels play a role in the cascade of events that mediate hypoxic injury. Antagonism of the voltage-sensitive calcium channels can act synergistically with glutamate antagonists to protect the brain.

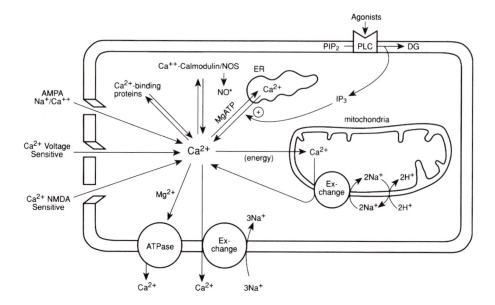

FIGURE 2–4.   A diagram of a neuron with both voltage-sensitive and glutamate-sensitive calcium channels. One effect of calcium entry is to stimulate production of the toxic chemical, nitric oxide (NO), by activation of nitric oxide synthetase (NOS). Agonists including glutamate can also activate phospholipase C (PLC) to produce IP_3. The mitochondria produce energy for ion pumps and also sequester calcium.

Special Role of NMDA Receptors in Learning and Memory

The special features of the NMDA receptor/channel complex allow it to play special roles in learning and memory. As shown in Figure 2–5, the NMDA receptor can serve as a "coincidence detector" by opening only when it senses glutamate/glycine occupancy and membrane depolarization together. This enables the neuron to respond differently to coincident threshold activation than to single stimuli by opening the NMDA channel.

NMDA receptor channels appear to play a role in encoding paired associative memories, as occurs when a neuron is affected by coincident activation by two neurons from different areas of the nervous system. Paired stimuli that open the NMDA channel allow a strong pulse of calcium to enter the neuron, triggering changes that may lead to encoding memories. Long-term potentiation (LTP), an important correlate of memory function in physiologic preparations, is dependent in part on NMDA receptor activity.[25] One effect of the calcium influx triggered by NMDA channel opening can be to stimulate production of messengers, such as the free radical nitric oxide, that may retrogradingly enhance neurotransmitter release. Both presynaptic

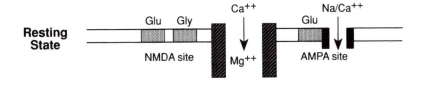

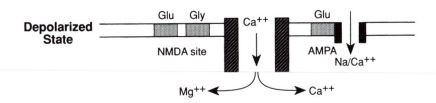

FIGURE 2–5. An illustration of how NMDA receptors can act as coincidence detectors. Glutamate acting at non-NMDA receptors depolarizes neuronal membranes, allowing magnesium to leave the channel. A combination of glycine and glutamate activation plus membrane depolarization is needed to pass calcium. Energy deficiency makes it easier to open the channel by depolarizing membranes.

and postsynaptic changes mediated by NMDA channel opening can enhance LTP and associative memory storage.

Receptors and Development

In the developing brain, neurotransmitter circuits have trophic or regulatory influences on brain circuitry as well as a message-carrying role.[6] Activity at excitatory receptors helps to determine which of the connections will be maintained as the developing brain is pruning synapses. Glutamate's involvement in LTP appears to be closely linked to the roles it plays in shaping and sculpting the brain's axonodendritic circuitry. Excitatory amino acid receptors have been shown to play a role in neuronal migration,[6,26] in mediating visual-evoked responses in kittens, in ocular dominance plasticity in the visual cortex, in activity-dependent matching of tectal maps in amphibians, and in synapse elimination in the cerebellum.[27]

Glutamate is a major neurotransmitter in the geniculocalcarine visual pathway to the visual cortex. Tsumoto's work showed that NMDA receptors in the visual cortex of young kittens are more effective in mediating visual responses than are NMDA receptors in adult cats.[28] In these experiments, microelectrodes were placed in the visual cortex of cats and kittens.

After wakening, the animals were shown a bar moving in the visual field. A visual-evoked potential that was sensitive to NMDA blockers could be detected in the visual cortex and the amplitude of the response was much greater in kittens than in adult cats. This suggests that the function of NMDA receptors and channels is enhanced during the period of cortical visual plasticity.

Hubel and Wiesel's experiments in primates examined the phenomenon of ocular dominance plasticity in which the organization of the visual cortex into ocular dominance columns is influenced by the relative visual activity in each eye.[29] One can study this by injecting tritiated amino acids into one eye and making tangential sections on the surface of the cortex when the amino acids have been transported in a retrograde fashion into the visual cortex. Normally, autoradiograms prepared from this material show alternating bands of dark and light, corresponding to alternating domination by each eye. When one eye is covered for some time during the period of development, the opposite eye gains a dominant influence over the visual cortex, claiming more territory because it is more active while the other eye is inactive. The activity-dependent shifts in connections in the visual cortex are limited by age, which is about 6 years in children. These activity-dependent shifts in eye dominance, termed "ocular dominance plasticity," appear to utilize the special features of the NMDA receptors and are blocked by NMDA antagonist drugs.[30]

The experiments on the visual cortex indicate that NMDA receptors are important for synapse stabilization. NMDA receptors also appear to be important in synapse elimination during cerebellar development.[27] Normally each circuit in the cerebellum has twice as many synapses during development as it will need. If NMDA receptor stimulation does not occur, the circuit will maintain too many synapses. Thus, NMDA receptor activity is important, not only in maintaining some synapses, but in eliminating others, probably related to the specific electrical code that it is subjected to.

Ontogeny of Glutamate Receptors

The ontogeny of excitatory receptors in the brain can be studied by autoradiography. An autoradiogram of the rat brain shows that at day 14 there is actually more binding to NMDA receptors than there is earlier or later.[31] Quantitative autoradiography reveals that at day 7 in the rat there is the beginning of a rapid rise in the binding of receptors, followed by an overshoot and then a return to the normal range. Thus the binding of glutamate receptors in the hippocampus has an overshoot, which is very similar to the overshoot in synapses seen in the human cortex.

In 1986 we described a study in which a series of adult human brains and a series of infant brains were examined by autoradiography to demonstrate binding to glutamate receptors within the brain.[32] We found that many of the areas of the brain of the infant had more glutamate receptors than the adult. Certain regions, such as the basal ganglia, showed an intense degree of binding. In contrast to many of the neurotransmitter systems in which the infant is deficient compared with the adult, in this example the infant is actually over-supplied with glutamate receptors compared with the adult. Recently a similar developmental overshoot in NMDA binding sites in the human brain has been reported.[33] It is now known from molecular genetic studies that these immature receptors are primed to flux calcium more than the adult, so that the system is "turned on" to perform functions such as modulating ocular dominance plasticity and carrying out a host of other developmental activities in the brain.[34]

Selective Vulnerability, Age, and Receptors

Overstimulation of glutamate receptors can cause neuronal injury through a process called excitotoxicity. The immature brain appears to have enhanced vulnerability to overstimulation of NMDA receptors compared with the adult brain.[6] At postnatal day 7, injection of 25 nmoles of NMDA results in a large hemisphere lesion whereas a week earlier, there is much less toxicity. By day 21, a dose that virtually destroys the hemisphere at day 7 does very little to the hemisphere. Thus there is enhanced sensitivity that correlates with enhanced physiologic activity of these receptors at this age. In fetal lambs, intracerebral injection of NMDA produces changes in cerebral blood flow and produces neurotoxicity resembling ischemic lesions.[35]

In contrast to NMDA, kainic acid, which was shown a number of years ago to cause extensive necrosis of the basal ganglia in the adult rodent brain, does not cause damage in the immature brain.[6,36] Even though kainic acid will induce seizures in rodents at 7 days of age, it does not produce prominent injury.[37] The vulnerability of the immature brain to excitatory amino acid receptor overstimulation is very different from the adult. Figure 2–6 illustrates the time-related changes in sensitivity to the various agonists. The spectrum of vulnerability, and probably the related neuropathology that could be mediated by this mechanism, changes during development.

Relationship to Hypoxic-Ischemic Injury

Receptor-mediated excitotoxicity can be triggered by a variety of insults such as hypoxia/ischemia, status epilepticus, and hypoglycemia, alone or in combination.[6,15,16] These insults can trigger the NMDA mechanism, triggering those coincidence detectors and producing injury to the very parts of the brain that are most plastic and are undergoing the most rapid development. The brain has complicated protective mechanisms to deal with calcium entry, enhanced through both voltage-sensitive calcium channels and glutamate channels. The mitochondria work very hard to sequester calcium and supply energy to pump the calcium out (Figure 2–4).[38] But in the context of an event like hypothermic circulatory arrest, in which there may be reduced mitochondrial function and perhaps enhanced glutamate stimulation of these receptors, it is possible for receptor stimulation to reach toxic levels.

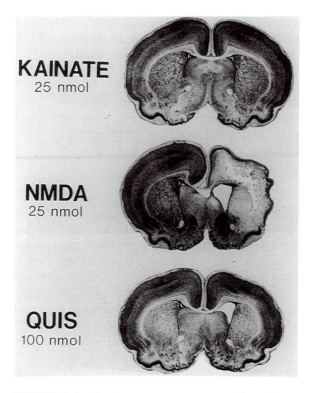

FIGURE 2–6.   Age has a major impact on the vulnerability of the brain to overstimulation of specific glutamate receptor subtypes. In this experiment, 7-day-old
rats received direct unilateral intracerebral injections
of the glutamate agonists shown. When examined 5
days later, the NMDA-injected brain was very damaged, but the kainate injected brain was not injured. In
adulthood, kainate is highly toxic but NMDA is much
less so. NMDA-mediated injury is a more important
pathogenic mechanism in the postnatal brain than are
non-NMDA mediated mechanisms.

A receptor mechanism that usually functions in the brain to accomplish normal development can become a disadvantage for an infant during periods of
metabolic stress.[39]

Summary

In summary, the nervous system—especially the immature nervous system—needs stimulation which is normally maintained by excitatory amino
acid neurotransmitters. However, too much excitement is not a good thing.

In infants, excitatory amino acid receptors play important roles in brain plasticity, that is, stabilizing some circuits and pruning others. Excessive activation of the excitatory mechanism is capable of producing what might be referred to colloquially as a "synaptic power surge" analogous to a power surge in a computer. In a computer, the electricity is carried by electrons. In the brain, much of the electricity is carried by ions such as calcium. In the brain, as in the computer, the power surge is capable of destroying neurons in a regionally selective fashion.[40] These concepts suggest that therapeutic interventions that block glutamate receptors might be efficacious, but that care must be taken because reduced activation of these receptors for a prolonged time is also capable of producing developmental abnormalities.[41] The theory of excitotoxicity has clarified a number of issues related to the pathogenesis of brain injury and supplied hypotheses for therapeutic studies.

References

1. Volpe JJ. Hypoxic-ischemic encephalopathy: Neuropathology and pathogenesis. In Volpe JJ (ed.), *Neurology of the newborn*, 3rd ed. Philadelphia: Saunders, 1994.
2. Tarplan KL. Brain changes in newborns, infants and children with congenital heart disease in association with cardiac surgery. *J Neurol* 1976;212:225–36.
3. Penn AA, Enzmann DR, Hahn JS, Stevenson DK. Kernicterus in a full-term infant. *Pediatrics* 1994;93:1003–1006.
4. Kandt RS, Johnston MV, Goldstein GW. The central nervous system: Basic concepts. In Gregory GA (ed.), *Pediatric anesthesia*. New York: Churchill Livingstone, 1989, p. 161.
5. Leviton A, Gilles FH. Acquired perinatal leukoencephalopathy. *Annals Neurol* 1984;16:1–8.
6. Conel J. *The postnatal development of the human cerebral cortex*, Vols. 1–8. Cambridge, MA: Harvard, 1939–1967.
7. Huttenlocher PR, deCourten C. The development of synapses in striate cortex of man. *Hum Neurobiol* 1987;6:1–9.
8. McDonald JW, Johnston MV. Physiological and pathophysiological roles of excitatory amino acids during central nervous system development. *Brain Res Rev* 1990;15:41–70.
9. Fagg GE, Foster AC. Amino acid neurotransmitters and their pathways in the mammalian central nervous system. *Neuroscience* 1983;91:701–719.
10. Wuarin FP, Kim YI, Cepeda C, et al. Synaptic transmission in human neocortex removed for treatment of intractable epilepsy in children. *Ann Neurol* 1990;28:503–508.
11. Cooper JR, Bloom FE, Roth RN. *The biochemical basis of neuropharmacology*, 2nd ed. New York: Macmillan, 1980.
12. Foster AC, Wills CL, Bakker MHM, Tridgett R. The pharmacology of NMDA receptors in relationship to neuronal degeneration. *Clinical Neuropharmacology* 1991;13:160–166.
13. Olney JW. Neurotoxicity of excitatory amino acids. In McGeer EG, Olney JW, and McGeer PL (eds.), *Kainic acid as a tool in neurobiology*. New York: Raven Press, 1978, pp. 95–121.

14. Choi DW, Rothman SW. The role of glutamate neurotoxicity in hypoxic-ischemic neuronal death. *Ann Rev Neurosci* 1990;13:171–182.
15. Simon RP, Swan JH, Griffiths T, Meldrum BS. Blockade of NMDA receptors may protect against ischemic damage in the brain. *Science* 1984;226:850–852.
16. Lipton SA, Rosenberg PA. Excitatory amino acids as a final common pathway for neurologic disorders. *N Engl J Med* 1994;300:613–622.
17. Mayer ML, Westbrook GL. The physiology of excitatory amino acids in the vertebrate central nervous system. *Prog Neurobiol* 1987;28:197–276.
18. Siesjo BK. Historical overview: Calcium, ischemia and death of brain cells. *Ann NY Acad Sci* 1988;522:638–661.
19. Seeburg PH. The molecular biology of mammalian glutamate receptor channels. *Trends in Neuroscience* 1993;16:359–365.
20. Ishii T, Mariyoshi K, Sugihara H, Sakurada K, Kadotani H, Yokoi M, Akazawa C, Shigemoto R, Mizuno N, Masu M, Nakanishi S. Molecular characterization of the family of NMDA receptor subunits. *J Biol Chem* 1993;268:2836–2843.
21. Hollman M, Martley M, Heinemann S. Ca^{2+} permeability of KA-AMPA-gated receptor channels depends on subunit composition. *Science* 1991;252:851–853.
22. Monyer H, Burnashev N, Laurie DJ, Sakmann B, Seeburg PH. Development and regional expression in the rat brain and functional properties of four NMDA receptors. *Neuron* 12:529–540.
23. Johnson JW, Ascher P. Voltage dependent block by intracellular Mg^{2+} of NMDA activated channels. *Biophys J* 1990;57:1085–1090.
24. Uematsu D, Araki N, Greenberg JH, Sladky J, Reivich M. Combined therapy with MK-801 and nimodipine for protection of ischemic brain damage. *Neurology* 1991;41:88–94.
25. Collingridge GL, Bliss TV. NMDA receptors—their role in long term potentiation. *Trends in Neurosci* 1987;10:288–293.
26. Komuro H, Rakic P. Modulation of neuronal migration by NMDA receptors. *Science* 1993;28:517–527.
27. Rabacchi S, Bailly Y, Delhaye-Bouchaud N, Miariani J. Involvement of the NMDA receptor in synapse elimination during cerebellar development. *Science* 1992;256:1823–1825.
28. Tsumoto T, Hagihara K, Soto H, Hata Y. NMDA receptors in the visual cortex of young kittens are more effective than those of adult cats. *Nature* 1987; 327:513–514.
29. Hubel DH, Wiesel TN. The period of susceptibility to the physiological effects of unilateral eye closure in kittens. *J Physiol* (Lond) 1970;206:419–436.
30. Kleinschmidt A, Bear MF, Singer W. Blockade of NMDA receptors disrupts experience dependent plasticity of kitten striate cortex. *Science* 1987;238: 355–358.
31. McDonald JW, Johnston MV, Young AB. Differential ontogenic development of three receptors comprising the NMDA receptor/channel complex in the rat hippocampus. *Experimental Neurology* 1990;110:237–247.
32. Greenamyre JT, Penney JB, Young AB, Hudson C, Silverstein FS, Johnston MV. Evidence for a transient perinatal glutamatergic innervation of globus pallidus. *J Neuroscience* 1987;7:1022–1030.
33. D'Souza SW, McConnell SE, Slater P, Barson AJ. NMDA binding sites in neonatal and adult brain. *Lancet* 1992;339:1240–1242.

34. Sheng M, Cummings J, Rolau LA, Jan YN, Jan LY. Changing subunit composition of heteromeric NMDA receptors during development of rat cortex. *Nature* 1994;368:144–147.
35. Taylor GA, Trescher WH, Traystman RJ, Johnston MV. Acute experimental neuronal injury in the newborn lamb: Ultrasound characterization and demonstration of hemodynamic effects. *Pediatr Radiol* 1993;23:260–275.
36. Campochiaro P, Coyle JT. Ontogenetic development of kainate neurotoxicity; correlates with glutamatergic innervation. *Proc Natl Acad Sci* (USA) 1978;75: 2025–2029.
37. Stafstrom CE, Thompson JL, Holmes GL. Kainic acid seizures in the developing brain; satus epilepticus and spontaneous recurrent seizures. *Dev Brain Res* 1992;65:227–236.
38. Coyle JT, Puttfarcken P. Oxidative stress, glutamate and neurodegenerative disorders. *Science* 1993;262:689–695.
39. Pellegrini-Giampietro DE, Zukin RS, Bennett MV, Cho S, Pulsinelli WA. Switch in glutamate receptor subunit gene expression in CA1 subfield of hypocampus following global ischemia in rats. *Proc Natl Acad Sci* (USA) 1992;89: 10499–10503.
40. Sugimoto A, Takeda A, Kogure K, Onodera H. NMDA receptor (NMDARI) expression in the rat hippocampus after forebrain ischemia. *Neuroscience Letters* 1994;170:39–42.
41. McDonald JW, Silverstein FS, Johnston MV. MK-801 pretreatment enhances NMDA mediated brain injury and increases brain NMDA recognition sites in rats. *Neuroscience* 1990;38:103–113.

CHAPTER 3

Maturation of Brain ATP Metabolism

David Holtzman
Miles Tsuji

Introduction

With the increasing use of cardiopulmonary bypass (CPB) and deep hypothermic circulatory arrest (DHCA) to support cardiac surgery in the newborn period, it is critical to understand the acute and late effects of hypothermia and complete or partial ischemia on energetics and cell viability in the developing brain. Protection of the neonatal brain under these conditions has been effective but is still incomplete.[1,2] Improved support for children during and after DHCA will be critical in improving neurological outcome.

Increased understanding of the physiology of energy regulation in the immature brain will be the basis for rational development of effective supportive regimens for neonatal cardiac surgery. The physiological bases and the efficacies of such supportive interventions in protecting brain cell viability and improving functional brain recovery will require close interactions in designing animal and clinical research protocols.

In this chapter, the physiology of energy in the mature and developing brain is reviewed. Human studies and studies from other altricial species are emphasized. These species are characterized by extensive post-natal brain growth and development. Most studies of brain metabolic development use newborn rats and piglets, though they are not the only altricial newborns used. For the purposes of this review, energy metabolism is considered to be ATP metabolism. The synthesis of ATP occurs in the pathways of aerobic glycolysis and in the creatine kinase (CK) catalyzed reaction (Figure 3–1). The utilization of ATP in the brain is predominantly by ATPases coupled to the regulation and distribution of electrolytes, metabolites, and water. Recent *in vivo* studies have shown that the maintenance of brain ATP

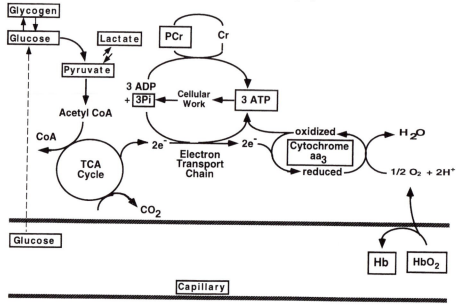

Energy Metabolites measured by *in vivo* spectroscopy and PET

FIGURE 3–1. Diagram of brain ATP metabolism. Those metabolites enclosed in rectangles can be measured noninvasively using nuclear magnetic resonance (NMR), near infrared spectroscopy, and positron emission tomography (PET).

concentration is effective under conditions of high energy demand (e.g., seizures) and energy deficit (e.g., hypoxia). These *in vivo* studies, using magnetic resonance spectroscopy (MRS), demonstrate that phosphocreatine (PCr) is partially lost before large decreases in ATP occur in the mature brain (Figure 3–2).[3–5] With hypoxia and ischemia, PCr and ATP are lost together.[6,7] This complex coupling of PCr and ATP suggests that understanding the function(s) of the PCr/CK system is important in understanding the physiology of ATP metabolism in the brain.

Because this chapter is specifically concerned with the newborn, ATP metabolism in the developing brain is described in detail. The relatively slow maturational increase in capacity for aerobic ATP synthesis has been studied extensively in the rat brain.[8] More space is devoted to the recently described maturation of the coupling of ATP synthesis to the large and rapid fluctuations in energy demand, which are characteristic of the mature brain. A possible central role of this coupled metabolism and of the PCr/CK system in adaptation to states of decreased energy availability, such as hypoxia and deep hypothermia, also are discussed. Finally, because ATP metabolism

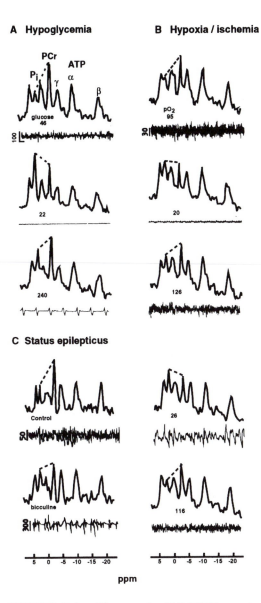

A Hypoglycemia

B Hypoxia / ischemia

C Status epilepticus

ppm

FIGURE 3–2. Changes in 31P-NMR spectra
and EEGs during hypoxia [A] and seizures [B].
The inorganic phosphate (P_i) and PCr peaks are
joined by dotted lines. Arterial oxygen tension
and administration of the convulsant, bicu-
culline, are indicated below the respective
NMR tracings. Also shown are 20 s EEG tracings obtained with the spectra above them.
(Reprinted with permission from Prichard J, Alger J, Behar K, Petroff O, Shulman R. Cerebral
metabolic studies in vivo by 31P-NMR. *Proc
Natl Acad Sci* (USA) 1983; 80: 2746–2751.)

and pathological changes in response to hypoxia show regional and cellular heterogeneity, the physiological differences between cerebral cortex and deep white matter are emphasized.

ATP Regulation in the Adult Brain

The physiology of ATP metabolism and regulation in the mature brain, as shown diagrammatically in Figure 3–1, has been reviewed recently.[9,10] The adult human brain, which is approximately 2% of body mass, accounts for 20% of body O_2 consumption. With cortical activity, the cerebral blood flow may increase as much as 3 to 5 times. Under most conditions, glucose is the ultimate source of carbon atoms for the production of CO_2. Glucose carbon atoms contribute to pools of glycogen, lipids, amino acids, and lactic acid to extents which may depend upon the region and physiological state. Approximately 15% of glucose carbons go to lactate even when the brain is well oxygenated. The turnover rates of these pools generally are high, suggesting that these carbons ultimately are available for mitochondrial aerobic metabolism. The regulatory enzyme steps in the utilization of glucose carbons appear to be the same in the brain as in other organ systems.[9,11]

Cellular and regional heterogeneity characterizes brain ATP metabolism. As shown in Table 3–1, respiratory rates and coupling of respiration to oxidative phosphorylation with glucose as substrate are greater in astrocytes than in neurons in primary culture.[12,13] Astrocytes also contain about twice the ATP concentration present in neurons from the cerebellum or cerebral cortex. The PCr/ATP ratio in astrocytes is about 1 while the ratio in neurons is closer to 2 . Even though astrocytes contain a large portion of the cortical mitochondria, neurons generally are thought to have higher

TABLE 3–1

Respiratory Rates Measured in Neurons and Astrocytes from Primary Culture (adapted from Holtzman D, Olson J. Developmental changes in brain cellular energy metabolism in relation to seizures and their sequelae. In Jaspers H, van Gelder N (eds.), *Basic mechanisms of neuronal hyperexcitability*. New York: Liss, 1983.)

| | *Primary Cultures* | |
Respiratory Rate	*Granular neurons*	*Astrocytes*
DNP-stimulated respiration (% of basal rate)	146 ± 6 (n = 8)	205 ± 8 (n = 17)
Respiratory control (DNP-stimulated rate/ Oligomycin-inhibited rate)	2.8 ± 0.4 (n = 4)	6.6 ± 0.4 (n = 12)

$p < .0001$

aerobic metabolic activities closely coupled to electrical activity.[10] Distributions of glycolytic and mitochondrial enzymes also suggest compartmentation of ATP metabolism in the cortex.[10,14-16] Neuronal glycolytic enzyme activity appears to be in higher concentration in the cell bodies and proximal dendrites, while the distal dendrites contain large numbers of mitochondria. This distribution is analogous to the relative concentrations of glycolytic and aerobic enzymes in white and red muscle fibers. Histochemical studies show stable increases in regional cytochrome oxidase activity with sustained electrical activity, while positron emission tomographic (PET) studies suggest that seizure foci in the human brain have decreased interictal glucose consumption.[17-19] These observations suggest both heterogeneity of aerobic and anaerobic metabolic pathways and an adaptation of these activities to increased ATP requirements, again analogous to those seen in exercised skeletal muscle. However, such analogies must be tentative since there is little known of the distributions and kinetics of these pathways and of multiple forms of critical regulatory enzymes, which couple anaerobic and aerobic glycolysis.

As in other tissues with rapidly changing, high rates of ATP metabolism, there are cytosolic and mitochondrial isoenzymes in the brain.[20,21] The CK isoenzymes are not uniformly distributed in brain tissue and do not consistently co-localize.[5] Little mitochondrial creatine kinase (Mi-CK) is found in cerebellar white matter while the brain isoenzyme (B-CK) is present in high concentrations in cerebellar white matter and gray matter. Regional concentrations of CK reactants in the brain—including ATP, PCr, and Cr—are not known with certainty.[10,22] The ATP concentration generally is thought to be about 3 mM in cerebral white and gray matter. Three physiological roles have been proposed for the heart muscle PCr/CK system with the Mi-CK isoenzyme complexed with the ATP-ADP translocase as shown diagrammatically in Figure 3–3.[21] First, PCr may act as a temporal buffer for the ATP concentration, as suggested by the loss of PCr before ATP in working or hypoxic skeletal muscle, and by the rapid CK-catalyzed reaction rate compared to oxidative phosphorylation.[23,24] Second, the PCr/CK system acts to facilitate transport of high-energy bonds from sites of ATP synthesis to sites of its utilization. The third proposed role is to maintain concentrations of CK reactants, particularly ADP, while closely coupling ATP synthesis to demand.

Less is known about localization and regulation of ATPases compared to ATP-synthesizing pathways in the brain.[10,13,25] Approximately 60% to 70% of brain ATP is consumed by Na,K-ATPases.[26] Three isoenzymes of Na,K-ATPase have been found in brain.[25] Cytochrome oxidase is localized in regions of high ATPase activities in the brain.[10] In primary cultured cells, small increases in extracellular K^+ produce increased oxygen consumption in both astrocytes and neurons.[13] In brain slices and astrocytes, but not in neurons, increased extracellular K^+ results in increased Na,K-ATPase activity and K^+ uptake.[13] Similarly, cell volume regulation in astrocytes is

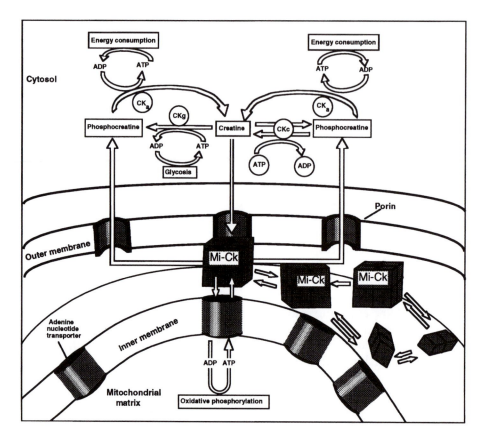

FIGURE 3–3.   A model for the cellular compartmentation of the kinase (CK) isoenzymes is shown diagrammatically. It is proposed that the soluble CK (CKc) catalyzes the free equilibration of the cytosolic ratios of phosphocreatine (PCr)/creatine (Cr) and ATP/ADP; cytosolic creatine kinase (CKg) couples glycolysis to phosphocreatine production; 'cytosolic creatine kinase' (CKa) is associated with subcellular sites of high and fluctuating ATP consumption. The mitochondrial creatine kinase (Mi-CK) is thought to function in regulating and coupling mitochondrial ATP synthesis to energy requirements of the cell. Although proposed for muscle, this model is relevant to interpreting results of studies of ATP regulation in brain. Like muscle, the physiology of energy metabolism is different in different cells and/or subcellular organelles.

coupled to a Na,K-ATPase-mediated Na$^+$ transport.[27] These studies suggest that heterogeneity of ATP consumption is due to heterogeneity in the physiological coupling of energy to cell-specific functions, including regulation of extracellular water and ions.

It has long been recognised that brain ATP metabolism must be studied *in situ* with intact cerebral blood flow (CBF), substrate transport, functioning interneuronal connections, and the interdependence of ATP utilization and synthesis.[9] Higher rates of aerobic glycolysis are measured in the intact brain than *in vitro*. *In vitro* measures of the effects of pre-mortem conditions always are plagued by the uncertain assumption that post-mortem changes do not alter morphologic and biochemical characteristics present at the time of sacrifice. These methodological weaknesses are avoided by noninvasive *in situ* measurement and imaging of brain ATP metabolic systems. The electroencephalogram (EEG) may provide an index of gross changes in ATP use during high energy demand (e.g., seizures) and energy deficit (e.g., hypoxia) states.[7,28] Regional measurements of glucose and oxygen consumption and of blood flow are possible using nonmetabolized, radio-labelled physiological analogues in animal and human studies.[9,29–31] These studies, including PET, provide localization of brain function because of the close coupling of large changes in localized ATP metabolism and CBF to physiological events.[9,31]

In vivo nonlocalized 31P-MRS allows measurement of changes in ATP, PCr, and phosphate concentrations and changes in pH relatively quickly averaged over cerebral gray and white matter in the human or animal brain.[32,33] With longer experimental times, these signals may be acquired from brain regions. Similarly, lH spectra provide measures of local blood flow, total creatine, and lactate, particularly under pathologic conditions. Glucose and glycogen metabolism also may be studied using 13C-MRS.[34] Recent developments in fast imaging techniques provide localized imaging of function-coupled changes in CBF.[35,36]

Although powerful techniques, PET and MRS suffer from the requirement for siting at a distance from clinical locations such as operating rooms and intensive care units. Near infrared spectroscopy (NIRS), the recently developed technique for measurement of cerebral blood volume and oxygenated and deoxygenated hemoglobin, can be performed at the bedside and provides excellent time resolution.[37] This technique also provides a measure of cytochrome oxidase redox state, potentially useful as an index of changes in cellular oxygenation.[38]

These noninvasive metabolic imaging and spectroscopic techniques have demonstrated close regulation of ATP in the presence of large and rapid changes in brain energy demand. Nonlocalized 31P spectra (see Figure 3–2) from the adult rat brain show a small decrease in ATP concentration with a 30% to 50% loss of PCr during reversible hypoxia and seizures.[3,4] The resting metabolic rates for glucose and oxygen and CBF are 2 to 3 times higher in cerebral gray matter than in white matter in rat and monkey.[39,40] These measures of ATP metabolism increase 2 to 4 times in the brain during seizures.[10,19,29] The CK-catalyzed flux increases during seizures.[28] Small decreases in ATP concentration are associated with loss of EEG activity during hypoxia.[38] These changes in ATP metabolism during hypoxia or seizures have not been compared in cerebral cortex and white matter.

In summary, there are many unanswered questions concerning the physiology of ATP metabolism in mature brain. Careful application of new, noninvasive spectroscopic techniques will allow approaches to these questions of regional and cellular energy regulation in the brain in animal models and in the human. Answering these questions will be important in understanding mechanisms of maintaining cell viability and function in critical clinical conditions.

Maturational Increase in Pathways of ATP Metabolism

The time courses of cellular and metabolic development vary in different brain regions.[8,41-45] In this and the following section, we shall concentrate on ATP metabolism in the cerebral hemispheres, contrasting gray matter and white matter. In both cortex and white matter, total wet weight increases about five times from birth to 40 days while total protein increases from 5 to 30 days.[41,46] Water concentration decreases to adult values in gray matter (82%) and white matter (72%) during this period.[47]

Results of human PET studies and the analogous autoradiographic animal studies have shown regional brain development of oxygen and glucose metabolism and blood flow.[44,48-50] In preterm human newborns (26 to 32 weeks gestation), blood flow is about five times higher in the cerebral gray matter than in white matter.[48] Blood flow values increase between birth and adulthood in both regions. Cerebral cortical metabolic rates for glucose generally double in the human brain from shortly after birth to around 8 months.[49] In the newborn cat, metabolic rates for oxygen and glucose are similar in cortical gray and white matter.[44] This metabolic rate increases 2 to 3 times in the gray matter but changes little in white matter between the neonatal period and adulthood in this species, which has extensive prenatal brain maturation (i.e., precocial).

Nonlocalized MRS (Figure 3–4) shows doubling of the PCr/NTP ratio over the first month of life in the rat and mouse brain.[5,51] Since the nucleoside triphosphate (NTP) concentration, of which 60% to 70% is ATP, is constant over this period in the rat brain,[22,52] the PCr concentration probably doubles in the altricial rodent cerebral hemispheres in the first month of life. *In vitro* measures of these concentrations in cerebral white matter in the developing brain are not available. A smaller maturational increase in the PCr/NTP ratio occurs in the human neonatal brain between 28 weeks post conception to about 10 months post term (Figure 3–5)[53,54] and in the piglet brain between 3 days and 4 weeks of age (unpublished results). These analogous maturational PCr changes in the human brain and the neonatal altricial animal brain suggest that matching these developmental time courses will enhance the usefulness of immature animal models for studying the physiology of brain ATP metabolism.

In the altricial rodent brain (e.g., rat, mouse, rabbit), the capacity for aerobic ATP synthesis increases postnatally.[8,12,55] As shown in Figure 3–6,

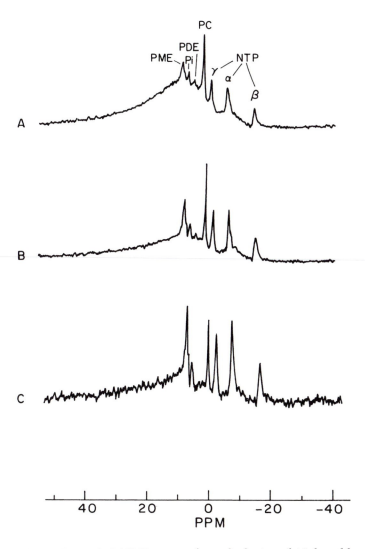

FIGURE 3–4.   31P-NMR spectra from the brains of 40-day-old
(A), 17-day-old (B), and 3-day-old (C) mice acquired with a surface coil. The spectra are shown without any baseline flattening
or normalizing applied. Resonance assignments are shown, including the three phosphorus nuclei of the nucleoside triphos-
phates (NTP), phosphocreatine (PC), inorganic phosphate (Pi),
and peaks generally assigned to phosphomonoesters (PME) and
phosphodiesters (PDE). The broad signal underlying the spectrum from the adult brain is generally attributed to phosphorus
nuclei in bone. The maturational increase in the PCr/NTP ratio is clearly seen in these spectra and is shown over this developmental period in the graph shown on page 38. (Reprinted
with permission from Holtzman D, McFarland E, Jacobs D,
Offutt M, Neuringer L. Maturational increase in mouse brain
creatine kinase reaction rates shown by phosphorus magnetic
resonance. *Dev Brain Res* 1991;58:181–188.)

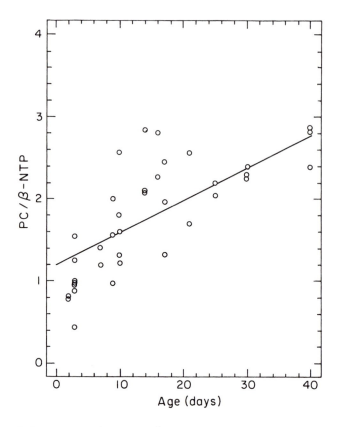

FIGURE 3–4.   (*continued*)

rates of aerobic and anaerobic glycolysis increase to a greater extent in cerebral cortex than in other regions over the first month of life.[56,57] Over this same time course, there is a marked increase in glucose carbon incorporation into amino acids in the rat brain.[58] Activities of glycolytic enzymes, such as hexokinase and aldolase, and of citric acid cycle enzymes, including citric acid synthetase, isocitrate dehydrogenase, and fumarase, increase 5 to 6 times over this period in the rat cerebral cortex.[41,42] There is a coincident 2-fold increase in the number of mitochondria per cell cortex, but the number of mitochondria per wet weight does not change.[59,60] The respiratory enzyme content per mitochondrion increases 3- to 4-fold. The total CK activity, made up mostly of the B-CK isoenzyme, increases about 4-fold from birth to 30 days in whole cerebral hemispheres of the rat.[5,61] In contrast, lactate dehydrogenase and pyruvate dehydrogenase, the regulatory enzymes coupling anaerobic and aerobic metabolism, increase over a shorter period, reaching adult levels by 20 days in rat cerebral cortex (Figure 3–7).[41,42]

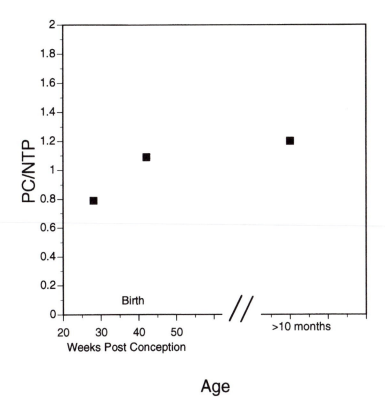

FIGURE 3–5.   Maturational increase in human brain PCr/NTP ratio. The increase in the PCr/NTP ratio has been observed between about 7 months post conception and about 10 months post term. (Modified from Azzopardi D, Wyatt J, Hamilton P, Cady E, Delpy D, Hope P, Reynolds E. Phosphorus metabolites and intracellular pH in the brains of normal and small for gestational age infants investigated by magnetic resonance spectroscopy. *Pediatr Res* 1989;25:440–444 and van der Knaap M, van der Grond J, van Rijen P, Faber J, Valk J, Willemse K. Age-dependent changes in localized proton and phosphorus MR spectroscopy of the brain. *Radiology* 1990;176:509–515.)

The development of cerebral ATPases in rat brain has been studied less than the ATP synthetic pathways. In the adult rabbit hippocampus, there are regional differences in the activity of Na,K-ATPase, the predominant ATPase of brain.[62] Within each region, there is a maturational increase in activity between days 8 and 15. The Na,K-ATPases from rabbit cerebral cortical neurons, glial-enriched fraction, and synaptosome-enriched fraction show the same kinetic properties, suggesting that the same enzyme is

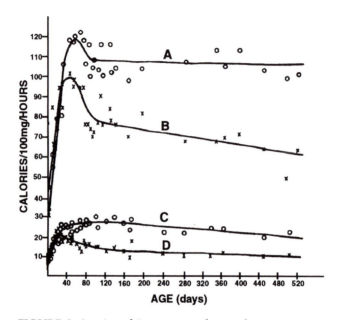

FIGURE 3–6.   A and B represent the aerobic energy production of the cerebral cortex and brain stem in the developing rat brain. C and D represent the anaerobic energy
production of these same brain regions. (Reprinted with
permission from Chesler A, Himwich H. Comparative
studies of the rates of oxidation and glycolysis in the cerebral cortex and brain stem of the rat. *Am J Physiol*
1944;141:513–517.)

present in these sites.[63] However, a recent developmental study demonstrates three Na,K-ATPase isoenzymes which are present throughout the
brain in different relative concentrations.[64] Only one of these isoenzymes
increases during the first month of life in the rat brain. Neurons contain all
three isoenzymes while glia contain only two, but both cell groups contain
the isoenzyme that increases with postnatal brain metabolic maturation.[65]
The subcellular localizations and physiological functions of these ATPases
are unknown.

These *in vitro* and *in vivo* developmental studies of brain ATP metabolism again leave many questions to be answered. Regional PET studies
of glucose metabolic rates suggest marked differences in ATP metabolism in mature cerebral gray and white matter.[11,43,44] *In vivo* maturational
time courses, particularly for white mattter, have not been studied in
detail. Similarly, regional comparisons of the relative concentrations of
PCr and NTP can be measured with localized 31P-MRS.[66] Such studies
in the piglet are currently underway. With poorer temporal resolution,

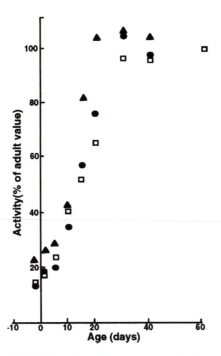

FIGURE 3–7. Comparative development of hexokinase (open squares), aldolase (solid circles), and lactate dehydrogenase (solid triangles) in the rat cerebral cortex. Enzyme activities are expressed as a percentage of the 60-day-old adult values. (Reprinted with permission from Leong S, Clark J. Regional enzyme development in rat brain: Enzymes associated with glucose utilization. *Biochem J* 1984; 218:131–138 and Leong S, Clark J. Regional enzyme development in rat brain; enzymes of energy metabolism. *Biochem J* 1984;218: 139–145.)

regional measurements of glucose and glycogen, and of their turnover in brain, can be made with 13C-MRS techniques.[33,35] Regional maturational changes in ATPases may further localize differences in ATP metabolism. Molecular biological techniques are being applied to these questions. However, multiple isoenzymes, regional and cellular heterogeneity, and independent maturational time courses make these studies very complex.

Development of ATP Metabolic Coupling in Brain

In contrast to the relatively slow postnatal increase in cerebral hemisphere capacity for ATP synthesis, related changes in ATP metabolism appear in a much shorter developmental time period. These metabolic changes suggest that during this period the physiology of ATP metabolism adapts to the large and rapid variations in ATP demand, which are characteristic of the mature cerebral cortex.[11]

Between 12 and 17 days of age, rat cerebral cortical tissue develops the capacity to increase rates of aerobic glycolysis 60% to 100% in response to rapid increases in ATP use. Metabolic stimulation, designed to model *in vivo* physiological and pathological conditions, includes electrical pulses (Figure 3–8A), increased extracellular KCl (Figure 3–8C), hyperthermia (Fig-

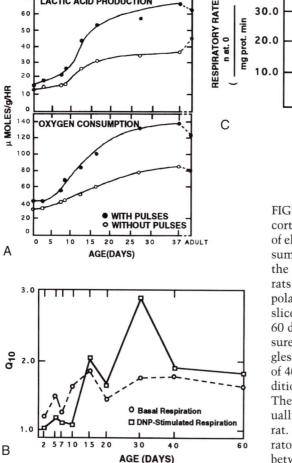

FIGURE 3–8.   Maturation of cerebral cortical respiratory control. A. Effects of electrical pulses on the oxygen consumption and lactic acid production of the cerebral cortical slices of young rats. B. Respiratory rates measured polarographically in cerebral cortical slices from rat pups and adults (50 to 60 days of age). Respiration was measured under basal conditions (triangles) and when stimulated by addition of 40 mM K^+ (closed circles) or by addition of dinitrophenol (open circles). The basal respiration increases gradually over the first month of life in the rat. In contrast, the stimulated respiratory rates approximately doubles between 10 and 15 days of age.

ure 3–C). In contrast to the slower development of glycolytic and most tricarboxylic acid cycle enzymes described in the previous section, the brief maturational time course also is seen in the increasing pyruvate and lactate dehydrogenase activities in rat cerebral cortex.[41,42] These regulatory enzymes couple glycolysis with pathways of aerobic metabolism. The maximal respiratory capacity and the fraction of respiration coupled to ATP synthesis in rat cerebral cortical tissue also increase markedly in this brief developmental period.[68]

As shown in Figure 3–9, the *in vivo* CK-catalyzed reaction rate increases 4-fold between about 13 and 17 days of age in the rat and mouse brain.[5] The Mi-CK activity increases much more than B-CK activity between days 12 and 25 in the rat brain (Figure 3–10). These results suggest that the appearance of the Mi-CK contributes to the increased CK-catalyzed reaction rate. In the cerebellum, the MiCK isoenzyme is mostly, or even entirely, present in gray matter while the B-CK is present in both gray and white matter.[5] Thus, the Mi-CK may be localized in brain regions with higher rates of aerobic glycolysis and blood flow. A compartmentalized distribution of Mi-CK also is suggested by the appearance of a subpopulation of rat cerebral mitochondria, which show resistance to separation of inner and outer membranes between 10 and 20 days of age.[69,70] This new fraction

---

FIGURE 3–8 continued. C. Temperature dependence of respiration, expressed as the Q10 for the temperature range 34°C to 44°C, in cerebral cortical tissue from rats 2 to 60 days of age. Respiration is measured polarographically. The Q10 is the slope of the log of the respiratory rate versus the temperature over the 10° temperature range. Each value is the mean of at least six experiments. SEMs are less than the symbol size for each point. (Modified from Greengard P, McIlwain H. Metabolic response to electric pulses in mammalian cerebral tissues during development.[67] In Waelsch H (ed.), *Biochemistry of the developing nervous system*. New York: Academic Press, 1955, pp. 251–260 and Holtzman D, Nguyen H, Zamvil S, and Olson J. In vivo cellular respiration at elevated temperatures in developing rat cerebral cortex. *Dev Brain Res* 1982;4: 401–405.)

Age vs. Kf

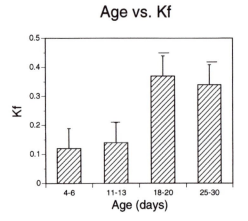

FIGURE 3–9.   The pseudo-rate constants (Kf) for the forward CK-catalyzed reaction rate in the developing rat brain are shown. The reaction rates were measured using the 31P-NMR saturation transfer experiment. Each value is the mean ± SEM for 5 to 6 animals at each of the ages indicated. Compared to the oldest group, the rate constants for the two younger groups are significantly smaller. The CK-catalyzed flux for the developing rat brain increases 4-fold in the narrow age period from about 13 to 17 days of age. Similar maturational increase in the CK-catalyzed reaction rate *in vivo* is seen in the mouse brain. (Reprinted with permission from Holtzman D, Tsuji M, Wallimann T, Hemmer W. Functional maturation of creatine kinase in rat brain. *Develop Neurosci* 1994;15:261–270.)

of cerebral mitochondria—approximately 50% of the mitochondria from cerebral gray plus white matter—shows contact sites between inner and outer membranes, the location of Mi-CK.[71] Rat cerebral mitochondria also show increased efficiency of oxidative phosphorylation during this brief maturational period.[72,73] These observations are consistent with the proposal that the PCr/CK system, including Mi-CK, contributes to close coupling of ATP synthesis and demand.[21,71]

Further support for a central role of the PCr/CK system in the regulation of brain ATP is suggested by recent studies of the hypoxic developing rat brain.[7] Spectra were acquired every minute before, during, and after 6 min

CK-Isoenzymes vs. age

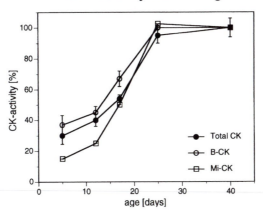

FIGURE 3–10. The developmental increase in whole brain total CK activity (solid circles), B-CK activity (open circles), and Mi-CK activity (squares) expressed as a percentage of the values measured in brains of adult rats. Activities were measured by densitometric scanning after separation of isoenzymes. In the adult rat brain, Mi-CK is about 5% of the total CK activity. Note that all CK-related parameters increase markedly between days 5 and 25 with Mi-CK showing the steepest maturational increase between 12 and 17 days of age. (Reprinted with permission from Holtzman D, Tsuji M, Wallimann T, Hemmer W. Functional maturation of creatine kinase in rat brain. *Develop Neurosci,* in press.)

of hypoxia (Figure 3–11). At all ages PCr decreases rapidly. At 4 and 10 days, PCr is almost fully depleted while ATP remains at 70% to 80% of the pre-hypoxic concentration, as calculated from the B-NTP signal. Thus in the immature hypoxic brain, the CK-catalyzed reaction may function as an energy reserve. At 25 days, PCr initially decreases to 50% while ATP decreases to about 80% of the pre-hypoxic concentration. Then, PCr and ATP decrease simultaneously (Figure 3–12). The close temporal coupling of PCr and ATP losses in the hypoxic mature brain suggests a metabolic regulatory role for the PCr/CK system. Of interest, the EEG activity was lost when ATP was about 30% depleted at all ages. Thus, ATP may be critical in sustaining electrocortical activity in the hypoxic brain at all ages.

These coincident changes in the physiology of ATP metabolism in the developing brain are summarized in Table 3–2. These results suggest a

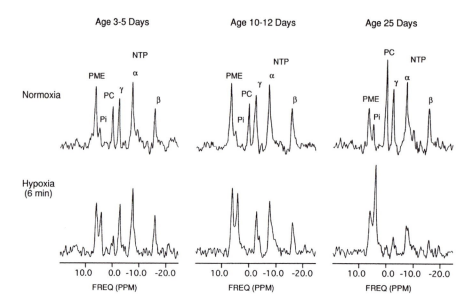

FIGURE 3–11. In vivo brain 31P-NMR spectra from rats of different ages under conditions of normoxia (top row) and after 6 min of hypoxia (bottom row). PCr decreased almost completely in all three animals. However, ATP loss as assessed from the β-NTP peak was much greater in the 25 day rat than at other ages.

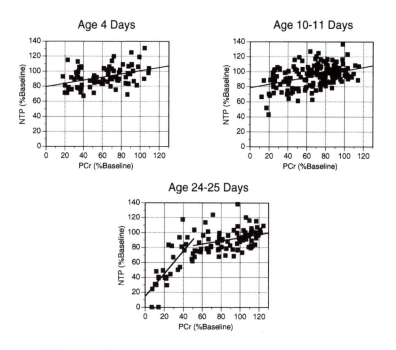

FIGURE 3–12. Losses of brain NTP versus PCr in hypoxic developing rats. The 4 and 10 to 11 day pups showed similar slopes of NTP loss versus PCr loss. In the 24 to 25 day rats, NTP loss was similar to that seen in younger animals until PCr was decreased about 50%, when PCr and ATP losses were simultaneous.

TABLE 3–2

Maturational changes in rat cerebral cortical mitochondrial and tissue properties which are temporarily and, hypothetically, functionally related to increased *in vivo* creatine kinase activity (Reference numbers refer to the references in this chapter.) (Adapted from Holtzman D, Tsuji M, Wallimann T, Hemmer W. Functional maturation of creatine kinase in rat brain. *Develop Neurosci* 1994; 15:261–270.)

Metabolic Changes	*Preparation*
Increased Mi-CK[5]	Whole brain homogenates
Mitochondrial intermembrane contact sites[69,70]	Isolated cerebral hemisphere mitochondria
Increased mitochondrial respiratory control[73]	
Increased mitochondrial ADP/O ratios[13,72]	
Increased stimulated aerobic glycolysis[11,12,67,68]	Cerebral cortical slices
Increased stimulated lactate production[67]	
Increased Q10 for hyperthermia stimulated tissue respiration[65]	
Simultaneous loss of brain PCr and ATP with hypoxia[7]	*In vivo* brain NMR spectroscopy (not localized)

two-compartment model of the mature brain PCr/CK system characterized by slow and fast CK-catalyzed reaction rates. This proposal also explains results of earlier studies in which mice were fed an analogue of creatine.[74] The hypothesized regional differences in CK reaction rates and in regulation of brain ATP are being tested using volume-localized 31P-NMR spectroscopy in the piglet. A second hypothesis in this model is that Mi-CK is a marker for the close coupling of PCr and ATP concentrations in the hypoxic brain. The maturational changes in localization and in physiological role(s) of the CK-catalyzed reaction rates may be important in understanding regional ATP regulation in the human newborn brain.

Animal Studies of Hypothermia and Energy Deficit

Hypothermia alters many, if not all, measures of mature cerebral ATP metabolism.[11] Oxygen consumption decreases with a Q10 of about 4 to 5 between 38° and 22°C (Figure 3–13). Some mechanisms contributing to the decreased oxidative glycolysis are suggested in a recent study of piglets on CPB with brain ATP metabolism measured by nonlocalized 31P-MRS, NIRS, and radiolabeled microspheres (unpublished results). When body and brain temperatures decrease from 35° to about 15°C, brain and blood pH increase

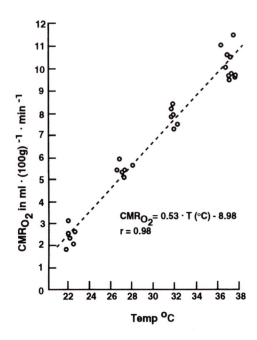

FIGURE 3–13. The temperature dependence of the cerebral metabolic rate for oxygen (CMRO$_2$) in rat cerebral cortex *in vivo*. (Reprinted with permission from[75] Hagerdal M, Harp J, Nilsson L, Siesjo B. The effect of induced hypothermia upon oxygen consumption in the rat brain. *J Neurochem* 1975;24:311–316.)

due to the temperature dependence of the dissociation constant of water. The ATP concentration is stable while the PCr concentration rises perhaps secondarily to the mass action effect of decreased H$^+$ concentration. Cerebral cytochrome oxidase becomes reduced while the oxygenated hemoglobin increases, consistent with the effect of hypothermia on the oxygen-hemoglobin dissociation curve.[76] The stable ATP indicates that glycolysis is sufficient to maintain brain cellular energy even when blood flow is markedly decreased.[77,78]

Normothermic regulation of PCr and ATP has been studied in brains of hypoxic 4-week-old piglets.[79] The ventilated animals were exposed to 7 min periods of increasing hypoxia (inspired O$_2$ concentrations were 12%, 8%, 6%, 4%, and 0%) with full recovery in 25% oxygen between each hypoxic period. In addition to systemic cardio-respiratory monitoring, brain ATP metabolism was measured using nonlocalized 31P-MRS and NIRS during and after the hypoxic periods. Moderate degrees of hypoxia produced an increase in brain blood volume and in cellular oxygenation as indicated by increased oxidation of cytochrome oxidase (Cytaa3). In many of these hypoxic episodes, brain pH became more alkalotic. More severe hypoxia produced a reduction in Cytaa3 which was always associated with decreased PCr (Figure 3–14). Reductions of PCr and ATP did not correlate with hemoglobin deoxygenation but correlated closely with reduction in Cytaa3. Both the reductions in PCr and ATP and the decrease in Cytaa3 oxidation state were closely correlated with decreased mean arterial pressure, supporting the proposal that maintaining increased cerebral perfusion is a critical compensatory mechanism in the hypoxic brain.[11] The decreases in PCr and ATP were the same as seen in the hypoxic rat in which PCr decreased about 50% before ATP began to fall. The two CK reactants then decreased together.

This complex relationship of PCr and ATP losses again suggests that understanding the function(s) of the PCr/CK systems in brain will be important in understanding the regulation of ATP metabolism during hypoxia. As already described, the temporally coincident losses of PCr and ATP, and the maturational increase in CK activity, appear at the same age.[5] Interpretation of the relationship of the CK-catalyzed reaction to regulation of ATP in hypoxic brain is complicated by the observation that the reaction

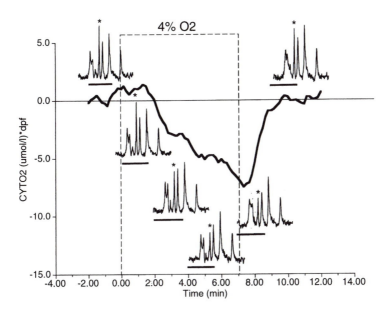

FIGURE 3–14. Time course of the oxidized Cytaa3 concentration changes during a hypoxic period in the piglet (4% O_2 for 7 min). The zero value for the oxidized Cytaa3 is the value just before the first hypoxic exposure. An initial increase in the oxidation state of Cytaa3 was frequently seen. The 31P-NMR spectra acquired during the same hypoxic period are shown.

rate decreases more than 50% after the first hypoxic episode (i.e., 12% inspired O_2), before any consistent changes in PCr or ATP are observed.[79] A similar result was observed in mice reversibly poisoned with cyanide.[80] The CK-catalyzed reaction rate varies 8-fold after cyanide poisoning (Figure 3–15). Low doses produce no measurable changes in brain pH or in PCr and ATP concentrations, but the CK-catalyzed reaction rate increases about 75%. Higher cyanide doses produce a 40% to 50% decrease in PCr, a decrease in pH, and a small decrease in ATP. After recovery of reactant concentrations, the CK-catalyzed reaction rate is decreased 50% to 80% to a rate similar to that found in the very immature mouse brain. The decreased

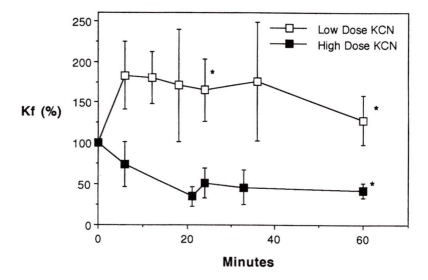

FIGURE 3–15.   Changes in pseudo-rate constants (Kf) for the creatine kinase-catalyzed phosphorus exchange from PC to ATP in brains of mice injected with low doses (1 to 3 mg/kg body weight, closed squares) or with moderate doses (4 to 5 mg/kg, open squares) of cyanide. The saturation transfer experiments were performed before the cyanide injection and after recovery of all metabolite concentrations after the injection. The post-injection values are expressed as a percent of the pre-cyanide value calculated for each experiment. Each point is the mean ± SD of at least three experiments. The differences between the pre-cyanide values and the total post-cyanide time courses were highly significant for both dosage groups. Significance values <.05 for differences between pre-cyanide value and individual post-cyanide times are indicated by asterisks. (Reprinted with permission from Holtzman D, Offutt M, Tsuji M, Neuringer L, Jacobs D. Creatine kinase reaction rates in the cyanide poisoned mouse brain. *J Cereb Blood Flow Metab* 1993;13:153–161.)

CK activity persists at least 90 min. Thus, in the post-hypoxic brain, CK activity increases after mild hypoxia and decreases for a prolonged period after moderate, reversible hypoxia.

These results suggest that the CK-catalyzed reaction reflects, or is a mechanism in, the metabolic adaptation of mature brain ATP metabolism to cellular energy deficit. In addition to the very early changes in CK activity in the hypoxic brain, ultraviolet/visible spectroscopy has shown marked changes in the regulation of cellular oxidation/reduction after ischemia. There is an increase in the resting oxidation state of Cytaa3. With electrical stimulation Cytaa3 becomes reduced rather than further oxidized as in normal animals.[81] These post-ischemic changes in regulation of the electron transport chain oxidation-reduction suggest that the Mi-CK, ATP-ADP translocase complex is important in the regulation of ATP synthesis in the mature brain.[5,21] Hypoxia also reduces brain Na,K-ATPase activity about 20% in the mature guinea pig.[82] This effect may be dependent on the developmental stage of the brain, because in the fetal guinea pig (50 days post conception) maternal hypoxia does not change ATPase rates, while at 60 days maternal hypoxia produces a 50% decrease in these reaction rates.

From this brief review of the physiology of ATP metabolism in the hypothermic, hypoxic, and ischemic brain, it is clear that very little is known about ATP regulation during and following these conditions. This lack of information is true particularly in the immature brain. Of great clinical importance will be systematic study of the physiology of brain ATP metabolism after hypothermia or ischemia. Ongoing studies of a piglet model of CPB and DHCA already have shown that recovery of high energy phosphates in brain is affected by variables such as blood pH, vasoactive drugs, removal of cerebral blood prior to the arrest of circulation, excitatory neurotransmitters, and nitric oxide synthetase inhibitors.[83–87] Use of this animal model will facilitate evaluations of potential clinical interventions and will inform the efforts to understand the adaptation of human brain ATP metabolism to these conditions.

Future Directions for Research

The success of cardiac repair in the neonatal period and the incomplete success in protecting the immature brain during these procedures dictate the need for further animal and human research related to the pathogenesis of cellular injury during and following DHCA. Understanding the regulation of ATP metabolism in the immature brain under these conditions is a necessary foundation for designing and evaluating interventions aimed at protecting the neonatal brain during cardiac repair. Our current understanding of the physiology and vulnerability of these pathways suggests further studies including:

1. Developmental studies of ATP metabolism could be compared in the human neonate and in altricial animals using faster 31P-NMR techniques that are becoming available.
2. The physiology of brain ATP regulation and the pathophysiology of brain injury must be studied further in an animal model under conditions of deep hypothermia with and without circulatory arrest.
3. Similarly, regulation of brain ATP must be studied after hypothermia and circulatory arrest. These studies should model the conditions of the human neonate in the period after cardiac repair.
4. Animal models of deep hypothermic circulatory arrest should be used to develop and rationally apply new bedside noninvasive techniques for measuring relevant parameters of ATP metabolism and cellular functions in the human brain after cardiac surgery and other relevant clinical conditions.
5. The piglet model of DHCA should continue to be used to assess potential means of improving brain protection under these experimental conditions.
6. These scientific and technical advances must be combined with rigorous, prospective long-term studies of the neurologic outcome in children who undergo cardiac repair as neonates.

References

1. Ferry P. Neurologic sequelae of open heart surgery in children. *Am J Dis Child* 1990; 144:369–373.
2. Newburger JW, Jonas RA, Wernovsky G, Wypij D, Hickey PR, Kuban KCK, Farrell DM, Holmes GL, Helmers SL, Constantinou J, Carrazana E, Barlow JK, Walsh AZ, Lucius KC, Share JC, Wessel DL, Hanley FL, Mayer JE, Castaneda AR, Ware JH. A comparison of the perioperative neurologic effects of hypothermic circulatory arrest versus low flow cardiopulmonary bypass in infant heart surgery. *N Engl J Med* 1993;329:1057–1064.
3. Petroff O, Prichard J, Behar K, Alger J, Shulman R. In vivo phosphorus nuclear magnetic resonance spectroscopy in status epilepticus. *Ann Neurol* 1984;16:169–177.
4. Prichard J, Alger J, Behar K, Petroff O, Shulman R. Cerebral metabolic studies in vivo by 31P-NMR. *Proc Natl Acad Sci (USA)* 1983;80:2746–2751.
5. Holtzman D, Tsuji M, Wallimann T, Hemmer W. Functional maturation of creatine kinase in rat brain. *Develop Neurosci,* 1994;15:261–270.
6. Lowry O, Passonneau J, Hasselberger F, Schulz D. Effect of ischemia on known substrates and cofactors of the glycolytic pathway in brain. *J Biol Chem* 1964; 239:18–30.
7. Tsuji M, Allred E, Jensen F, Holtzman D. Sequential loss of phosphocreatine and ATP in hypoxic immature rat brain. *Pediatr Res* 1993;33:376A.
8. Himwich H. Historical review. In Himwich WA (ed.), *Developmental neurobiology.* Springfield: Thomas, pp. 22–44.
9. Clarke D, Sokoloff L. Circulation and energy metabolism of the brain. In Siegel G, Agranoff B, Albers R, Molinoff P (eds.), *Basic neurochemistry,* 5th ed. New York: Raven Press, pp. 645–680.

10. Erecinska M, Silver I. ATP and brain function. *J Cereb Blood Flow Metab* 1989; 9:2–19.
11. Siesjo B. *Cerebral energy metabolism.* Chichester, UK: Wiley, 1978.
12. Holtzman D, Olson J. Developmental changes in brain cellular energy metabolism in relation to seizures and their sequelae. In Jaspers H, van Gelder N (eds.), *Basic mechanisms of neuronal hyperexcitability.* New York: Liss, 1983.
13. Hertz L, Peng L. Energy metabolism at the cellular level of the CNS. *Can J Physiol Pharmacol* 1992;70:S145–157.
14. Friede, R. *Topographic brain chemistry.* New York: Academic Press, 1966.
15. Kao-Jen J, Wilson J. Localization of hexokinase in neural tissue: Electron microscopic studies of rat cerebellar cortex. *J Neurochem* 1980;35:667–678.
16. Nafstad P, Blackstad T. Distribution of mitochondria in pyramidal cells and boutons in hippocampal cortex. *J Zellforsch* 1966;73:234–245.
17. Wong-Riley M. Changes in the visual system of mono-nuclearly sutured or enucleated cats demonstrable with cytochrome oxidase histochemistry. *Brain Res* 1979;171:11–28.
18. Kageyama G, Wong-Riley M. Histochemical localization of cytochrome oxidase in the hippocampus: Correlation with specific neuronal types and afferent pathways. *Neuroscience* 1982;7:2337–2361.
19. Engel J, Kuhl D, Phelps M. Patterns of human local cerebral glucose metabolism during epileptic seizures. *Science* 1982;218:64–66.
20. Jacobus W, Lehninger A. Creatine kinase of rat heart mitochondria. *J Biol Chem* 1973;248:4803–4810.
21. Wyss M, Smeitink J, Wevers R, Wallimann T. Mitochondrial creatine kinase: A key enzyme of aerobic energy metabolism. *Biochim Biophys Acta* 1992;1102: 119–166.
22. Chapman A, Westerberg E, Siesjo B. The metabolism of purine and pyrimidine nucleotides during insulin-induced hypoglycemia and recovery. *J Neurochem* 1981;36:179–189.
23. McGilvery R, Murray T. Calculated equilibrium of phosphocreatine and adenosine phosphates during utilization of high energy phosphates by muscle. *J Biol Chem* 1974;249:5849–5857.
24. Holtzman D, McFarland E, Jacobs D, Offutt M, Neuringer L. Maturational increase in mouse brain creatine kinase reaction rates shown by phosphorus magnetic resonance. *Dev Brain Res* 1991;58:181–188.
25. Sweadner K. Overlapping and diverse distribution of Na-K ATPase isozymes in neurons and glia. *Can J Physiol Pharmacol* 1992;70:S255–S259.
26. Mata M, Fink D, Gainer H, Smith CB, Davidsen L, Savaki H, Schwartz WJ, Sokoloff L. Activity-dependent energy metabolism in rat posterior pituitary primarily reflects sodium pump activity. *J Neurochem* 1980;34:213–215.
27. Olson J, Sankar R, Holtzman D, James A, Fleischhacker D. Energy dependent volume regulation in primary cultured cerebral astrocytes. *J Cell Physiol* 1986; 128:209–215.
28. Sauter A, Rudin M. Determination of creatine kinase kinetic parameters in rat brain by NMR magnetization transfer. *J Biol Chem* 1993;268:13166–13171.
29. Sokoloff L. Relation between physiological function and energy metabolism in the central nervous system. *J Neurochem* 1977;29:13–26.
30. Frey K. Positron emission tomography. In Siegel G, Agranoff B, Albers W, Molinoff P (eds.), *Basic neurochemistry,* 5th ed. New York: Raven Press, 1994, pp. 935–956.

31. Phelps M, Mazziotta J, Huang S. Study of cerebral function with positron computed tomography. *J Cereb Blood Flow Metab* 1982;2:113–162.
32. Cady, E. *Clinical magnetic resonance spectroscopy.* New York: Plenum, 1990.
33. Gadian D. *Nuclear magnetic resonance and its application to living systems.* Oxford: Clarendon, 1982.
34. Badar-Goffer R, Bachelard H, Morris, P. Cerebral metabolism of acetate and glucose studied by 13C-NMR spectroscopy: A technique for investigating metabolic compartmentation in the brain. *Biochem J* 1990;266:133–139.
35. Belliveau J, Kennedy D, McKinstry R, Buchbinder B, Weisskoff R, Cohen M, Vevea J, Brady T, Rosen B. Functional mapping of the human visual cortex by magnetic resonance imaging. *Science* 1991;254:716–719.
36. Cohen M, Bookheimer S. Localization of brain function using magnetic resonance imaging. *Trends Neurosci* 1994;17:268–277.
37. Reynolds E, Wyatt J, Azzopardi D, Delpy D, Cady E, Cope M, Wray S. New non-invasive methods for assessing brain oxygenation and haemodynamics. *Br Med Bull* 1988;44:1052–1075.
38. Tsuji M, Naruse H, Volpe J, Holtzman D. Cerebral hemoglobin and cytochrome oxidase reduction during hypoxic energy loss. *Pediatr Res* 1994;35:388A.
39. Sokoloff L, Reivich M, Kennedy C, DesRosiers M, Patlak D, Pettigrew K, Sakurada O, Shinohara M. The [14C] deoxyglucose method for the measurement of local cerebral glucose utilization: Theory, procedure, and normal values in the conscious and anesthetized albino rat. *J Neurochem* 1977;28:897–916.
40. Kennedy C, Sakurada O, Shinohara M, Jehle J, Sokoloff L. Local cerebral glucose utilization in the normal conscious Macaque monkey. *Ann Neurol* 1978;4:293–301.
41. Leong S, Clark J. Regional enzyme development in rat brain: Enzymes associated with glucose utilization. *Biochem J* 1984a;218:131–138.
42. Leong S, Clark J. Regional enzyme development in rat brain; enzymes of energy metabolism. *Biochem J* 1984b;218:139–145.
43. Chugani H, Phelps M, Mazziotta J. Positron emission tomography study of human brain functional development. *Ann Neurol* 1987;22:487–497.
44. Chugani H, Hovda D, Villablanca F. Metabolic maturation of the brain: A study of local cerebral utilization in the developing cat. *J Cereb Blood Flow Metab* 1991;11:35–47.
45. Tennyson V. The fine structure of the developing nervous system. In Himwich W (ed.), *Developmental neurobiology.* Springfield, Thomas, 1970, pp. 47–116.
46. Himwich H. *Brain metabolism and cerebral disorders.* Baltimore: Williams & Wilkins, 1951.
47. Agranoff B, Hajra A. Lipids. In Siegel G, Agranoff B, Albers R, Molinoff P (eds.), *Basic neurochemistry,* 5th ed. New York: Raven Press, 1994, pp. 97–116.
48. Altman DI, Powers WJ, Perlman JM, Herscovitch P, Volpe SL, Volpe JJ. Cerebral blood flow requirement for brain viability in newborn infants is lower than in adults. *Ann Neurol* 1988;24:218–226.
49. Chugani H, Phelps M. Maturational changes in cerebral function in infants determined by [18] FDG positron emission tomography. *Science* 1986;231:840–843.
50. Kennedy C, Grave G, Jehle J, Sokoloff L. Changes in blood flow in the component structures of the dog brain during postnatal maturation. *J Neurochem* 1972;19:2423–2433.

51. Tofts P, Wray S. Changes in brain phosphorus metabolites during the postnatal development of the rat. *J Physiol* 1985;359:417–429.
52. Lolley R, Balfour W, Samson F. The high energy phosphates in developing brain. *J Neurochem* 1961;7:289–297.
53. Azzopardi D, Wyatt J, Hamilton P, Cady E, Delpy D, Hope P, Reynolds E. Phosphorus metabolites and intracellular pH in the brains of normal and small for gestational age infants investigated by magnetic resonance spectroscopy. *Pediatr Res* 1989;25:440–444.
54. van der Knaap M, van der Grond J, van Rijen P, Faber J, Valk J, Willemse K. Age-dependent changes in localized proton and phosphorus MR spectroscopy of the brain. *Radiology* 1990;176:509–515.
55. McIlwain H, Bachelard H. *Biochemistry and the central nervous system.* Edinburgh: Churchill-Livingstone, 1985, pp. 406–444.
56. Tyler D, Van Harreveld A. The respiration of the developing brain. *Am J Physiol* 1942;136:600–603.
57. Chesler A, Himwich H. Comparative studies of the rates of oxidation and glycolysis in the cerebral cortex and brain stem of the rat. *Am J Physiol* 1944;141:513–517.
58. Gaitonde M, Richter D. Changes with age in the utilization of glucose carbon in liver and brain. *J Neurochem* 1966;13:1309–1316.
59. Dahl D, Samson F. Metabolism of rat brain mitochondria during postnatal development. *Am J Physiol* 1959;196:470–472.
60. Gregson N, Williams P. A comparative study of brain and liver mitochondria from new-born and adult rats. *J Neurochem* 1969;16:617–626.
61. Booth R, Clark J. Studies on the mitochondrial bound form of rat brain creatine kinase. *Biochem J* 1978;170:145–151.
62. Haglund M, Stahl W, Kunkel D, Schwartzkroin P. Developmental and regional differences in the localization of Na,K-ATPase activity in the rabbit hippocampus. *Brain Res* 1985;343:198–203.
63. Averet L, Arrigoni E, Loiseau H, Cohadon F. Na,K-ATPase activity of glial, neuronal, and synaptosomal enriched fractions from normal and freezing injured rabbit cerebral cortex. *Neurochem Res* 1987;17:607–612.
64. Urayama O, Shutt H, Sweadner K. Identification of three isozyme proteins of the catalytic subunit of the Na,K-ATPase in rat brain. *J Biol Chem* 1992;264:8271–8280.
65. Holtzman D, Nguyen H, Zamvil S, Olson J. In vivo cellular respiration at elevated temperatures in developing rat cerebral cortex. *Dev Brain Res* 1982;4:401–405.
66. Cadoux-Hudson T, Blackledge M, Radda, G. Imaging of human brain creatine kinase activity in vivo. *FASEB J* 1989;3:2660–2666.
67. Greengard P, McIlwain H. Metabolic response to electric pulses in mammalian cerebral tissues during development. In Waelsch H (ed.), *Biochemistry of the developing nervous system.* New York: Academic Press, 1955, pp. 251–260.
68. Holtzman D, Olson J, Samvil S, Nguyen H. Maturation of potassium stimulated respiration in rat cerebral cortical slices. *J Neurochem* 1982;39:274–276.
69. Holtzman D, Lewiston N, Herman M, Desautel M, Brewer E, Robin E. Effects of osmolar changes in isolated brain versus liver mitochondria. *J Neurochem* 1978;30:1409–1419.
70. Holtzman D, Herman M, Desautel M, Lewiston N. Effects of altered osmolarity on respiration and morphology of mitochondria from the developing brain. *J Neurochem* 1979;33:453–460.

71. Wallimann T, Wyss M, Brdiczka D, Nicolay K, Eppenberger HM. Intracellular compartmentation, structure and function of creatine kinase isoenzymes in tissues with high and fluctuating energy demands: The 'phosphocreatine circuit' for cellular homeostasis. *Biochem J* 1992;281:21–40.
72. Holtzman D, Moore C. Oxidative phosphorylation in immature rat brain mitochondria. *Biol of the Neonate* 1973;22:230–242.
73. Holtzman D, Magruder C. Effects of oligomycin on respiration in developing rat brain mitochondria. *Brain Res* 1977;120:373–378.
74. Holtzman D, McFarland E, Moerland T, Koutcher J, Kushmerick M, Neuringer L. Brain creatine phosphate and creatine kinase in mice fed an analogue of creatine. *Brain Res* 1989;483:68–77.
75. Hagerdal M, Harp J, Nilsson L, Siesjo B. The effect of induced hypothermia upon oxygen consumption in the rat brain. *J Neurochem* 1975;24:311–316.
76. Barcroft J, King W. The effect of temperature on the oxygen dissociation curve of blood. *J Physiol* 1909;39:374–384.
77. Swain J, McDonald T, Griffith P, Robbins R, Balaban R. Low flow hypothermic cardiopulmonary bypass protects the brain. *J Thoracic Cardiovasc Surg* 1991; 102:76–83.
78. Kawata H, Fackler J, Aoki M, Tsuji M, Sawatari K, Offutt M, Hickey P, Holtzman D, Jonas R. Recovery of cerebral blood flow and energy state in piglets after hypothermic circulatory arrest versus recovery after low-flow bypass. *J Thoracic Cardiovasc Surg* 1993;106:671–685.
79. Tsuji M, Naruse H, Holtzman D. Hypoxia decreases brain creatine kinase reaction rate *in vivo. Biophys J* 1994;66:A344.
80. Holtzman D, Offutt M, Tsuji M, Neuringer L, Jacobs D. Creatine kinase reaction rates in the cyanide-poisoned mouse brain. *J Cereb Blood Flow Metab* 1993; 13:153–161.
81. Duckrow F, LaManna J, Rosenthal M. Disparate recovery of resting and stimulated oxidative metabolism following transient ischemia. *Stroke* 1981;12:677–685.
82. Mishra O, Delivoria-Papadopoulos M. Na, K-ATPase in developing fetal guinea pig brain and the effect of maternal hypoxia. *Neurochemical Res* 1988;13: 765–770.
83. Aoki M, Nomura F, Stromski M, Tsuji M, Fackler J, Hickey P, Holtzman D, Jonas R. Effects of pH strategy on recovery of piglet brain energetics after hypothermic circulatory arrest. *Ann Thorac Surg* 1993;55:1093–1103.
84. Aoki M, Nomura F, Stromski M, Tsuji M, Fackler J, Hickey P, Holtzman D, Jonas R. Effects of MK-801 and NBQX on recovery of cerebral metabolism after hypothermic circulatory arrest. *J Cerebr Blood Flow Metab* 1994;14:156–165.
85. Hiramatsu T, Miura T, Forbess J, duPlessis A, Holtzman D, Jonas R. L-NAME blocks recovery of cerebral energy state after deep hypothermic circulatory arrest in piglets. In Krieglstein J, Oberpichler-Schwenk J (eds.), *Pharmacology of cerebral ischemia.* Stuttgart: Med Pharm Medical Publishers, 1994.
86. Aoki M, Jonas RA, Nomura F, Stromski ME, Tsuji MK, Hickey PR, Holtzman D. Effects of aprotinin on acute recovery of cerebral metabolism with hypothermic circulatory arrest. *Ann Thorac Surg* 1994;58:146–153.
87. Aoki M, Jonas RA, Nomura F, Stromski ME, Tsuji MK, Hickey PR, Holtzman D. Effects of cerebroplegic solutions during hypothermic circulatory arrest and short-term recovery. *J Thorac Cardiovasc Surg* 1994;108:291–301.

Acknowledgments

Recent studies cited in this review were supported by grants from the Cerebral Palsy Foundation (R-4010) and the National Institutes of Health (NS 26371). The animal cardiopulmonary bypass studies were supported by the Cardiac Surgery Research Foundation of the Children's Hospital, Boston, MA. MT is supported in part by a grant from the National Institute of Child Health (K11 HD 01010). We dedicate this review to the memory of Dr. Leo Neuringer who provided enthusiastic and critical advice in applying NMR spectroscopy to the study of cardiopulmonary bypass in the piglet.

CHAPTER 4

EEG Maturation with Special Reference to Epileptogenic Effects of Hypoxia

Frances E. Jensen

EEG Activity during Brain Maturation

There are established patterns in the maturation of EEG activity in both animals and humans. For infants undergoing cardiac bypass, the EEG is a practical method of assessing brain function and maturation and, perhaps, risk for perioperative complications. In both animals and humans, stages of EEG development can be approximately related to brain maturation. In addition, observations from human neonates and data from animal models provide evidence that there are age-dependent responses of the brain and of EEG activity to hypoxia and ischemia. Age-dependent differences seen in some of the animal model systems might provide an indication as to where age-specific therapy can be directed, especially for neonatal patients.

The pattern of EEG activity changes most dramatically in the neonatal period and first year of life, a period of development characterized by multiple maturational events in the brain. In the human, neuronal proliferation and migration occur throughout gestation. At about 6 months conceptual age, there are rapid increases in axonal arborization, dendritic elaboration, and synaptogenesis. The peak of synaptogenesis actually occurs in the early postnatal period.[1] Myelination occurs somewhat later, starting perinatally and continuing until the end of childhood.[2,3] The prolonged development of myelinated fibers is likely to affect EEG activity. In fact, the frequency and amplitude of background activity progressively increases until mid to late childhood, at which point it stabilizes at the 9 Hz alpha activity that is seen in adults.[4]

Several features of the normal EEG can be used for comparisons across development: continuity, synchrony, sleep pattern, and reactivity. In addition, there are patterns that occur as normal phenomena during early development that would be considered abnormal in the mature EEG. An example of such a phenomenon is the tracé discontinu pattern, which is present in preterm infants and is characterized by extremely low amplitude EEG activity punctuated intermittently by higher voltage bursts.[5] As the infant matures to term, there is a shift to a pattern of increased continuity in the baseline frequency alternating with intervals of higher voltage activity, termed tracé alternant.[6,7]

Synchrony of EEG activity is another feature that increases during development. Synergy of activity between the hemispheres is largely complete by term. Interhemispheric synchrony is thought to relate to the level of myelination in the corpus callosum, which is known to occur over the same time period.[3,8] Sleep patterns also undergo pronounced changes in the perinatal period. The preterm infant spends 60% to 70% of its time in rapid eye movement (REM) sleep, or active sleep. With increasing postnatal age, the time spent in REM sleep decreases and a better differentiation of these sleep states is seen by 1 month of age.[4,9]

There are other transient features in EEG activity in infancy that would be considered abnormal in the EEG of the adult or older child. For example, spike activity can be seen in the infant EEG and does not necessarily indicate an epileptic condition. During 33 to 44 weeks of conceptual age, there is an increase in this kind of activity, which disappears by the second postnatal month.[9] This conceptual age overlaps with a period of intense synaptogenesis.[1] In the human, the relationship of these phenomena to seizure susceptibility or excitotoxicity is unknown. Hence, in evaluating the neonatal EEG, it is important to monitor for deviations from the normal pattern and to see whether the developmental stage of the EEG matches the conceptual age of the infant. The term dysmature refers to the presence of an EEG feature that is appropriate to an earlier stage of development but would not normally be seen at the chronologic age of the infant being studied.[4,9,10]

Developmental Changes in Seizure Susceptibility

Clinical observations indicate that the perinatal period represents a window of development in which there is heightened seizure susceptibility. It has long been recognized that the vast majority of cases of status epilepticus occur in the first year of life, particularly in the neonatal period (Figure 4–1).[11] Many different pathologic conditions are observed to cause seizures in the immature brain that are infrequently associated with seizures in the adult, including hypoxia and hypoxia/ischemia.[12–15] Seizures in the neonate are multifocal and migratory.[10] Notably, these multifocal and migratory seizures are occurring at a developmental stage characterized by incomplete myelination and a high rate of synaptogenesis.

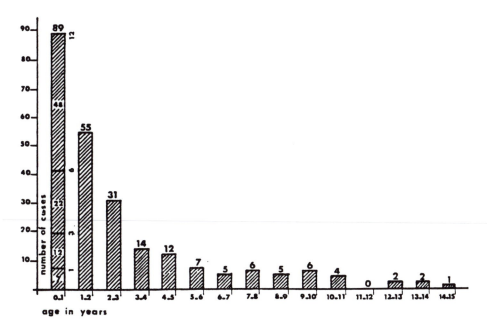

FIGURE 4–1. Incidence of status epilepticus is highest in the first year of life. Age distribution of 239 children with status. The figures in the first bar show the numbers in 4 subgroups (0 to 1 month, 1 to 3 months, 3 to 6 months, 6 to 12 months). (Reprinted with permission from Aicardi J, Chevrie JJ. Convulsive status epilepticus in infants and children. A study of 239 cases. *Epilepsia* 1970;11:187–197.)

Neonatal seizures are associated with a variety of conditions, including hypoxia/ischemia, metabolic derangements, intraventricular hemorrhage, and infection.[15,16] In the presence of intercurrent pathologic processes, the EEG can be used as a prognostic tool. The degree of background abnormality can be related to prognosis.[17,18] A clear correlation exists between the presence of a burst suppression pattern and poor outcome in the term infant, but the relationship is less clear in premature infants.[7,17,18]

In the population of neonates undergoing planned cardiopulmonary bypass, there is an opportunity to obtain EEG information preoperatively, which may give important information about the state of brain maturation and relative risk for adverse neurologic complications. In addition, the postoperative EEG may be an important tool in assessing neurologic outcome.

Experimental Evidence for Heightened Seizure Susceptibility in the Newborn and the Age-Dependent Epileptogenic Effect of Hypoxia

Given these human correlates between brain maturation and EEG activity patterns, we and others have developed animal models to evaluate pathophysiologic mechanisms underlying age-dependent differences in EEG to hypoxic/ischemic injury.[19] Using a perinatal rat model, we have demonstrated age-dependent differences in EEG response to hypoxia and subsequent outcome.[20-22] There appears to be a window of vulnerability to the epileptogenic effects of hypoxia. In the animal model, this developmental window can be identified by patterns of baseline EEG activity. Furthermore, EEG response to hypoxic stress can be used as an indicator of prognosis. As in the human, the rat undergoes a series of changes in EEG background activity during development.

In the early postnatal life of the rat (postnatal day (P) 0 to 5), the EEG baseline is very flat with some punctuation of higher voltage activity (Figure 4–2A),[20,23] and this resembles the tracé discontinu of the preterm human. By 10 to 12 days of age, there is an increase in background (Figure 4–2B), with periodic alternations of amplitude and perhaps this EEG may be analogous to the tracé alternant state seen in the term human. In fact, the brain of the 10 to 12 day rat has been thought to be analogous to that of the human at term according to a number of parameters and EEG features as well as degree of myelination.[24-26] Finally, the rat EEG progressively matures with a gradual increase of amplitude and frequency from 15 days to adult (P60)(Figure 4–2C,D,E).

Using a model of global hypoxia, we have previously demonstrated that hypoxia induces seizure activity in immature rats but not in adults.[20] In the rat, this seizure susceptibility occurs between postnatal days (P)5 to 17, with peak seizure frequency and severity occurring around P10 with exposure to moderate hypoxia (3% to 4% O_2) (see Figure 4–3). Electroencephalographic (EEG) and electrocardiographic (ECG) activity were measured while animals were exposed to hypoxia (0%, 2%, 3%, or 4% O_2); animals were resuscitated with room air at the onset of apnea. Hypoxia resulted in seizure activity in the immature animals but not in adults. The peak effect was seen at 10 days of age, with the window extending between P5 and P17. In contrast, more severe O_2 deprivation (0% to 2% O_2) resulted in depression of EEG activity to an isoelectric state in all ages. The administration of hypoxia to P5 to 17 animals resulted in a high incidence of epileptiform EEG activity during hypoxia (Figure 4–3B). At these ages, 80% to 100% of the animals exhibited epileptiform EEG changes. Controlling for O_2 concentration, the incidence of epileptiform activity was significantly higher in the three younger age groups (P5 to 7, P10 to 12, P15 to 17) (Figures 4–3A, B, C) compared to the older groups (P25 to 27, P50 to 60) (Figure 4–3D, E) ($p<.0001$). In contrast, the older animals exhibited only rare isolated EEG spikes before reaching an isoelectric EEG. This age dependence was not related to differences in blood gases between these groups. Furthermore, we have demonstrated persistent seizures for hours to days into recovery from hypoxia in animals exposed at P5 to 17 but not at older ages (Figure 4–4).

In addition to the acute epileptogenic effect of hypoxia, the long term outcome also appears to be dependent upon the age of exposure to hypoxia.

Prehypoxic Baseline EEG

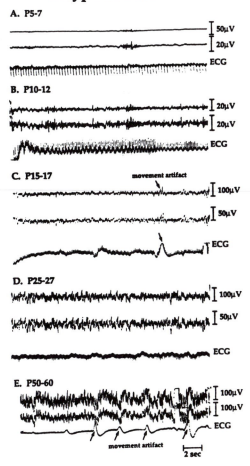

FIGURE 4–2.   Baseline EEG activity in the developing rat. There is a gradual increase in the amplitude and frequency of EEG activity with maturation. (A) EEG at postnatal days (P) 5 to 7 reveals low amplitude baseline punctuated by bursts of high voltage slowing; (B) at P10 to 12, baseline frequency and amplitude are increased, but there are still episodes of high voltage activity; and (C through E) between P15 to adult, there is a progressive increase in EEG amplitude and frequency. (Reprinted with permission from Jensen FE, Applegate CD, Holtzman D, Belin TR, Burchfiel JL. Epileptogenic effects of hypoxia on immature rodent brain. *Ann Neurol* 1991;29:629–637.)

Acute Hypoxia EEG

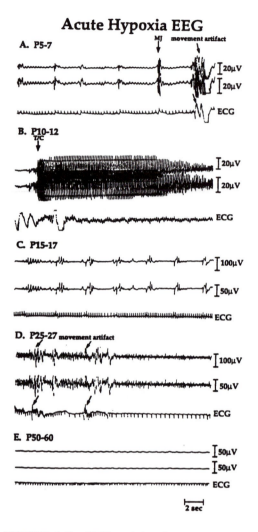

FIGURE 4–3. EEG activity during exposure to 3% oxygen in rats in each age group. (A) Spike discharges are seen in isolation, and in association with a myoclonic jerk (MJ) in the P5 to 7 group. (B) At P10 to 12, hypoxia induces trains of spike discharges in association with tonic-clonic head and trunk activity (T/C). (C) Rhythmic spike discharges are seen during hypoxia at P15 to 17, without behavioral seizures. (D) At P25 to 27, low amplitude spike activity occurs without behavioral seizures. (E) In the adult, hypoxia results in the gradual decline of EEG activity to an isolelectric state, without seizure activity. (Reprinted with permission from Jensen FE, Applegate CD, Holtzman D, Belin TR, Burchfiel JL. Epileptogenic effects of hypoxia on immature rodent brain. *Ann Neurol* 1991;29:629–637.)

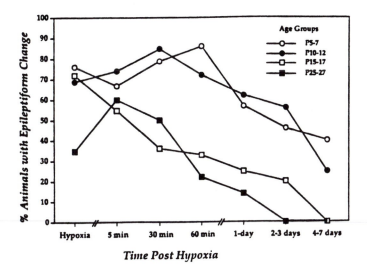

FIGURE 4–4.   Frequency of epileptiform EEG changes in animals from 4 age groups sampled at 5, 30, and 60 min, and at 1 to 7 days following hypoxia. Data are represented as the frequency of epileptiform events during hypoxia. (Reprinted with permission from Jensen FE, Applegate CD, Holtzman D, Belin TR, Burchfiel JL. Epileptogenic effects of hypoxia on immature rodent brain. *Ann Neurol* 1991;29:629–637.)

Seizure susceptibility is permanently increased in the animals rendered hypoxic at P10 and not in animals made hypoxic at younger ages (P5) or older ages (P60) (Figure 4–5).[21,22] No significant histopathologic damage was noted by light microscopy after hypoxia alone at any age. In the rats previously rendered hypoxic at P10, more severe seizure activity during hypoxia appeared to increase their seizure susceptibility as adults. Taken together, these experiments therefore identified a window of development in the rat during which exposure to hypoxia results in both acute and long-term brain hyperexcitability.

In the same age window, an epileptiform response similar to that seen during hypoxia alone can also be evoked by hypoxia in combination with ischemia. Rat pups exposed to hypoxia after undergoing unilateral carotid ligation exhibit EEG spike discharges ipsilateral to the ligation, but not in the nonligated hemisphere. These epileptiform events can be seen for 48 hours into the recovery period. In contrast, no sustained behavioral or EEG epileptiform activity is observed in either hemisphere of adult animals undergoing unilateral carotid ligation. When severe hypoxia/ischemia resulting from bilateral carotid ligation and hypoxia is administered to P10 to 12 rat pups, prolonged generalized seizure activity is observed during the insult as well as in recovery. A positive correlation between infarct size and seizure

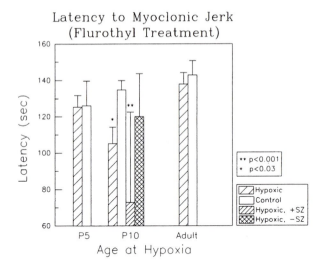

FIGURE 4–5.   Differential effects of hypoxia administered at P5, P10, or P60 (adult) rat on subsequent seizure
threshold to flurothyl-induced epileptiform activity
tested 60 days after hypoxia. Latency to flurothyl-
induced myoclonic jerk was significantly reduced only
in the group of rats exposed to hypoxia at P10 and not
after hypoxia at younger (P5) or older (P60) ages. The
most significant reduction in threshold was in the group
of rats that had exhibited severe seizures during hypoxia
at P10 (double hatched bars). (Reprinted with permission from Jensen FE, Holmes GH, Lombroso CT, Blume
HK, Firkusny IR. Age-dependent long-term changes in
seizure susceptibility and neurobehavior following hypoxia in the rat. *Epilepsia* 1992;33:971–980.)

severity and duration was found in these experimental animals (Jensen, unpublished results). The presence of severe seizure activity during hypoxia in
the pups with bilateral carotid ligation predicted infarct size, and to a lesser
extent morbidity, within the 48 hours following the insult.

The Role of Glutamate Receptors in the
Pathophysiology of Stroke and Epilepsy

There is much evidence to suggest that excessive release of excitatory amino
acid (EAA) neurotransmitters mediates neuronal damage in the setting of
hypoxia/ischemia.[27,28] The predominant EAA in the brain is glutamate,
and certain glutamate antagonists prevent glutamate-induced neurotoxic-

ity.[19,29–31] *In vitro* studies have shown that direct application of glutamate to neuronal cells in culture results in a primary phase of swelling followed by a delayed phase of toxicity over the next 24 hours, which is dependent upon Ca^{2+} influx, primarily via activation of the N-methyl-D-aspartate (NMDA) glutamate receptor subtype.[32,33] This Ca^{2+} influx initiates a cascade of biochemical events, including activation of proteases and lipases, free radical formation, membrane breakdown, and ultimately cell death.[27] The existence of this delayed phase may present a window for therapeutic intervention following stroke. EAA receptor activity has been implicated in seizures,[34] and EAAs are elevated in epileptic foci of humans.[35] Furthermore, EAA antagonists have also been shown to have anticonvulsant properties.[36]

EAAs Are Essential for Normal Development, Plasticity, and Learning

EAAs have been shown to have trophic influences on neurons during development[37–40] and to regulate activity-dependent growth.[41] Long-term potentiation (LTP) is an enduring increase in synaptic efficacy following brief tetanic stimulation and is postulated to be involved in memory.[42] The induction of LTP requires the activation of NMDA receptors.[43] NMDA receptors are also implicated in experience-dependent plasticity, and this plasticity can be blocked with NMDA receptor antagonists such as MK-801.[44,45]

Maturational Changes Responsible for the Predominance of Excitation over Inhibition in the Developing Brain

The age window during which hypoxia and hypoxia/ischemia cause dramatic epileptiform responses in the rat occurs at a maturational stage in which excitatory mechanisms predominate over those which are inhibitory. The maturational curve for densities of the different EAA receptors exhibits a transient overshoot in density for both the N-methyl-D-aspartate (NMDA) and the amino-3-hydroxy-5-methyl-4-isoxazole proprionic acid (AMPA) receptor subtypes. For both receptor subtypes, this overshoot occurs around the second postnatal week in the rat.[19,46] Under normal conditions, the NMDA calcium channel is blocked by magnesium, but under conditions of excess neuronal activity and depolarization, Mg^{2+} is displaced from the channel, allowing calcium to enter intracellularly. The configuration of this channel is controlled by its subunit composition, and these subunits are known to change with development. During the second postnatal week, the NMDAR2c subunit is expressed,[47] and the presence of this subunit is thought to confer Mg^{2+} insensitivity.[48] In fact, it is precisely during this age window in the rat that the NMDA receptor is shown to be less sensitive to Mg^{2+} blockade than in the adult.[49]

In addition to the conformational changes in the NMDA receptor, there is also differential subunit expression in the non-NMDA AMPA receptor that predisposes it to neuronal hyperexcitability. In the adult rat, only the

NMDA receptor is permeable to calcium. However, like the NMDA receptor, the permeability of the AMPA receptor to calcium is governed by subunit composition. During the first and second postnatal weeks in the rat, the ratio of the AMPA receptor subunits GluR1 and GluR3 to GluR2 is high, in contrast to a low ratio in the adult.[50] The GluR2 subunit encodes for calcium impermeability of the AMPA related ion channels, and hence the increased ratio of GluR1 and GluR3 to GluR2 is thought to underlie the calcium permeability observed in neurons from immature animals.[50] In addition, Wasterlain, et al. have demonstrated that during the same developmental window immature hippocampal neurons lack adult levels of the calcium binding protein, calbindin D28K.[51] The cumulative effect of these maturational changes in receptor densities and subunit composition, as well as ion metabolism, may increase intracellular calcium concentration. Because increases in intracellular calcium mediate excitotoxicity and activation of second messenger systems and gene regulation,[32,52,53] the immature brain is more vulnerable than the adult to functional and structural consequences of conditions that may alter seizure susceptibility.

The Relative Anticonvulsant Efficacy of EAA Antagonists and Conventional Anticonvulsants during Experimental Perinatal Hypoxia

Given the central role of EAA activation in excitotoxicity and epileptogenesis, we compared the anticonvulsant efficacy of the NMDA antagonist MK-801 and the non-NMDA antagonist NBQX versus conventional anticonvulsants, such as lorazepam, phenytoin, and phenobarbital, on seizures induced in the rat model of perinatal hypoxia.[54] Clinically, seizures associated with hypoxia/ischemia are difficult to treat and can often be refractory to conventional therapies.[13,14] Compared to saline, pretreatment with MK-801 or NBQX significantly reduced seizures, while lorazepam did not.[54] A further study has evaluated whether seizure suppression with EAA antagonists (the NMDA antagonist MK-801 or the AMPA antagonist NBQX) or the anticonvulsant lorazepam prevented long-term seizure susceptibility (Figure 4–6).[55] Long Evans rats (P10) were exposed to hypoxia after pretreatment with normal saline (NS), MK-801, NBQX), or lorazepam, and seizure thresholds to flurothyl were tested at P70 for comparison with nonhypoxic littermates. Hypoxic, NS-treated rats had significantly lowered seizure thresholds compared to nonhypoxic controls. While MK-801 significantly suppressed acute seizures at P10, latencies to flurothyl seizures in adulthood were not different from NS-treated animals. In contrast, NBQX pretreatment significantly reduced acute seizures and delayed latency to flurothyl-induced myoclonic jerk in adulthood. Animals treated with lorazepam did not differ from saline treated rats. In conclusion, EAA antagonists and conventional anticonvulsants may have differential effects on perinatal hypoxic seizures and on subsequent adulthood seizure susceptibility.

TREATMENT EFFECT DURING HYPOXIA

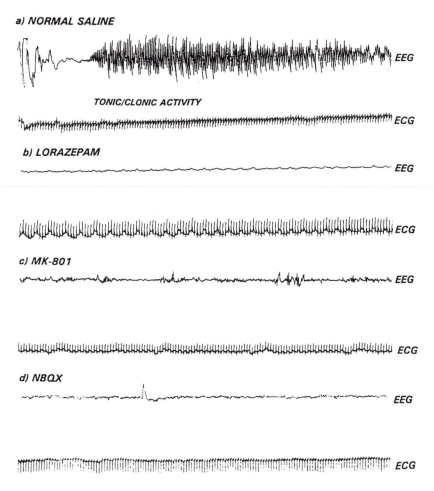

FIGURE 4–6.   The relative effects of the agents administered as treatment prior to hypoxia in the P10 rat. (A) Tonic/clonic seizure activity in rats treated with normal saline (NS, control). (B) Lorazepam (1 mg/kg) suppressed tonic clonic seizures in most cases, but myoclonic jerks persisted. In contrast, both (C) MK-801 (1 mg/kg) and (D) NBQX (20 mg/kg) significantly suppressed hypoxia-induced seizure activity.

To better describe underlying mechanisms, we have evaluated the age-dependence of the effect of hypoxia administered either *in vivo* or *in vitro*. Extracellular recordings of evoked and spontaneous activity in area CA1 of the hippocampus was performed in slices from adult versus P10 to 15 rats either after hypoxia *in vivo* or during hypoxia *in vitro*. Slices from previously hypoxic rat pups showed enhanced LTP compared to controls and more prolonged evoked responses, suggesting an enhancement of NMDA-mediated activity.[56] In the second part of this study, normal slices were exposed to hypoxia in 0 Mg^{2+} medium. Hypoxia/0 Mg^{2+} induced ictal discharges more frequently in immature slices than in adult slices. Both 0 Mg^{2+} and hypoxia/0 Mg^{2+} induced ictal discharges were suppressed by the NMDA receptor blocker APV and the non-NMDA antagonist CNQX.[57] These results are consistent with the previous *in vivo* experiments and suggest that neuronal excitability is altered by hypoxia in an age-dependent manner that may involve the EAA receptors.

Conclusion

These results support the hypothesis that EAA antagonists may be protective in hypoxic/ischemic perinatal injury and that they may prevent both the neuronal damage as well as the epileptic response. However, as discussed earlier, EAA blockade in the immature brain may not be tolerated because the activity at the EAA receptors, particularly the NMDA receptor, is likely to be critical for normal brain development. Some EAA antagonists have been shown to have neurobehavioral side effects such as sedation and impaired learning.[31] In addition, recent studies have shown that MK-801 produces early vacuolization within the cytosol of neurons, although this appears to be reversible.[31,58] More recently, it has been demonstrated that chronic daily treatment with the NMDA antagonist MK-801 in the first 2 postnatal weeks of life in the rat results in increased seizure susceptibility later in life.[59]

A better understanding of the mechanisms underlying the increased susceptibility of the immature neuron to epileptogenesis and hypoxic/ischemic injury will lead to the development of more specific therapy directed only at the pathologic actions of EAA receptors. Further studies of potential therapeutic agents will have to directly address their impact on the development of the nervous system as well as their neuroprotective potency. Physiologic parameters, including EEG activity, can be used to establish markers of human maturation that coincide with those shown in animal studies to represent periods of heightened vulnerability to hypoxic injury and epileptogenesis.

REFERENCES

1. Huttenlocher PR, deCourten C, Garey LJ, Van der Loos H. Synaptogenesis in human visual cortex—evidence for synapse elimination during normal development. *Neurosc Lett* 1982;33:247.
2. Rorke LB, Riggs HE. *Myelination of the brain in the newborn.* Philadelphia: Lippincott, 1969.

3. Gilles FH. Myelination in the neonatal brain. *Hum Pathol* 1976;7:244–248.
4. Niedermeyer E. Maturation of the EEG: Development of waking and sleep patterns. In Niedermeyer E, Lopes Da Silva F (eds.), *Electroencephalography*, 3rd ed. Baltimore: Williams and Wilkins, 1993, pp. 167–191.
5. Dreyfus-Brisac C, Peschanski N, Radvanyi MF, Cukier-Hemeury F, Monod N. Convulsions in neonates. Clinical, electrophysiologic, etiopathogenic and prognostic aspects. *Rev Electroencephalogr Neurphysiolo Clin* 1981;11:367–378.
6. Dreyfus C, Curzi-Dascalova L. The EEG during the first year of life. In Redmond A (ed.), *Handbook of electroencephalography and clinical neurophysiology*, Vol. 6. Amsterdam: Elsevier, 1975, pp. 24–30.
7. Holmes GL, Lombroso CT. Prognostic value of background patterns in the neonatal EEG. *J Clin Neurophysiol* 1993;10:323–352.
8. Yakovlev PI, Lecours AR. The myelogenetic cycles of regional maturation of the brain. In Minkowski A (ed.), *Regional development of the brain in early life*, 3rd ed. Philadelphia: F.A. Davis, 1967.
9. Stockard-Pope JE, Werner SS, Bickford RG, Curran JS. *Atlas of neonatal electroencephalography*, 2nd ed. New York: Raven Press, 1994.
10. Lombroso CT. Neonatal EEG polygraphy in normal and abnormal newborns. In Niedermeyer E, Lopes Da Silva F (eds.), *Electroencephalography*, 3rd ed. Baltimore: Williams and Wilkins, 1993, pp. 803–876.
11. Aicardi J, Chevrie JJ. Convulsive status epilepticus in infants and children. A study of 239 cases. *Epilepsia* 1970;11:187–197.
12. Bergamasco B, Benna P, Ferrero P, Gavinelli R. Neonatal hypoxia and epileptic risk: A clinical prospective study. *Epilepsia* 1984;25:131–146.
13. Volpe JJ. *Neurology of the newborn*, 2nd ed. Philadelphia: W.B.Saunders, 1987.
14. Volpe JJ. Neonatal seizures: Current concepts and revised classifications. *Pediatrics* 1989;84:422–428.
15. Holmes GL. Neonatal seizures. In Pedley TA, Meldrum BS (eds.), *Recent advances in epilepsy*, 2nd ed. New York: Churchill Livingstone, 1985, pp. 207–237.
16. Holmes GL, Kull LL. Neonatal seizures. *Am J EEG Technol* 1990;30:281–308.
17. Lombroso CT, Holmes GL. Value of the EEG in neonatal seizures. *J Epilepsy* 1993;6:39–70.
18. Rowe JC, Holmes GL, Hafford J, Baboval D, Robinson S, Phillips A, Rosenkrantz T, Raye J. Prognostic value of the electroencephalogram in term and preterm infants following neonatal seizures. *Electroencephalogr Clin Neurophysiol* 1994; 60:183–196.
19. McDonald JW, Johnston MV. Physiological and pathophysiological roles of excitatory amino acids during central nervous system development. *Brain Res Rev* 1990;15:41–70.
20. Jensen FE, Applegate CD, Holtzman D, Belin TR, Burchfiel JL. Epileptogenic effects of hypoxia on immature rodent brain. *Ann Neurol* 1991;29:629–637.
21. Jensen FE, Applegate CD, Burchfiel JL, Lombroso CT. Differential effects of perinatal hypoxia and anoxia on long term in seizure susceptibility in the rat. *Life Sci* 1991;49, 399–407.
22. Jensen FE, Holmes GH, Lombroso CT, Blume HK, Firkusny IR. Age dependent long term changes in seizure susceptibility and neurobehavior following hypoxia in the rat. *Epilepsia* 1992;33:971–980.
23. Himwich W. *Developmental neurobiology*. Springfield, IL: Charles Thomas Publishers, 1970.

24. Romijn HJ, Hofman MA, Gramsbergen A. At what age is the developing cerebral cortex of the rat comparable to that of the full-term newborn human baby? *Early Hum Dev* 1991;26:61–67.

25. Vanier MT, Holm M, Ohman R, Svennerholm L. Developmental profiles of gangliosides in human and rat brain. *J Neurochem* 1971;18:581–592.

26. Mares P, Maresova D, Schickova R. Effect of antiepileptic drugs on metrazol convulsions during ontogenesis in the rat. *Physiologia Bohemoslovacoa* 1981; 30:113–121.

27. Choi DW, Rothman SM. The role of glutamate neurotoxicity in hypoxic-ichemic neuronal death. *Ann Rev Neurosci* 1990;13:171–182.

28. Meldrum B, Garthwaite J. Excitatory amino acid neurotoxicity and neurodegenerative disease. *Trends Pharmacol Sci* 1990;11:379–387.

29. Hattori H, Morin AM, Schwartz PH, Fujikawa DG, Wasterlain CG. Posthypoxic treatment with MK-801 reduces hypoxic-ischemic damage in the neonatal rat. *Neurology* 1989;39:713–718.

30. McDonald JW, Silverstein FS, Cardona D, Hudson C, Chen R, Johnston MV. Systemic administration of MK-801 protects against N-methyl-d-aspartate-neurotoxicity in perinatal rats. *Neuroscience* 1990;36:589–599.

31. Olney JW, Labnuyere J, Wang G, Wozniak DF, Price MT, Sesma MA. NMDA antagonist neurotoxicity: Mechanism and prevention. *Science* 1991;254: 1515–1518.

32. Michaels RL, Rothman SM. Glutamate toxicity in vitro: Antagonist pharmacology and intracellular calcium concentrations. *J Neuroscience* 1990;10:283–292.

33. Choi DW. Excitatory cell death. *J Neurobiol* 1992;23:1261–1276.

34. Rogawski MA. The NMDA receptor, NMDA antagonists and epilepsy therapy: A status report. *Drugs* 1992;44:279–292.

35. Scherwin AL, Val Gelder NM. Amino acid and catecholamine markers of metabolic abnormalities in human focal epilepsy. In Delgado-Escueta AV, Ward, Jr. AA, Woodbury DM, Porter RJ (eds.), *Advances in neurology* New York: Raven Press, 1994, pp. 1011–1032.

36. Thomson AM, West DC. N-methyl-d aspartate receptors mediate epileptiform activity evoked in some, but not all, conditions in rat neocortical slices. *Neuroscience* 1986;19:1161–1177.

37. Aruffo C, Ferszt R, Hildebrandt AG, Cervox-Nararro J. In vitro neuronal plasticity triggered by subtoxic doses of monosodium glutamate. *Prog Clin Biol Res* 1987;253:229–237.

38. Cline HT, Constantine-Paton M. NMDA receptor antagonists disrupt the retinotectal topographic map. *Neuron* 1989;3:413–426.

39. Pearce IA, Cambray-Deakin MA, Burgoyne RD. Glutamate acting on NMDA receptors stimulates neurite outgrowth from cerebellar granule cells. *FEBS Lett* 1987;223:143–147.

40. Collingridge GL, Singer W. Excitatory amino acid receptors and synaptic plasticity. *Trends Pharmacol Sci* 1990;11:290–296.

41. Mattson MP. Neurotransmitters in the regulation of neuronal cytoarchitecture. *Brain Res* 1988;13:179–212.

42. Baudry M, Davis JL. *Long term potentiation: A debate of current issues.* Cambridge: MIT Press, 1991.

43. Harris EW, Ganong AH, Cotman CW. Long term potentiation in the hippocampus involves activation of the NMDA receptors. *Brain Res* 1984;323: 132–137.

44. Kleinschmidt A, Bear MF, Winger W. Blockage of NMDA receptors disrupts experience-dependent plasticity of kitten striate cortex. *Science* 1987;238: 355–358.
45. Rauschecker JP, Hahn S. Ketamine-xylazine anaesthesia blocks consolidation of ocular dominance changes in kitten visual cortex. *Nature* 1987;326:183–185.
46. Insel TR, Miller L, Gelhard RE. The ontogeny of excitatory amino acid in the rat forebrain: I N-methyl-d-aspartate and quisqualate receptors. *Neuroscience* 1990; 35:31–43.
47. Pollard H, Khrestchatisky M, Moreau J, Ben Ari Y. Transient expression of the NR2C subunit of the NMDA receptor in developing rat brain. *NeuroReport* 1993;4:411–414.
48. Monyer H, Sprengel R, Schoepfer R, Herb A, Higuchi M, Lomeli H, Burnashev N, Sakmann B, Seeberg PH. Heteromeric NMDA receptors: Molecular and functional distinction of subtypes. *Science* 1992;256:1217–1221.
49. Bowe MA, Nadler JV. Developmental increase in the sensitivity to magnesium of NMDA receptors on CA1 hippocampal pyramidal cells. *Dev Brain Res* 1990;56:55–61.
50. Pellegrini-Giampietro DE, Bennett MV, Zukin RS. Are Ca^{2+} -permeable kainate/ AMPA receptors more abundant in immature brain?. *Neuroscience Letters* 1992; 144:65–69.
51. Wasterlain CG, Hattori H, Yang C, Schwartz PH, Rujikawa DG, Morin AM, Dwyer BE. Selective vulnerability of neuronal subpopulations during ontogeny reflects discrete molecular events associated with normal brain development. In Wasterlain CG, Vert P (eds.), *Neonatal seizures.* New York: Raven Press, 1991.
52. Dubinsky JM, Rothman SM. Intracellular calcium concentrations during "chemical hypoxia" and excitotoxic neuronal injury. *J Neuroscience* 1991;11: 2545–2551.
53. Choi DW. Glutamate neurotoxicity and diseases of the nervous system. *Neuron* 1988;1:623–634.
54. Jensen FE, Firkusny IR, Blume HK. Improved anticonvulsant efficacy of EAA antagonists over conventional AEDs in a rat model of perinatal hypoxia-induced seizures. *Epilepsia* 1992;33:20
55. Jensen FE, Alvarado SP, Firkusny IR, Blume H, Geary C. NBQX blocks acute and late epileptogenic effects of perinatal hypoxia. *Epilepsia,* in press.
56. Jensen FE, Wang CD, Stevens MC. Enhanced LTP in hippocampal slices following in vivo perinatal hypoxia. *Society for neuroscience meeting* 1994, (abstract).
57. Wang C, Jensen FE. Increased seizure susceptibility to low magnesium and hypoxia in immature hippocampal slices is suppressed by APV, a NMDA receptor antagonist. *Society for neuroscience meeting* 1994, (abstract).
58. Olney JW, Labruyere J, Price MT. Pathological changes induced in cerebrocortical neurons by phencyclidine and related drugs. *Science* 1989;244:1360–1362.
59. Facchinetti F, Ciani E, Dall'Olio R, Virgili M, Contestable A, Fonnum F. Structural, neurochemical and behavioural consequences of neonatal blockade of NMDA receptor through chronic treatment with CGP 39551 or MK-801. *Dev Brain Res* 1993;74:219–224.

CHAPTER 5

Programmed Cell Death: The Biology of Cell Death in the Nematode *Caenorhabditis elegans* and Implications for the Understanding and Treatment of Human Brain Injury after Cardiac Surgery

H. Robert Horvitz

Nerve cell death is responsible for the clinical symptoms of many neurologic disorders, including the brain damage that occurs subsequent to traumatic challenge and stroke as well as after cardiac surgery.[1] Nerve cell death is also a basic feature of the neurodegenerative diseases—including Alzheimer's disease, Parkinson's disease, Huntington's disease, and amyotrophic lateral sclerosis—all of which are characterized by the deaths of specific classes of neurons. In addition, abnormalities in cell death can cause cancerous growth, which results from a loss of control over cell number and can be a consequence of either too much cell division or too little cell death.[2] Thus, abnormal cell deaths, and abnormalities in the control of which cells live and which cells die, are associated with a great variety of human disorders, including those that are the focus of this book.

Cell death not only is a basic feature of many disease processes but also is a completely normal aspect of the development of all animals that have been studied, including humans.[3] For example, during development of the human immune system, more than 95% of the cells that are generated die. During the development of the mammalian central nervous system, in certain areas and at certain times, as many as 90% of the neurons that are made die. Naturally-occurring cell death thus constitutes a fundamental aspect of animal development and a fundamental problem in the field of developmental biology. These observations raise the possibility that human disorders in which cells that should live instead die might be consequences of an ectopic activation of an otherwise normal process of cell death. In such disorders, the cells that are dying could be undergoing a fundamentally normal process but could be of the wrong cell type or could be dying at the wrong time.

Recent studies of the biology of cell death have revealed that, at least in many cases, cell death is an active process on the part of the cells that die. In other words, many cell deaths appear to be cellular suicides. For example, it has been shown in a variety of experimental systems that the cell death process requires gene expression because inhibitors of RNA or protein synthesis prevent cell death. In some systems it has been found that there are changes in the expression of specific genes, with certain new genes being expressed in cells that are undergoing cell death. In addition, in the neurologic disorders characterized by nerve cell deaths that occur in response to insults or injury, it appears that many of these cell deaths are not immediate events but rather are delayed, secondary responses to the initiating challenges.

Together these various findings lead to the hypothesis that in many human disorders, including in the brain damage that can occur after cardiac surgery, the cell death events that occur are active cellular suicides that involve specific cell-death genes and proteins. If so, and if we can understand the biological process of cell death and can determine the identity and functions of the genes and proteins that regulate and cause cell death, we might well have new targets for therapy and new approaches toward treatments that could help prevent the cell deaths and the disorders they cause.

The Nematode *Caenorhabditis elegans*

We have been studying the biology of cell death, focusing not on the human brain or even on a vertebrate. Instead, we have been analyzing the animal that has the simplest nervous system that has been described in biology, the nematode *Caenorhabditis elegans*. This roundworm is only one millimeter in length, and it grows on Petri plates, just like bacteria, which it eats. Because of its small size and a variety of other features that make it highly tractable for experimental analysis,[4] this nematode has proved to be exceptionally well suited for the study of the biology of cell death.

Will a knowledge of the biology of cell death in a microscopic round-worm help us understand the cell deaths that occur in human development and disease? Recent findings strongly suggest that the answer to this question will be "yes." Studies of such basic cellular processes as the cell cycle and signal transduction from many laboratories have revealed a striking biological universality, namely, that the same classes of genes and proteins function in organisms as diverse as yeast, nematodes, insects, and mammals. For example, signal transduction pathways that are involved in human oncogenesis can be matched, gene by gene, with signal transduction pathways that function during the development of the eye of the fruit fly *Drosophila melanogaster* as well as during the development of the sexual organs of *C. elegans*, the nematode we study.[5-7] In each of these pathways—human oncogenesis, fly eye development, worm sex organ development—there is a protein growth factor, for example, of the EGF family, an EGF receptor type molecule, a signal transduction molecule that is an adapter protein with SH3 and SH2 *src*-homology domains, a RAS protein, a RAF protein, an MAP kinase, and an ETS family transcription factor. It seems plausible that a comparable universality will apply to many biological processes. Indeed, our studies to date indicate that many features of the biology of cell death, like many features of the biology of signal transduction, are conserved between nematodes and humans.

C. elegans is a free-living nonparasitic nematode.[4] There are two sexes: male and hermaphrodite, the latter of which makes both sperm and eggs and is capable of reproducing either by self-fertilization or by mating with males. These animals are cellularly very simple. For example, the adult hermaphrodite contains a total of 959 cells, 302 of which are neurons. The complete connectivity of the nervous system has been determined by the analysis of serial-section electron micrographs. The neurotransmitters in this nervous system have also been characterized, and about 40% of the 302 neurons now have defined neural transmitters associated with them. These neurotransmitters are familiar and include acetylcholine, serotonin, octopamine, dopamine, and GABA. The cell lineage of *C. elegans*, which describes the pattern of cell divisions and cell fates that occur as the single-celled egg generates the 959-celled adult, has also been determined in its entirety.

Programmed Cell Death

During *C. elegans'* development, in addition to the 959 cells that are generated to form the adult body, there are 131 cells generated that undergo naturally-occurring, or programmed, cell death.[3] Thus, about 14% of the cells made in this organism die during the normal course of development. Of the 131 programmed cell deaths, 105 are in the nervous system. In other words, the programmed cell deaths that occur during worm development are primarily events in neural development.

These cell deaths are rapid. Cells normally die within about an hour of the time that they are formed and, in most cases, before the onset of differentiation. The cells that undergo these programmed deaths have a highly characteristic flat, disc-like appearance when viewed with a light microscope using Nomarski differential contrast optics.

When viewed with an electron microscope, these dying cells display a variety of ultrastructural features. For example, dying cells become very electron-dense. Based on morphology, the programmed deaths that occur in *C. elegans* have a number of characteristics similar to cell deaths that occur during the normal development of mammals and that are said to undergo the process of "apoptosis."

The Genetic Program for Programmed Cell Death

To analyze the molecular genetic control of programmed cell death, we have used the approach of classical genetics. Specifically, we have identified mutations affecting the pattern of programmed cell deaths that occur or the process of programmed cell death itself. These mutations define specific genes involved in programmed cell death. By studying these genes using methods of genetics, developmental biology, and molecular biology, we have defined a genetic program for programmed cell death in *C. elegans*.

This program consists of three general steps (Figure 5–1). The first step is "kill" and involves three genes, called *ced-3*, *ced-4* and *ced-9* (*ced, cell death abnormal*). Once a cell is killed and a cell corpse has been generated, that corpse is removed from the body by the process of engulfment or phagocytosis by a nearby cell. The activities of six genes (*ced-1*, *ced-2*, *ced-5*, *ced-6*, *ced-7*, *ced-10*) are involved in this process of phagocytosis. Finally, residual material from the cell corpse is degraded. One gene, *nuc-1*, that acts in the process of degradation has been identified.

Seven Genes Act to Remove and
Degrade Cell Corpses

The gene *nuc-1* controls the activity of a DNAase that degrades the DNA in dying cells.[8] If that nuclease is defective, the DNA is not degraded. Nonetheless, cells still die and still are engulfed. These observations indicate that although the nuclease acts in the pathway of programmed cell death, it is not causally involved. In other words, action of the *nuc-1*-controlled nuclease is not what kills cells during programmed cell death.

The six genes that control the process of engulfment appear to act in two parallel pathways that are mostly redundant in function.[9] If only one of these pathways is disrupted by mutation, most cell corpses are still engulfed,

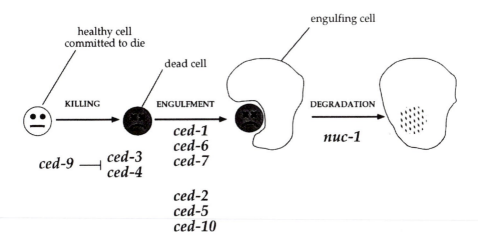

FIGURE 5–1. The genetic program for programmed cell death in *C. elegans*. (Modified from Ellis RE, Yuan J, Horvitz HR. Mechanisms and functions of cell death. *Ann Rev Cell Biol* 1991;7:663–698.)

but if both pathways are disrupted in appropriate double mutants, engulfment is blocked. If engulfment is blocked, cells still die. Thus, phagocytosis, although again an important step in the cell death process, is not what is killing cells. What, then, kills?

The Genes ced-3 and ced-4 Function to Kill Cells

The activities of the genes *ced-3* and *ced-4* are necessary for killing cells by the process of programmed cell death.[10] If either of these genes is inactivated by mutation, all 131 cells that should undergo programmed cell death instead survive. Not only do these cells survive; they differentiate and, in at least those cases that have been tested, become sufficiently normal to be capable of functioning.[11]

How do *ced-3* and *ced-4* cause cells to undergo programmed cell death? To address this question, we first asked whether these genes act within dying cells or act elsewhere in the body of the animal, perhaps controlling a humoral factor that triggers cell death. We used the technique of genetic mosaic analysis, in which animals are constructed with cells of different genotypes, and then the phenotype of a given cell is analyzed to see whether it is determined by its own genotype with respect to a given gene or by the genotype of some other cell or cells. Our findings indicate that both *ced-3* and *ced-4* act cell-autonomously, i.e., act within the cells that die, causing them to undergo programmed cell death.[12]

ced-3 *Encodes a Cysteine Protease Similar to the Human Enzyme ICE*

To determine how *ced-3* and *ced-4* function as apparent cell suicide genes, we characterized both of these genes molecularly.[13,14] Each encodes a single messenger RNA that is expressed primarily during embryonic development, the time when 113 of the 131 cell deaths occur. Thus, both of these genes are expressed at the time when cells are dying.

Based upon DNA sequence, the *ced-4* gene encodes a protein unlike any in the available databases. By contrast, the *ced-3* gene encodes a protein with marked similarity to the human enzyme *interleukin-1-beta-converting en*zyme (ICE), which was purified based upon its ability to generate the cytokine interleukin-1-beta from an inactive pro-protein by proteolytic cleavage. The CED-3 and ICE proteins are 29% identical over their entire lengths and 43% identical over a 115 amino acid region that includes a completely conserved pentapeptide (QACRG), within which is located the active-site cysteine of ICE.

These observations strongly suggest that the CED-3 protein causes programmed cell death in *C. elegans* by acting as a cysteine protease, presumably either by activating other killer proteins or by inactivating proteins that protect cells from dying. These observations also suggest that members of the CED-3/ICE family of cysteine proteases, perhaps even ICE itself, might function in causing programmed cell death in other organisms, including humans. This hypothesis has been strongly supported by the findings that expression of either *ced-3* or ICE in rat fibroblasts can cause these cells to undergo apoptotic cell death[15] and that a viral protein inhibitor of ICE, *crmA*, can block the apoptotic death of chick dorsal root ganglion cells that have been deprived of nerve growth factor.[16] Thus, a CED-3/ICE-like cysteine protease can cause mammalian cell death, and an inhibitor of such a protease can block a normal pathway of vertebrate cell death, indicating that an endogenous protease of this class functions in this pathway.

ced-9 *Protects Cells Against Programmed Cell Death*

What regulates the activities of the killer genes *ced-3* and *ced-4*? One candidate is the gene *ced-9*, which we discovered because of a mutation in this gene. Like mutations in *ced-3* and *ced-4*, this mutation, called *ced-9(n1950)*, prevents programmed cell death.[17] Despite its similar consequences, *n1950* is fundamentally different from the *ced-3* and *ced-4* mutations that prevent programmed cell death. First, based on genetic mapping, *n1950* is located in a different gene. Second, whereas the effects of mutations in *ced-3* and *ced-4* are recessive, the effects of *n1950* are dominant. That *n1950* results in a dominant phenotype suggests that its effects might not simply be to reduce or eliminate the activity of *ced-9*. Most mutations that reduce or eliminate gene function are recessive as a consequence of the gene activity provided by the wild-type gene on the homologous chromosome.[18]

To test the hypothesis that *n1950* does not reduce or eliminate *ced-9* gene activity and to determine the consequences of reducing *ced-9* activity, we sought and identified mutations that eliminated the dominant effects of the mutation *n1950*. Such mutations proved to reduce *ced-9* function and allowed us to analyze the role of this gene. We discovered that animals with reduced *ced-9* function are missing cells and that these cells are missing because they undergo programmed cell death. Specifically, the cells undergo a process that looks morphologically like programmed cell death (displaying the characteristic flat, disc-like appearance) and that depends on the activities of the cell death genes *ced-3* and *ced-4*; e.g., in mutants with reduced *ced-9* activity and also lacking *ced-3* or *ced-4* activity, cells are not missing. If *ced-9* activity is reduced even further, development arrests at an early stage of embryogenesis, with many of the cells in the embryo undergoing programmed cell death.

These observations reveal that if *ced-9* function is reduced, cells that should live instead undergo programmed cell death. In other words, the activity of *ced-9* protects cells against programmed cell death. Interestingly, since a strong reduction in *ced-9* activity causes massive cell death, it seems that most, and perhaps all, cells in the animal are poised, ready to self-destruct by programmed cell death, and it is the activity of *ced-9* that prevents them from doing so. The consequence of the *ced-9* mutation *n1950* is precisely the opposite of that of mutations that reduce *ced-9* activity: *n1950* causes cells that should die to live. Thus, it seems plausible that *n1950* causes not too little, but rather too much *ced-9* activity. These findings reveal that *ced-9* is a developmental switch gene, controlling the very important binary choice between cell (and organismal) life and death. If *ced-9* is off, cells undergo programmed cell death. If *ced-9* is on, cells do not undergo programmed cell death and, instead, survive. Normally during development the activity of *ced-9* must be regulated so those 131 cells that should die do so because *ced-9* is off, whereas other cells have *ced-9* on and so are protected from dying.

The *ced-9* Protein Is Similar to the Human Oncoprotein *bcl-2*

How does *ced-9* protect cells from dying? Molecular characterization of this gene revealed that *ced-9* is a member of a family of genes, the prototype of which is *bcl-2*, a human oncogene.[19] *bcl-2* causes B-cell lymphoma in patients in which this gene is ectopically expressed in B cells of the immune system. This ectopic expression occurs as a consequence of a chromosome 14; 18 translocation that brings the *bcl-2* gene under the control of an enhancer of the immunoglobulin heavy chain locus.[20]

How does *bcl-2* cause cancerous growth? The answer appears to be that it does so by preventing programmed cell deaths, thereby allowing an abnormal increase in cell number.[21] Over-expression of a normal *bcl-2* protein has been found to retard or prevent cell death in a variety of experimental systems; furthermore, the *bcl-2* gene is highly expressed in progenitor and long-lived cells—cells that might be specifically marked for survival. Thus, *ced-9* and *bcl-2* are similar not only in sequence but also in terms of their biological function of protecting cells from programmed cell death.

To explore further the similarity between the worm *ced-9* gene and the human *bcl-2* gene, both we[19] and others[22] constructed transgenic *C. elegans* that expressed a *bcl-2* transgene under the control of a heat-shock promoter and found that human *bcl-2* can block the process of programmed cell death in *C. elegans*. In additional experiments, we found that human *bcl-2* can substitute for the worm's *ced-9* gene. Ectopic cell deaths that occur as a consequence of a lack of *ced-9* function can be prevented by the expression of the human *bcl-2* gene. Thus, *bcl-2* and *ced-9* are similar in sequence, have similar biological functions in protecting against cell death, and are at least in part functionally interchangeable within the organism.

The Mechanisms of Programmed Cell Death Appear to be Evolutionarily Conserved

It is striking that human *bcl-2* can act in *C. elegans*. Genes and their protein products do not work in isolation. Rather, every gene must interact with other genes to exert its biological effects. That *bcl-2* can act in *C. elegans* to prevent cell death, and can do so apparently by substituting for worm *ced-9*, suggests that in humans *bcl-2* functions by interacting with genes similar to those that interact with *ced-9* in worms, for example, genes similar to *ced-3* and *ced-4*. The findings that cysteine proteases similar to CED-3 control programmed cell death in vertebrates strongly support the hypothesis that genes similar to *ced-3* and *ced-4* interact with *bcl-2* in the process of programmed cell death in humans.

One implication of this hypothesis is that the genes and proteins we have identified in *C. elegans* can provide access to the genes and proteins that function in the pathway of cell death that occurs in humans. If, indeed, abnormal expression of such a cell-death pathway is responsible for at least some of the neurologic disorders characterized by cell death, then by identifying, for example, agonists of genes like *ced-9/bcl-2* or antagonists of genes like *ced-3/ICE* or *ced-4*, we might define novel approaches to therapy, approaches based upon intervening with the biology of cell death.

References

1. Choi D. Glutamate neurotoxicity and diseases of the nervous system. *Neuron* 1988;1:623–634.
2. Vaux DL, Cory S, Adams JM. *bcl-2* gene promotes haemopoietic cell survival and cooperates with *c-myc* to immortalize pre-B cells. *Nature* 1988;335:440–442.

3. Ellis RE, Yuan J, Horvitz HR. Mechanisms and functions of cell death. *Ann Rev Cell Biol* 1991;7:663–698.
4. Wood W, the Community of *C.* elegans Researchers (eds.). *The nematode* Caenorhabditis elegans. Cold Spring Harbor, New York: Cold Spring Harbor Laboratory, 1988.
5. Clark SG, Stern MJ, Horvitz HR. Genes involved in two *Caenorhabditis elegans* cell-signaling pathways. *Cold Spring Harbor Symp Quant Biol* 1992;57: 363–373.
6. Greenwald I, Rubin GM. Making a difference: The role of cell-cell interactions in establishing separate identities for equivalent cells. *Cell* 1992;68:271–281.
7. Lackner MR, Kornfeld K, Miller LM, Horvitz HR, Kim SK. A MAP kinase homolog, *mpk-1*, is involved in *ras*-mediated induction of vulval cell fates in *C. elegans*. *Genes Dev* 1994;8:160–173.
8. Hedgecock EM, Sulston JE, Thomson JN. Mutations affecting programmed cell deaths in the nematode *Caenorhabditis elegans*. *Science* 1983;220:1277–1279.
9. Ellis RE, Jacobson DM, Horvitz HR. Genes required for the engulfment of cell corpses during programmed cell death in *C. elegans*. *Genetics* 1991;129:79–94.
10. Ellis HM, Horvitz HR. Genetic control of programmed cell death in the nematode *C. elegans*. *Cell* 1986;44:817–829.
11. Avery L, Horvitz HR. A cell that dies during wild-type *C. elegans* development can function as a neuron in a *ced-3* mutant. *Cell* 1987;51:1071–1078.
12. Yuan J, Horvitz HR. The *Caenorhabditis elegans* genes *ced-3* and *ced-4* act cell-autonomously to cause programmed cell death. *Develop Biol* 1990;138:33–41.
13. Yuan J, Horvitz HR. The *C. elegans* cell death gene *ced-3* encodes a novel protein and is expressed during the period of extensive programmed cell death. *Development* 1992;116:309–320.
14. Yuan J, Shaham S, Ledoux S, Ellis H, Horvitz HR. The *C. elegans* cell death gene *ced-3* encodes a protein similar to mammalian interleukin-1-beta-converting enzyme. *Cell* 1993;75, 641–652.
15. Miura M, Zhu H, Rotello R, Hartwieg E, Yuan J. Induction of apoptosis in fibroblasts by IL-1-beta-converting enzyme, a mammalian homolog of the *C. elegans* cell death gene *ced-3*. *Cell* 1993;75:653–660.
16. Gagliardini V, Fernandez PA, Lee RK, Drexler HC, Rotello RJ, Fishman MC, Yuan J. Prevention of vertebrate neuronal death by the *crmA* gene. *Science* 1994;263:826–828.
17. Hengartner MO, Ellis RE, Horvitz HR. *C. elegans* gene *ced-9* protects cells from programmed cell death. *Nature* 1992;356:494–499.
18. Park EC, Horvitz HR. Mutations with dominant effects on the behavior and morphology of the nematode *Caenorhabditis elegans*. *Genetics* 1986;113: 821–852.
19. Hengartner MO, Horvitz HR. *C. elegans* cell survival gene *ced-9* encodes a functional homolog of the mammalian proto-oncogene *bcl-2*. *Cell* 1994;76:665–676.
20. Tsujimoto Y, Croce C. Analysis of the structure, transcripts, and protein products of *bcl-2*, the gene involved in human follicular lymphoma. *Proc Natl Acad Sci* (USA) 1986;83:5214–5218.
21. Korsmeyer SJ. *Bcl-2*: An antidote to programmed cell death. *Cancer Surv* 1992; 15:105–118.
22. Vaux DL, Weissman IL, Kim SK. Prevention of programmed cell death in *Caenorhabditis elegans* by human *bcl-2*. *Science* 1992;258:1955–1957.

PART II

Assessment of CNS Function

CHAPTER 6

The Neurological Examination

*Joseph J. Volpe**

Introduction

The clinical neurological examination remains the starting point in the assessment of the child who is thought to have suffered a neurological insult related to cardiac surgery. Evaluation by this method alone however is complicated by the rapid changes that occur in the young infant's neurological maturity as well as the plasticity, which allows a young infant or child to adapt remarkably to the loss of function in one area of the brain. For this reason it is essential to avoid unduly pessimistic prognostication in discussions with the child's parents based on the neurological examination alone.[1] The same caution should be exercised in interpreting the results of research studies such as the Boston Circulatory Arrest Study (see Part V).

This chapter will emphasize the examination of the newborn, which is based on the framework of the neurological examination of older infants and children but is supplemented and modified significantly for adaptation to the newborn (Table 6–1). Unfortunately, an organized and systematic approach to examination of the newborn in the intensive care unit is often omitted because of the tangle of catheters and leads surrounding the child.

Sensory Examination

Examination of the Head

Head circumference is a useful measure of intracranial volume and therefore also of brain volume and cerebrospinal fluid volume. It is important to make

*Adapted from The Neurological Examination: Normal and Abnormal Features, in Volpe JJ, Neurology of the Newborn, W. B. Saunders, 3rd edition, 1995.

TABLE 6–1
Neonatal Neurological Examination—Basic Elements

Examination of the Head
Level of Alertness
Cranial Nerves

Olfaction (I)
Vision (II)
Optic fundi (II)
Pupils (III)
Extraocular movements (III, IV, VI)
Facial sensation and masticatory power (V)
Facial motility (VII)
Audition (VIII)
Sucking and swallowing (V, VII, IX, X, XII)
Sternocleidomastoid function (XI)
Tongue function (XII)
Taste (VII, IX)

Motor Examination

Tone and posture
Motility and power
Tendon reflexes and plantar response

Primary Neonatal Reflexes

Moro reflex
Palmar grasp
Tonic neck response

allowance for the effects of scalp edema, subcutaneous infiltration of fluid, and cephalhematoma in taking this measurement. In spite of these limitations, head circumference remains one of the most readily available and useful means for evaluating the status of the central nervous system in the newborn period. Sequential measurements, in particular, provide valuable information.

Head circumference is influenced by head shape. The more circular the head shape, the greater the intracranial volume for the same circumference. This has important implications for infants with a skull deformity such as craniosynostosis. During the first 2 to 3 months of life, premature infants have a distinctive change in head shape, which is characterized by an increase in the occipital-frontal diameter relative to the parietal diameter[2] (Figure 6–1).

Even though normal rates of head growth during intrauterine development have been well defined, the normal rate of postnatal head growth is not

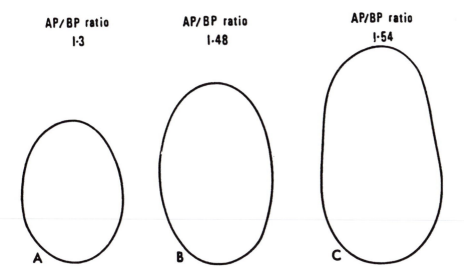

FIGURE 6–1.   Premature infants have a change in head shape during the first 2 to 3 months of life. It is important to note that the more circular the head shape, the greater the intracranial volume for the same circumference.

as well established, particularly for premature infants. Often there is a small amount of head shrinkage in the first 3 to 4 days of life correlating closely with postnatal weight loss and urinary sodium loss. Premature infants then demonstrate an increase in head circumference of 0.5 cm in the second week of life, 0.75 cm in the third week, and 1.0 cm per week thereafter in the neonatal period. Slower rates of head growth are observed in infants with serious systemic disorders.[3] The duration of suboptimal growth is directly related to the duration of caloric deprivation and to the duration of ventilation. This period may be followed by a period of catch-up growth. Premature infants who are calorically deprived for more than 4 weeks are likely to have developmental scores below normal at one year of corrected age.[4]

Apart from measurement of head circumference, examination of the head is important in defining the presence of dimples or tracts, subcutaneous masses (e.g. encephalocele, tumor), or cutaneous lesions such as port-wine stains. The latter are associated with abnormalities of choroidal vessels in the eye which may result in glaucoma, and of meningeal and superficial cerebral vessels which may result in cortical lesions with seizures and other neurological deficits.

Assessment of Level of Alertness

The general level of alertness is one of the most sensitive indices of global neurological function. It is dependent on the integrity of several levels of the central nervous system. The level of alertness of the normal infant will vary according to a number of factors including the time of last feeding, environmental stimuli, recent experiences, and gestational age. Prior to 28 weeks gestation it is difficult to identify periods of wakefulness. At approximately 28 weeks there is a distinct change in the level of alertness. Gentle stimuli result in several minutes of alertness and there may be spontaneous periods of wakefulness. By 32 weeks the eyes are frequently open and spontaneous roving eye movements appear. By 36 weeks increased alertness can be observed and vigorous crying appears during wakefulness. By term the infant exhibits periods of attention to visual and auditory stimuli, and it is possible to study sleep-waking patterns in detail.[5]

Cranial Nerves

I Olfaction

Although it is rarely evaluated in the newborn period, olfaction is present in the newborn period. Studies have demonstrated complex associative olfactory learning as well as olfactory discrimination in the first 48 hours of life. Olfactory function appears to be normal beyond 32 weeks gestation, but it is not consistently present between 29 and 32 weeks, and it is rarely present before 26 to 28 weeks.[6]

II Vision

Visual fixation can be identified by 32 weeks gestation and increases over the next 4 weeks. The neonate will follow a bright target through an arc of at least 30 degrees. Optico-kinetic nystagmus, elicited by a rotating drum, is present in the majority of infants at 36 weeks and is present consistently at term. Visual discrimination of a sensitive degree has been demonstrated in newborn infants. Infants as young as 35 weeks gestation exhibit a preference for patterns, particularly those with a greater number and size of details. Curved contours are favored over straight lines. Binocular vision and appreciation of depth appear at 3 to 4 months postnatally.

Fundoscopic examination is difficult in the newborn. The optic disc is pale, and retinal hemorrhages are observed in 20 to 40% of all newborn infants, particularly those born by vaginal delivery.

III Pupils

Reaction to light begins to appear at 30 weeks gestation but is not consistently present until 32 to 35 weeks[7] (Figure 6–2).

III, IV, VI Extraocular movements

As early as 25 weeks gestation, full ocular movement with the doll's eye maneuver can be elicited. It is important to note that although vertical

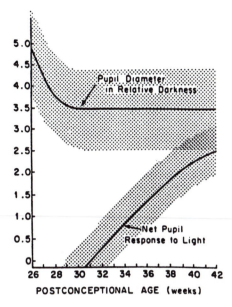

FIGURE 6–2. Diameter of pupil (mean ± SD) in term and pre-term neonates in relative darkness and after light stimulation. Note that reaction to light tends to appear at 30 weeks gestation but is not consistently present until 32 to 35 weeks.

oculovestibular responses are present at birth, voluntary upward gaze is not consistently present before 10 weeks of age.[8]

V Facial sensation and bite

The sensory component of the trigeminal nerve is best tested by pinprick. The resulting facial grimace begins on the stimulated side of the face. Note however that if the infant has a facial palsy the response will be impaired. The strength of the infant's bite will also be dependent on the function of the trigeminal nerve. This is best evaluated by placing a finger in the infant's mouth to see how strong the bite is.

VII Facial motility

Facial symmetry should be examined in the quiet resting state and in spontaneous movements and during crying. With the face at rest, attention should be paid to the vertical width of the palpebral fissure, the nasolabial fold, and the position of the corner of the mouth.

VIII Hearing

By 28 weeks the infant will startle or blink in response to a sudden loud noise.[5] As the infant matures, more subtle responses to auditory stimulation become evident, e.g. cessation of motor activity, change in respiratory pattern, opening of the mouth, and wide opening of the eyes. It is important to undertake the auditory examination in an appropriately quiet environment.

V, VII, IX, X, XII Bulbar function,
sucking and, swallowing

Feeding requires coordination of breathing, sucking and, swallowing.[9] Sucking and swallowing are coordinated sufficiently for oral feeding as early as 28 weeks gestation. However, synchronization with breathing is not well developed until 32 to 34 weeks gestation.

The gag reflex is tested by stimulating the posterior pharynx with a tongue blade or cotton-tipped swab. Active contraction of the soft palate, with upward movement of the uvula and the posterior pharyngeal muscles, should be observed.

XI Sternocleidomastoid function

The function of the spinal accessory nerve is best tested with the infant lying supine with its head slightly extended over the edge of the examination table. Flexion and lateral rotation movements can only be seen adequately if the short neck of the infant is extended. Passive rotation of the head reveals the configuration and bulk of the sternocleidomastoid muscle.

XII Tongue function

The size and symmetry of the tongue, as well as the presence of fasciculations and the coordination of movements, should be examined. Tongue movement is best assessed when the infant is sucking on the examiner's finger.

VII, IX Taste

The newborn infant is very responsive to variations in taste and is capable of fine discrimination. However, taste is rarely evaluated in the standard neurological examination.

Motor Examination

The most important features of the motor examination of the neonate and young infant are muscle tone, posture of the limbs, motility and muscle power, and the tendon reflexes and plantar response. The postnatal age and level of alertness will affect all of these features.

Muscle Tone

Tone in the limbs should be tested by passive movement of the limbs with the infant's head held forward in the midline. This is done to eliminate the tonic neck reflex. Besides moving the infant's limbs passively, the examiner should assess axial tone by grasping its hands and pulling the child from supine to sitting.

There is a caudal to rostral progression in the development of tone, particularly flexor tone, with maturation. At 28 weeks there is minimal resistance to passive manipulation in all limbs, but by 32 weeks distinct flexor tone becomes apparent in the lower extremities. By 36 weeks flexor tone is prominent in the lower extremities and can be detected in the upper extremities. By term strong flexor tone is present in all extremities.[5]

In the neonate, diminished tone may be a sign of either upper motor neuron or lower motor neuron pathology. The other components of the motor examination, namely power and myotactic reflexes, help to localize the cause of hypotonia to either central or peripheral mechanisms. A newborn with hypotonia due to disease in the cortex or corticospinal tracts usually has the ability to move the limbs against gravity. The patient with a disorder of anterior horn cells is generally hypotonic and too weak to overcome gravity with limb movements.

The posture of the infant reflects the developmental changes in tone. At 28 weeks the very quiet infant often lies with minimally flexed limbs whereas by 32 weeks there is distinct flexion of the lower limbs at the knees and hips. By term the infant assumes a flexed posture of all limbs. An interesting aspect of posture in the newborn is a preference for position of the head toward the right side. Prechtl et al.[10] demonstrated head position toward the right side 79% of the time, toward the left 19% of the time, and toward the midline 2% of the time. This preference apparently reflects a normal asymmetry of cerebral function at this age (Figure 6–3).

Motility and Power

The quantity, quality, and symmetry of motility and muscle power are important items in the motor examination. In the first 4 weeks of normal postnatal development, movements with a writhing quality predominate. In the period from 4 to 12 weeks, "fidgety" movements are prominent and after 8 to 12 weeks, rapid, large-amplitude swipes and swats are prominent. In general, preterm infants exhibit similar patterns of motor development when they attain comparable postmenstrual ages.[11]

In the preterm infant spontaneous movements are predominantly flexor at the hips and knees by 32 weeks gestation. Neck flexor and extensor power are negligible at this age. By 36 weeks the active flexor movements of the lower extremities are stronger, and definite neck extensor power can be observed for the first time. When the infant is supported in the sitting position, its head is lifted off the chest and remains upright for several seconds.

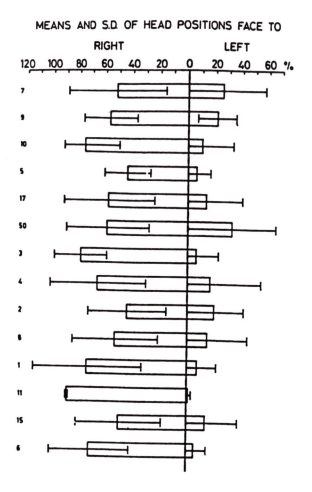

FIGURE 6–3. The normal newborn has a preference for head position toward the right side. The figure indicates the mean ± SD percentage of minutes that each of 14 infants faces to the right or left side (from Prechtl HFR, et al. Postures, motility and respiration of low risk, preterm infants. *Dev Med Child Neurol* 21:3:1979, with permission)

By term, neck flexor power becomes apparent; when the infant is pulled to a sitting position with a firm grasp of the proximal upper limbs, the head is held in the same plane as the rest of the body for several seconds.[5]

Significant asymmetry in both spontaneous and elicited movements of the limbs can give a strong clue to the location of nervous system pathology. The patient with upper motor neuron pathology is more likely to have a diaparesis or hemiparesis and should have exaggerated tendon reflexes. The

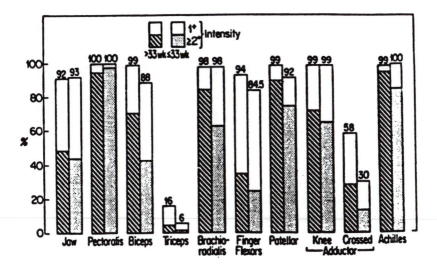

FIGURE 6–4. Percent of neonates either less than or greater than 33 weeks gestation in whom deep tendon reflexes can be elicited.

child with a lower motor neuron problem is more likely to be weak in all limbs and will have hypoactive tendon reflexes.

Tendon Reflexes and Plantar Response

The pectoralis, biceps, brachioradialis, knee, and ankle jerks are tendon reflexes that are readily elicited in the newborn[12] (Figure 6–4). Ankle clonus of 5 to 10 beats is a normal finding in the newborn if no other abnormal neurological signs are present and the clonus is not asymmetrical. Ankle clonus usually disappears with maturation and is abnormal beyond 1 to 2 months of age.

The plantar response is of limited value in the motor examination of the newborn.[13] There are at least four competing reflexes which can cause movement of the toes. Two reflexes that result in extension are nociceptive withdrawal and contact avoidance. Two responses that lead to flexion are plantar grasp and positive supporting reaction. The response is highly dependent on the manner in which the test is performed; for example, thumbnail drag along the lateral aspect of the sole is reported in toe flexion in more than 90% of newborns while other observers report that pin drag results in toe extension in more than 90%.

Primary Neonatal Reflexes

In addition to the tendon and myotactic reflexes described above, the "primary neonatal reflexes" are complex developmental reflexes that involve segmental vestibulospinal and diencephalic control of movement under certain conditions and with specific stimuli. The value of evaluating these reflexes is to determine if there is any developmental delay in their appearance or persistence suggesting focal neuropathology. Of the many reflexes of this nature which have been described, the most useful are the Moro reflex, the palmar grasp, and the tonic neck response. These reflexes are more valuable in the assessment of disorders of lower motor neuron, nerve, and muscle than of upper motor neuron.

Moro reflex

The Moro reflex is best elicited by sudden dropping (with immediate subsequent catching) of the baby's head relative to its trunk. The response is an opening of the hands and extension and abduction of the upper extremities, followed by anterior flexion of the upper extremities and an audible cry. Hand opening is present by 28 weeks, extension and abduction by 32 weeks, and anterior flexion by 37 weeks. Audible crying appears at 32 weeks. The Moro reflex disappears by 6 months of age in normal infants.[5]

Palmar grasp

Palmar grasp is clearly present at 28 weeks gestation, is strong at 32 weeks, and is strong enough and associated with enough extension of upper extremity muscles to allow the infant to be lifted from the bed at 37 weeks. The palmar grasp becomes less consistent after about 2 months of age.[5]

Tonic neck response

The tonic neck response, elicited by rotation of the head, consists of extension of the upper extremity on the side to which the face is rotated and flexion of the upper extremity on the side of the occiput ("fencing posture"). The response appears by 35 weeks gestation but is most prominent about 1 month post term. It disappears by 6 to 7 months of age.[5]

Placing, stepping

The placing and stepping reactions are elicited readily by 37 weeks. The former reaction is provoked by contacting the dorsum of the foot with the edge of a table. These reflexes are commonly elicited, but their significance is not clear.

Sensory Examination

Evaluation of sensory function is not a part of the usual neonatal neurological examination. The premature infant at 28 weeks gestation is able to discriminate touch and pain. Touch results in an increased level of alertness and slight motor activity, while pain results in withdrawal and cry response. The rooting reflex is established by 32 weeks gestation. By approximately 36 weeks there is rapid turning of the head away from pinprick over the side of the face.

It is useful to assess the response of the infant to multiple pinpricks over the medial aspect of the extremities.[14] Responses to be observed are latency, limb movement, facial movement, vocalization, and habituation. A lower level response is extremely rapid and is not accompanied by grimace or cry. A normal, higher level response has a recognizable latency and consists usually of an apparently purposeful avoidance maneuver, usually lateral withdrawal, and grimace or cry. The response dampens with repeated trials. Habituation is an important feature of the normal neonatal response.[15]

Examination of the Infant Between 1 Month and 6 Months

The structure of the examination at this age is similar to the neonatal examination described above. The infant is usually cooperative at this age. Differences in the cranial nerve examination relative to the neonate include the ability to visually fixate through 180 degrees by 8 to 10 weeks and the ability to track vertically by 10 to 12 weeks. The presence of strabismus should be distinguished from a cranial nerve palsy using tests of binocular vision and doll's eye movements. The motor examination at this age may reveal evidence of spasticity. The child tends to move the arms parallel to, but not in front of, the trunk. There should be no head lag by 4 to 5 months. Suspending the child by supporting it under the arms may reveal scissoring of the lower extremities with plantar flexion, leg adduction, and internal rotation of the hips if a spastic diaparesis is present. Assessment of early cerebellar function is possible toward the end of this time-frame by examining postural reflexes with the child in the sitting position.

Examination Between 6 Months and 2 Years

Examination at this age is complicated by a child's anxiety at separation from its parents as well as anxiety toward strangers. Observation of spontaneous activities, such as walking and using the fingers to grasp and pick up objects, provides important information regarding multiple systems. Motor tone is evaluated with the child being held by a parent. Table 6–2 lists specific abnormalities of the clinical neurological examination at 1 year of age which were defined for the Boston Circulatory Arrest Study.

Examination Between 2 and 4 Years

By this age the child is able to follow simple commands. Many tests can be demonstrated and then imitated. A very important aspect of the examination at this age is to allay the child's anxiety as much as possible. Skillful involvement of the parents in the examination is an essential ingredient for the success of the examination.

TABLE 6–2
Definitions of abnormalities on 1-year neurologic examination

I. *Definite Abnormalities*

A. Of Head
    1. head circumference > 97%
    2. head circumference < 3%
    3. bulging fontanel
B. Of Mental Status
    1. alteration of consciousness
    2. visual avoidance/lack of interaction (with normal vision and hearing)
    3. lack of vocalizations
C. Of Cranial Nerves
    1. any cranial nerve paresis/palsy
    2. II: lack of pupillary response or pupillary asymmetry (>2 mm)
                 lack of vision (with documentation)
                 abnormal fundoscopic examination
                 visual field inattention
    3. III, IV, VI: ptosis
                 abnormality of eye movement (motor paresis or paralysis)
                 nonpendular nystagmus (exclude strabismus)
                 gaze preference
    4. V, VII: absent corneal reflex
                 facial palsy
    5. VIII: lack of hearing (need documentation)
    6. IX, X: lack of gag reflex
                 abnormal phonation
    7. XII: tongue atrophy
D. Of Motor System
    1. weakness/hemiparesis
        quadriparesis
        monoparesis
        diparesis
        The above may be spastic, hypotonic, or dystonic
    2. trunkal incoordination
        lack of protective reflexes
        inability to maintain or attain sitting position
        inability to stand supported
        head lag on traction pull or poor head control
    3. appendicular incoordination
        persistent fisting
        inability to take Cheerios with either hand with thumb-finger grasp
        tremor on reach (when not crying and not on sympathomimetic)
        dysmetria on reach
    4. adventitious movements
        choreoathetosis
        myoclonus/excessive startling
E. Deep tendon reflexes: sustained clonus

TABLE 6–2
(continued)

II.	*Possible or Borderline Abnormalities*

A. Of Head: abnormal shape
               brachycephalic, dolicocephalic, phagiocephalic
B. Of Mental Status: inability to engage due to continuous crying
C. Of Cranial Nerves: pendular nystagmus
                            strabismus
                            drooling
                            torticollis
D. Of Motor System: stands on toes but without spasticity/upgoing toes/clonus
                            hypotonia without paresis
E. Deep tendon reflexes, plantars
   symmetric or asymmetric extensor plantars in isolate

Examination Beyond 4 Years

By 4 years of age it is generally possible to undertake a standard neurological examination that would be performed in an adult. An inability to cooperate may signify developmental delay or regression due to intercurrent illness.

Conclusion

Although there are definite limitations to the diagnostic and prognostic value of the neurological examination of the infant, neonate, and particularly premature neonates, it is essential that a trained pediatric neurologist be involved early in the assessment of a child who is suspected to have sustained an insult related to cardiac surgery. Preferably this person will have a close personal familiarity with specific issues pertinent to the use of cardiopulmonary bypass as well as an appreciation of the multitude of insults to which the child may have been exposed before surgery—including hypoxia and acidosis before diagnosis—as well as the risks inherent in catheterization procedures. Skillful interpretation of the neurological examination will allow the number of diagnostic studies to be minimized. Most importantly the neurologist should establish early contact with the family so that the family will have a realistic appreciation of the child's problems. More than any other personnel who are likely to speak to the family about the child's future, the pediatric neurologist, with knowledge of the lack of prognostic accuracy of both the clinical examination and diagnostic studies, will be able to avoid an unduly pessimistic outlook.

References

1. Korner AF. The scope and limitations of neurologic and behavioral assessments of the newborn. In Stevenson DK, Sunshine P (eds.), *Fetal and neonatal brain injury.* Toronto: B.C. Decker, 1989, pp 239–249.
2. Baum JD, Searls D. Head shape and size of newborn infants. *Dev Med Child Neurol* 1981;13:576.
3. Gross SJ, Eckerman CO. Normative early head growth in very low-birth-weight infants. *J Pediatr* 1983;103:946–949.
4. Georgieff MD, Hoffmann JS, Pereira GR, et al. Effect of neonatal caloric deprivation on head growth and 1-year development status in preterm infants. *J Pediatric* 1985;107:581–587.
5. Saint-Anne Sargassies S. *Neurological development in the full-term and premature eonates.* New York: Excerpta Medica, 1977.
6. Sarnat HB. Olfactory reflexes in the newborn infant. *J Pediatr* 1978;92:624–626.
7. Robinson J, Fielder AR. Pupillary diameter and reaction to light in premature neonates. *Arch Dis Child* 1990;65:35–38.
8. Weissman BM, DiScenna AO, Leigh RJ. Maturation of the vestibulo-ocular reflex in normal infants during the first 2 months of life. *Neurology* 1989;39:534–538.
9. Stevenson RD, Allair JH. The development of normal feeding and swallowing. *Pediatr Clin North Am* 1991;38:1439–1453.
10. Prechtl HFR, Fargel JW, Weinmann HM, et al. Postures, motility and respiration of low-risk pre-term infants. *Dev Med Child Neurol* 1979;21:3–27.
11. Hadders-Algra M, Prechtl HFR. Developmental outcome of general movements in early infants. 1. Descriptive analysis of change in form. *Early Hum Dev* 1992;28:201–215.
12. Kuban KC, Skouteli HN, Urion DK, et al. Deep tendon reflexes in premature infants. *Pediatr Neurol* 1986;2:266–271.
13. Rich E, Marshall R, Volpe J. Plantar reflex flexor in normal neonates (letter). *N Engl J Med* 1973;289:1043.
14. Rich EC, Marshall RE, Volpe JJ. The normal neonatal response to pin-prick. *Dev Med Child Neurol* 1972;317:1321–1329.
15. Moreau T, Birch HG, Turkewitz G. Ease of habituation to repeated auditory and somesthetic stimulation in the human newborn. *J Exp Child Psychol* 1980;9:193–207.

CHAPTER 7

Cognitive and Psychomotor Developmental Assessment

David Bellinger
Leonard A. Rappaport

As the survival of children undergoing corrective heart surgery has improved, end points reflecting children's quality-of-life are more frequently serving as the focus of outcomes research. A topic of particular interest is whether these patients bear an increased burden of cognitive and developmental morbidity, specifically whether they suffer functional impairments that jeopardize their success in school and beyond. In addition, it has become important to compare the contributions of alternative treatment modalities to morbidity.

In this chapter we discuss the strengths and weaknesses of the major approaches to the assessment of behavior and development, which can be viewed as the highest level of neurological organization. We limit our focus to the period of infancy because the methods available and the demands placed on the assessor are quite different from those germane to the preschool- or school-age child. Four specific differences are the following: (1) IQ tests designed to be administered to older children cannot be extended downward for use with infants by making the problems simpler. Many of the cognitive skills tested at older ages, such as language and quantitative abilities, are not developmentally accessible in a recognizable form in infancy. (2) What is measured in infancy is not IQ in the usual sense of an immutable characteristic of the child. Instead, the tests available document a child's progress in achieving developmental milestones, i.e., in doing what it is that infants typically do at particular ages. Intra-individual stability of current status defined in this way is not high in that the rate at which a child proceeds from milestone to milestone within a domain does not necessarily correlate highly with the level a child will achieve in that domain in later childhood. Accordingly, what is measured is generally referred to as "developmental quotient" or "mental development index" rather than IQ. (3) The test setting differs from that of the preschool- or school-age child because infants have no set for test-taking, i.e., they appear not to experience any social pressure to cooperate with an assessor. They will attend to a task only if it captures their interest. This tendency must be exploited in test construction by engineering the situation in such a way as to increase the likelihood that a particular response will be elicited (if it is in the infant's current behavioral repertoire). One of the primary tasks of an assessor is to draw inferences about the knowledge an infant must have to be able to respond in the fashion observed. These judgments are sometimes difficult to make. If an infant does not perform the behavior being sought, is it because he or she hasn't yet developed the requisite skill, or simply because of a lack of interest, or perhaps both? (4) The previous point highlights the important role played by the assessor. Developmental testing of an infant occurs in the context of an interaction between the assessor and the child and requires considerable clinical skill. If the assessor cannot establish a good rapport with the child, the validity of the test results must be questioned. Some individuals are better than others at eliciting specific behaviors from infants.

The two major approaches to the developmental assessment of infants involve sensory-motor and information-processing tests. These approaches are complimentary rather than mutually exclusive.

Sensory-Motor- (SM) Based Tests

Currently, SM tests are widely viewed as the "gold standard." These tests issue from what is referred to as the "psychometric" tradition. The selection of items for inclusion tends to be based on a statistical criterion, i.e., the ability of a test item to discriminate among children of a certain age, rather than on an organized system of hypotheses or principles about child development. Such tests provide a broad sampling of the types of behaviors children engage in at various ages, and as a result permit conclusions about whether a child's development is progressing at an age-appropriate pace and in an age-appropriate form. Because children's abilities change so rapidly as they age, the items contributing to such a test differ considerably in nature and difficulty as well. For example, items that are administered to a 3-month-old child are heavily weighted toward the assessment of object manipulation and visually directed reaching. When a child is around 12 months of age, the skills tested include imitation, language comprehension, and the emerging understanding of causal relationships. By 2 years of age, the most salient emerging skills include language production and the understanding of complex syntactic structures. In essence, the groups of items administered to children of different ages constitute qualitatively different tests, a characteristic that complicates the effort to interpret scores obtained over time as true repeated measures.

The best exemplar of SM tests is the recently revised and restandardized Bayley Scales of Infant Development,[1] which can be used to assess the development of children between the ages of 1 and 42 months. It has three components—Mental Development Index, Psychomotor Development Index, and Behavior Rating Scale.

The Mental Development Index, referred to as MDI, assesses what are usually thought of as "cognitive" skills, including "memory, habituation, problem solving, early number concepts, generalization, classification, vocalization, language, and social skills."[1] Table 7–1 provides examples of items that are administered to children of different ages. The child's performance on each item is scored simply as pass or fail.

The Psychomotor Development Index, or PDI, assesses children's gross motor planning, balance, ability to imitate different postures, visual-motor integration, and fine motor skills. Table 7–1 provides examples of items from this scale.

The numbers of Mental Scale and Psychomotor Scale items passed are converted to age-standardized scores (MDI and PDI, respectively) that are distributed with a mean of 100 and a standard deviation of 16. In addition to these global scores, separate scores can be calculated for different facets of development (i.e., cognitive, language, personal-social, and motor). Since the expected standard score at each age is 100, a child's developmental status relative to age-mates can be tracked over time (even though, as noted, the behaviors assessed at different ages are not the same).

The Behavior Rating Scale (called the Infant Behavior Record in the 1969 version of the Bayley Scales[2]), consists of a series of 5-point scales that enable the examiner to render clinical judgments about qualitative aspects of the child's performance. These judgments supplement MDI and PDI scores by providing information about a child's motor quality, attention/arousal, orientation/engagement, and emotional regulation (endurance, mood, reactivity). Cut-off scores are provided to identify children whose behavior is not within normal limits for age.

Limitations of Sensory-Motor-Based Tests

Two disadvantages of this type of infant test should be recognized. First, although they are satisfactory in terms of most criteria by which the adequacy of a psychological test is evaluated (e.g., test-retest reliability, split-half reliability, and concurrent validity), scores such as the MDI or PDI tend to have low predictive validity. In other words, they share little variance with the results of cognitive assessments conducted just a few years later. For example,

TABLE 7–1
Sample items from the Bayley Scales of Infant Development (2nd ed.).

Age	Mental	Motor

1 month	eyes follow ring (circular path)
	discriminates between bell
	  and rattle
	becomes excited in anticipation
		adjusts posture when held at
		  shoulder
		adjusts head to ventral suspension
		retains ring

3 months	reacts to disappearance of face
	reaches for suspended ring
	habituates to visual stimulus
		turns from back to side
		maintains head at 45° and lowers
		  with control
		sits with slight support for
		  10 seconds

6 months	retains 2 of 3 cubes for 3 seconds rings bell purposely looks for fallen spoon	sits alone for 30 seconds uses partial thumb opposition to grasp cube brings spoons or cubes to midline
12 months	puts 9 cubes in cup removes lids from box pats toys in imitation	grasps pencil at middle walks alone throws ball
18 months	places pegs in 25 seconds names one picture points to 3 of doll's body parts	walks backward stands alone on right foot jumps off floor (both feet)
24 months	names five pictures completes blue board in 75 seconds imitates a two-word sentence	laces three beads jumps distance of 4 inches swings leg to kick ball

30 months	understands concept of one
	imitates vertical and horizontal
	  strokes
	produces multiple-word utter-
	  ance in response to picture
	  book
		imitates hand movements
		buttons one button
		walks on tiptoe for 9 feet

40 months	solves bridge-building problem repeats 3-number sequences understands concept of more	traces designs imitates postures walks down stairs, alternating feet

the median correlation between 1 year scores on prior versions of the Bayley Scales and IQ at age 5 to 7 years in low-risk children is approximately 0.1,[3] although it may be considerably higher among children born prematurely or who are otherwise at medical risk.[4] This low predictive validity is not necessarily a flaw in SM tests, but it may reflect the fact that developmental trajectories are dynamic and that the speed at which a child achieves some criterion level of skill within one domain is not necessarily predictive of how quickly a criterion level will be achieved in a different domain or even in another aspect of the same domain. It is useful to view scores on SM tests as analogous to birth weight.[5] Although birth weight is not a strong predictor of school-age weight, neonatologists find it a useful marker of a newborn's current health. Similarly, Bayley scores provide reliable information about an infant's current developmental status. Because many items on SM tests require motoric responses, such tests are of limited utility in evaluating infants with motor handicaps, as scores tend to underestimate the children's cognitive abilities. In the extreme, this may result in a child being treated in a way that produces what has been called "iatrogenic mental retardation".[6]

Information-Processing (IP) Tests

The poor predictive validity of SM tests has been attributed by some to dissimilarities in the underlying cognitive domains assessed by these tests and by traditional tests of intelligence administered in the preschool period and later. One hypothesis is that greater continuity in development (and hence prediction from earlier measurements) would be apparent if infant assessment methods could be developed to tap the types of skills called upon by intelligence tests. Abilities considered likely candidates include aspects of information processing such as perception, discrimination, storage, retrieval, and classification. Many of these affect infants' performance on habituation and recognition memory tasks. As a result, the possibility that such processes provide windows onto cognitive development has been a topic of considerable basic research in child development since the 1960s.[7,8] In the past 10 years, several assessment procedures based on these findings have become available for use in clinical research. The best known among such tests is the Fagan test of Infant Intelligence (FTII),[9] although other researchers have developed similar methods based on both visual and nonvisual methods of information processing (e.g., cross-modal transfer of information).[4] These tests appear to be most applicable to the assessment of children during the last half of the first year of life.

The FTII is based on the principle that an infant will generally prefer to look at something novel than at something familiar. This test consists of 10 problems. The child is first allowed to view a photograph of a face for a familiarization period that depends on the child's age (10 to 20 seconds). In a novelty trial, this familiar picture is juxtaposed with a picture that is similar but in some way discrepant. Observing corneal reflections, an observer records the time the infant spends looking at each picture. Trials in which the left-right position of the novel and familiar pictures is counterbalanced are administered to eliminate the impact of the left-right preferences infants sometimes display. Summing over all 10 problems, a mean novelty preference score is computed (i.e., the percentage of time an infant looks at the novel picture). In the last half of the first year, infants tend to spend about 60% of the time looking at a novel picture. In an attempt to integrate SM and IP approaches to assessment, the recent revision of the Bayley

Scales[1] includes several new items that assess infants' visual recognition memory skills.

A recent meta-analysis of 31 studies that examined the predictive validity of IP tests found a weighted correlation between novelty preference score and preschool-age IQ of .36.[10] Scores obtained in the interval between 2 and 8 months were most predictive, and preschool IQs of at-risk children could be predicted more accurately from novelty preference scores than could the IQs of nonrisk infants. The predictive validity of IP tests was greater than that of SM tests for nonrisk infants but not for at-risk infants. Despite the statistical significance of the weighted correlation, however, a value of .36 means that indices of IP account for only about 15% of the variance in preschool IQ. This level of prediction is no better than what can be achieved using data that are less costly to obtain, such as parental education or socioeconomic status. Clearly, the search for signs in infancy that accurately predict later IQ has not been very successful, supporting a cautious approach in using the results of infant testing to draw inferences about the CNS consequences of early insult.

Limitations of IP Tests

Information-processing tests assess only a restricted set of infant behaviors, albeit ones that may underlie later reasoning and predict later performance in this domain reasonably well. They do not provide the clinically valuable broad characterization of an infant's current developmental status that SM tests do. In addition, currently available IP tests can only be administered within a rather narrow age window (approximately 9 months), further reducing the range of their clinical applications.

Issues in Using Development as an End Point in Cardiac Surgery Outcomes Research

Normative Drift

For reasons that are not clear, the norms for developmental and intellectual tests become increasingly inappropriate as the length of time since test standardization increases. For instance, as part of the recent revision of the Bayley Scales, both the 1969 and 1993 versions were administered to a group of 200 children. As expected, mean MDI and PDI scores on the 1993 version were approximately 100. Mean scores on the older version were 112 (MDI) and 110 (PDI), however, suggesting that a score of 100 on the 1969 version, typically interpreted as the population mean, is almost 3/4 of a standard deviation below the contemporary expected level.[1] This phenomenon has been noted by others[11,12] and illustrates the general principle that interpretation of test scores always requires consideration of how applicable published norms are to the specific sample under study. In some cases, use of histori-cal controls may not be appropriate, requiring the recruitment of compara-ble contemporaneous controls.

Timing of Developmental Assessments

In evaluating the developmental morbidity associated with a particular car-diac surgical intervention, testing within the first year is appealing for sev-eral reasons. First, many socioeconomic factors (e.g., parental education, occupation, and IQ) do not emerge as strong predictors of childhood cogni-tive status until the second year of life.[13] Thus, one might obtain a clearer picture of a factor's impact by conducting assessments before these poten-tially confounding factors come into play. On the other hand, other consid-erations dictate a different approach. First, unless the insult produced by the intervention or risk factor of interest is massive, its impact is generally more likely to be on a child's acquisition of new skills than on the performance of skills already acquired. The postoperative follow-up interval may thus need to be sufficiently long to allow this process to be expressed. Developmental assessments performed relatively soon after surgery would tend to reflect a mix of a child's preoperative status and any acute effects of surgery. Second, prior knowledge of the site or mechanism of surgery-related brain insult may lead to the expectation that the primary impact will be on a domain of func-tioning that cannot be assessed in infancy, such as language pragmatics, ab-stract reasoning, or executive functions (e.g., planning and organization skills). It may be most efficient to delay follow-up assessments until such time that the response modalities available to the children are sufficiently differentiated that valid information can be obtained on such domains. In some follow-up studies of at-risk children, group differences increased as the period of follow-up lengthened,[14] perhaps due in part to age-related differ-ences in test sensitivity. Like most research design issues, the decision about what developmental assessments to use and when to administer them de-pends on the question being asked and existing knowledge about the under-lying biological mechanisms of the hypothesized effect.

Conclusion

The field of infant developmental testing continues to evolve as investigators search for more sensitive markers of current function and more accurate pre-dictors of later function. The tools presently available provide reliable, valid, and comprehensive descriptions of infants' status and are useful in tracking progress over time. None of the techniques provides scores that predict fu-ture function with sufficient accuracy to obviate the need for long-term fol-low-up studies. Those remain the best option for identifying clinically significant intellectual handicaps associated with early brain insult.

References

1. Bayley N. *Bayley scales of infant development*, 2nd ed. San Antonio: The Psychological Corporation, 1993.
2. Bayley N. *Bayley scales of infant development*. New York: The Psychological Corporation, 1969.
3. Kopp C, McCall R. Predicting later mental performance for normal, at risk, and handicapped infants. In Baltes P, Brim O (eds.), *Life-span development and behavior*, Vol. 4. New York: Academic Press, 1982, pp. 33–61.
4. Rose SA, Feldman JF, Wallace IF, McCarton C. Information processing at 1 year: Relation to birth status and developmental outcome during the first 5 years. *Dev Psychol* 1991;27:723–737.
5. McCall RB. The development of intellectual functioning in infancy and the prediction of later I.Q. In Osofsky JD (ed.), *Handbook of infant development*. New York: John Wiley & Sons, 1979, pp. 707–741.
6. Kearsley RB. Iatrogenic retardation: A syndrome of learned incompetence. In Kearsley RB, Sigel IE (eds.), *Infants at risk: Assessment of cognitive functioning*. New York: Lawrence Erlbaum Associates, 1979, pp. 153–180.
7. Zelazo PR. Reactivity to perceptual-cognitive events: Application for infant assessment. In Kearsley RB, Sigel IE (eds.), *Infants at risk: Assessment of cognitive functioning*. New York: Lawrence Erlbaum Associates, 1979, pp. 49–83.
8. Fagan JF, Singer LT. Infant recognition memory as a measure of intelligence. In Lipsitt LP (ed.), *Advances in infancy research*, Vol. 2. Norwood, NJ: Ablex Publishing Corporation, 1983, pp. 31–78.
9. Fagan JF, Singer LT, Montie JE, Shepherd PA. Selective screening device for the early detection of normal or delayed cognitive development in infants at risk for later mental retardation. *Pediatrics* 1986;78:1021–1026.
10. McCall RB, Carriger MS. A meta-analysis of infant habituation and recognition memory performance as predictors of later IQ. *Child Development* 1993;64:57–79.
11. Flynn J. Massive IQ gains in 14 nations: What IQ tests really measure. *Psychological Bulletin* 1987;101:171–191.
12. Gross SJ, Slagle TA, D'Eugenio DB, Mettelman BB. Impact of a matched term control group on interpretation of developmental performance in preterm infants. *Pediatrics* 1992; 90:681–687.
13. Golden M, Birns B. Social class and infant intelligence. In Lewis M (ed.), *Origins of intelligence: Infancy and early childhood*, 2nd ed. New York: Plenum Press, 1983, pp.347–398.
14. Achenbach TM, Howell CT, Aoki MF, Rauh VA. Nine-year outcome of the Vermont intervention program for low birth weight infants. *Pediatrics* 1993;91:45–55.

CHAPTER 8

EEG Methods with Particular Reference to Neonatal Seizures

Gregory L. Holmes

Introduction

Despite being one of the oldest tests available, the EEG remains one of the most valuable tests in the armamentarium of the pediatric neurologist. While the neonatal EEG is very useful in the diagnosis of seizures, the true strength of the test lies in its ability to predict prognosis. Background patterns, more than epileptiform patterns, correlate with eventual neurological outcome. The power of the prognostic value of this study increases further if background patterns, whether normal or abnormal, are present on serial studies.

The neonatal EEG has been found to be a valuable tool in assessing or following a variety of neonatal neurological disorders including intracranial hemorrhages,[1-7] hydrocephalus,[8] brain abscesses,[9] metabolic diseases including phenylketonuria[10,11] and methylmalonic aciduria,[12] hyperinsulinema,[13] citrullinema,[14] urea cycle defects,[15] and hyperglycinemia.[16-20] The background of EEGs obtained following neonatal hypoxic-ischemic injuries have also been shown to be predictive of outcome.[20-34] Watanabe et al.[34] reviewed EEGs from 132 full-term infants with neonatal asphyxia, which was defined as an episode of fetal distress or an Apgar score of 5 or less at 1 or 5 min after delivery. Background EEG activity was found to be an excellent indicator of prognosis while paroxysmal epileptiform EEG abnormalities had far less prognostic significance.

The EEG is also used to assess the neurological status in infants who cannot be examined neurologically because of the need for paralysis. The EEG provides a noninvasive means of examining central nervous system functions. Tharp and Laboyrie[35] recognized that the great majority of curarized infants (93%) with markedly abnormal EEGs either died or had neurological deficits at follow-up. However, if the EEG was normal or only mildly abnormal the outcome was good for 80% of these infants. Similar observations on newborns with neuromuscular blockade were published by Staudt et al.,[36] by Goldberg et al.,[37] and by Eyre et al.,[38] the latter authors using EEG monitoring to detect seizure activity.

The EEG has been found to be useful in monitoring response to medications[39] and predicting recurrence risk of seizures following neonatal seizures.[40,41] Brod et al.[40] found that a normal initial EEG was a reliable predictor for discontinuing antiepileptic drugs in 18 of 22 term infants with neonatal seizures. Clancy and Legido[41] found that postnatal epilepsy occurred in 68% of patients with moderately or markedly abnormal EEG backgrounds but in only 25% of patients with normal background activity. It should be noted that this incidence of postnatal epilepsy in neonates with seizures is much higher than that found by other investigators,[32,42–49] who reported an incidence between 16% and 25%.

The EEG usually fails to reveal specific diagnostic conditions. However, there are exceptions. For example, an interhemispheric or regional asymmetry of background patterns is often the first clue for an underlying lesion, such as an intrauterine ischemic event unsuspected by history or examination. Several EEG features suggest clinically unsuspected etiologies—those seen in infants with various dysgenetic brain anomalies, those suggesting inborn errors of metabolism (like nonketotic hyperglycinemia or pyridoxine dependency), those suggesting viral CNS infections such as herpes simplex encephalitis, and the surface positive sharp waves found with pathologies that induce deep white matter lesions. The EEG is the essential tool to diagnose seizures that might be clinically unsuspected; conversely, it reduces the likelihood of treating nonseizure behaviors. In addition, the EEG is a useful technique to assess neurological status in neonates who need to be paralyzed. However, the primary value of neonatal electroencephalography is its powerful contribution to the assessment of short- and long-term prognosis. In effect, this noninvasive test is more valuable in this respect during the neonatal period than at other ages.

EEG and Prognosis

In the context of seizure disorders, the EEG has been shown to be an excellent predictor of outcome by the vast majority of prospective or retrospective investigations performed during almost three decades. For prognostic purposes the background EEG patterns are more significant than the patterns of EEG discharges. In a prospective study conducted about three decades ago on 137 full-term neonates with seizures, it was found that those who had a normal background EEG had an 86% change of good neurodevelopmental outcome at age 4, regardless of other clinical data, as compared with only a 7% change of good outcome for neonates whose EEG was classified as "flat" (i.e., inactive), "periodic" (i.e., burst-suppression), or "multifocal."[50,51] Similar correlations were found for neonates with seizures by Monod et al.[52] In a review of 691 EEGs of 270 neonates (gestational age, 36 to 40 weeks) recorded during the first month of age, Monod et al. found that normal EEGs were highly correlated with favorable outcome while low-voltage, inactive, or paroxysmal (i.e., burst-suppression) EEGs were highly prognostic of poor outcomes in both premature and full-term infants.

Rowe et al.,[53] in a prospective study of 74 neonates with seizures, found that in both premature and full-term infants the EEG background patterns correlated highly with outcome while the EEG discharges, interictally, were not as highly significant. Similar conclusions were reached by Holmes et al.[21] for a group of 38 full-term infants with hypoxic-ischemia encephalopathy. In this study, besides confirming that the background EEG activity was the important determining factor in the correlation with clinical follow-up, the authors also established that the efficiency using the EEG as a predictive test was significantly higher than the initial neurological examination. This is an important finding since the clinical repertoire of behavior in the neonate is narrow, making the neurological and developmental examination of rather limited value in the newborn.

In further support of the superiority of the EEG over examination Scher et al.[54] also reported more favorable outcomes when the ictal discharge was superimposed on normal background, regardless of the clinical status at the time of recording. More recently, Hrachovy et al.,[55] regardless of their classification of epileptic and nonepileptic seizures, reached similar conclusions about the prognostic correlations of both background and ictal patterns.

Effect of Drugs on the Neonatal EEG

Although studies on the effects of drugs on the neonatal EEG are few, it is clear that, as with older children, drugs, especially if in the toxic range, can alter background activity.[56–59] Some antiepileptic drugs, even in normal doses, may affect the infant's sleep cycles. Phenobarbital and benzodiazepines have been shown to decrease percentages of REM states,[57] but since newborns with seizures have been reported to also show a decreased REM time,[58] these effects need further study. Thoman and colleagues[60] reported that theophylline administration to premature infants altered the normal development of state organizations, reducing REM time. Denenberg and colleagues[61] found a similar disruption of sleep state development in rabbits given theophylline. These abnormalities persisted for weeks following discontinuation of the theophylline. Watanabe et al.[62] observed a decreased REM time in hypocalcemic neonates. The acute administration of antiepileptic drugs has also been noted to depress cerebral electrical activity.[63] Antiepileptic drugs, particularly barbiturates, are often administered to infants with seizures prior to their first EEG, making it difficult to assess the prognostic value of the recording. Staudt et al.[64] compared EEG background activity with phenobarbital blood levels. The phenobarbital plasma levels in the groups with severe or moderate suppression of background activity, mild suppression, and normal background activity were not statistically different. The authors concluded that with phenobarbital plasma levels of 13 to 59 μg/ml, background suppression does not occur. In support of this observation, Benda et al.,[65] in a study of 46 premature infants reported that mean phenobarbital levels at the time of the EEG failed to show a significant relationship with the duration of the inactive phase of discontinuous sleep.

However, phenobarbital levels greater than 25 μg/ml may, in sick or young neonates, suppress EEG activity.[66,67] A discordance between EEG activity and radionuclide uptake in infants with levels between 25 and 35 ug/ml was found. The lack of EEG activity with presence of cerebral blood flow suggested that the phenobarbital suppressed EEG activity. One infant, who met the clinical criteria for brain death and had absent cerebral activity with a phenobarbital level of 30 μg/ml, developed some cerebral activity when the phenobarbital level fell to zero. Pezzani et al.[68] also reported two patients with high antiepileptic drug levels that likely resulted in severely abnormal EEGs.

Medications other than antiepileptic drugs may also alter the EEG. Drugs consumed during pregnancy may alter the neonatal EEG. An excess of spikes and sharp waves were seen in 17 of 38 (45%) neonates born to mothers abusing cocaine during pregnancy.[69] The abnormalities were multifocal in 14 of 17 tracings. None of the infants had clinical seizures. Alcohol consumption during the first trimester of pregnancy was associated with disturbances in sleep and arousal in affected infants while marijuana affected sleep and motility, regardless of trimester used.[70] Loffe et al.[71] reported that newborn infants of mothers who abused alcohol during pregnancy had hypersynchronous EEGs with total power of spectral analysis higher in quiet, indeterminate, and rapid eye movement sleep (REM) than in control infants. In addition, we have made unpublished observations that opiates may depress background activity, increase the amount of discontinuity, and alter sleep cycles.

EEG Seizure Patterns

A striking difference between seizures in neonates and those of older subjects is seen in the features of ictal (seizure) EEG patterns and their correlations with peripheral manifestations. In neonates, ictal discharges may often be focal in the context of metabolic derangements (for instance in hypocalcemic seizures) or may correspond to an underlying focal lesion. They have erratic evolutions, shifting from one area to another or starting with multifocal expressions, regardless of the presence or diffuse of restricted pathologies or even in the absence of specific pathology. Neonatal ictal patterns may vary considerably at different times during the course of one event or from one to the next. The discharges vary in frequency, amplitude, morphology, and duration.

There is not yet an accepted definition of what constitutes an ictal discharge. To classify a discharge as ictal, some authors require that it last at least 10 s;[72-74] others require a duration of at least 20 s.[75] On the other hand, many well-documented clinical and electrical seizures have been described to last only a few seconds.[42,52,56, 76-82]

As Shewmon[83] points out, an arbitrary cut-off of 10 or 20 s required to define ictal discharges would result in great inter-rater inconsistencies in the EEG identification of ictal events. For example, a brief beta- or alpha-like discharge, occurring concomitantly with a clinical event, would not be accepted by some as an ictal EEG discharge. Shewmon[83] proposed the purposefully ambiguous, acronym of B.I.R.D., namely "brief ictal rhythmic discharges," for the short paroxysmal EEG events that accompany clinical seizures. The ambiguity of this B.I.R.D. acronym lies in the fact that the letter "I" may stand for either ictal or interictal. The same author had earlier proposed B.I.R.D. for "brief interictal rhythmic discharges."[84] This ambiguity exists as an occasional confounding issue for electroencephalography in general. For example, the bursts of spikes and waves which are called subclinical discharges can often be shown to have a clinical correlate with mental dysfunction.

Criteria for duration become necessary to classify as ictal some of the paroxysmal EEG events in neonatal EEGs. This applies for instance to the focal or multifocal discharges that arise from background activities. We have already mentioned that paroxysmal bursts of variable frequency and morphology occur often in neonatal records with no implication to suggest seizure conditions. They occur in normal infants though more frequently in neonates with various pathologies. The significance of paroxysmal bursts depends upon calcium level and states of the infants, which influence the morphology and topography of these events. It is rare to find that these brief paroxysmal events in the EEG of neonates with seizures have diagnostic clues similar to interictal discharges occurring in older patients with epilepsy. Thus, duration of some EEG discharge becomes meaningful as one of the criteria to define when these EEG discharges in the newborn are indeed ictal ones. As a practical guide, an old classification of the main ictal patterns seen in newborns with seizures[50,57,79-81,85] is still found useful.

Focal Spike or Sharp Wave Discharges

These consist of trains of rhythmic spikes or sharp waves that erupt focally out of the background activity, usually abruptly (Figure 8-1). At first the amplitude may be low, but soon it increases, often as the frequency decreases. The frequency of the discharge varies most commonly within the delta to alpha bands (from 4 to 10 Hz). Its most frequent location is in

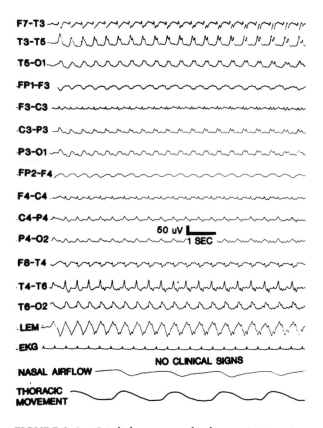

FIGURE 8–1.   Ictal sharp wave discharges in term infant with hypoxic-ischemic encephalopathy.

the Rolandic areas as noted by Rose and Lombroso.[51] The next most common location is in the temporal areas, less often in the posterior areas and rarely in anterior ones. The discharge may spread to adjacent cortex but usually at a much slower pace in neonates than in older subjects. It may appear in homotopic areas of the other hemisphere. In general, these types of focal patterns correlate well with the clinical manifestations that are usually clonic, but not invariably. Ictal focal EEG discharges do not necessarily indicate an underlying lesion because they often occur in the context of transient metabolic disorders or following a mild hypoxic event or a subarachnoid hemorrhage. In these situations the background activities and state organizations are usually normal and the prognosis generally good. On the other hand, similar focal ictal discharges occur in the presence of acquired or congenital brain lesions. In these infants EEGs often exhibit abnormalities of background. The type and degree of these abnormalities and, of course, the underlying pathology will dictate how guarded is the prognosis.

Generalized or Focal Pseudo-Delta/ Theta/Alpha/Beta Activities

These discharges consist of more or less prolonged runs of rhythmic monomorphic waves varying from 0.5 to 15 Hz, thus with a resemblance to normal background activities (Figure 8–2). Their amplitude varies from a low of 20 to 30 μV to a high of 200 μV, generally being higher for the slower frequencies. They may occur with a generalized or a focal distribution. Sometimes these discharges can appear in all states, but as they often occur in severely compromised neonates, state organization may be disrupted and background activities undifferentiated.

Although these patterns can be seen after severe hypoxic-ischemic insults, intraventricular hemorrhages, or in neonates with inborn metabolic defects, these patterns often suggest the presence of various chromosomal and dysgenetic brain abnormalities, such as migrational disorders. Similar periods of rhythmic activity within these frequency bands were previously described, together with other abnormalities in the EEGs of infants with holoprosencephaly.

Low-Frequency Discharge Pattern and Periodic Lateralized Epileptiform Discharge Pattern

Both are pathological patterns, occurring in encephalopathic conditions, and both exhibit paroxysmal features without necessarily implying ictal events.

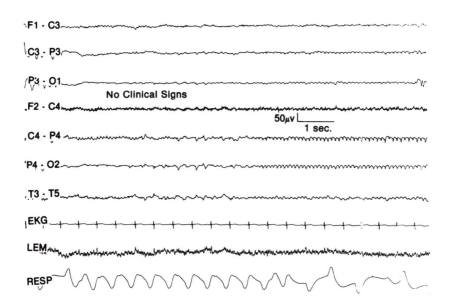

FIGURE 8–2. Pseudo-alpha discharge in term infant with hypoxic-ischemic encephalopathy.

The difference between the two patterns is at times difficult to define. Similarly there is some confusion regarding their relationships with ictal semiology. The patterns share similarities as both exhibit stereotyped, repetitive, rhythmic or quasi-rhythmic paroxysmal discharges consisting of sharp, broad-based waves occurring at low frequencies (around 0.5 to 1 Hz). They may be focal or may involve an entire hemisphere and at times may be multifocal. Almost invariably the patterns occur in the context of abnormal backgrounds, usually of the inactive or low-voltage patterns.

The Low-Frequency Discharge Pattern (LFD)

This pattern occurs in both full-term and premature neonates, the discharges often having a distinct contour, broad-based waves[42,57,85] (Figure 8–3). The pattern can be focal but also can appear independently at various locations. It may last from a few seconds to many minutes. It may at times evolve into more frequent discharges that then display morphological changes.[86] The clinical seizures observed in relation to this pattern are often subtle and at

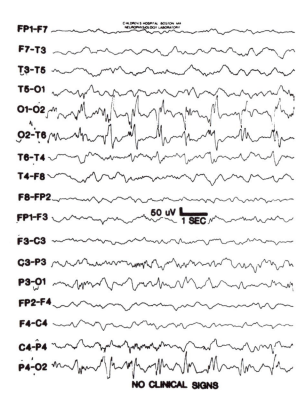

FIGURE 8–3.   Low-frequency discharge in term infant with seizures.

times the discharges appear time-locked with contralateral jerks. This pattern seems to correspond to the "depressed brain seizure" described by Kellaway and Mizrahi[87] and to the "periodic and quasi-periodic" multifocal electrical seizures described by Pettay et al.[88] and Mizrahi and Tharp[89] as characteristic for neonatal herpes simplex encephalitis. Although the LFD can occur in the course of this viral encephalitis, it is not by itself pathognomonic. LFD may develop after severe asphyxia[90] in the course of bacterial meningitis, after cerebrovascular insults, in some severe brain malformations, or with congenital metabolic disorders.[57,81,91]

Prognostically, the LFD pattern, occurring in conjunction with ictal manifestations, usually suggests a poor outcome. In a prospective study of a cohort of neonates with seizures, 14 of 152 infants showed this ictal pattern. At follow-up, 11 had severe outcomes, including 3 deaths, but 3 were considered normal.[56] A poor prognostic implication for this ictal pattern was previously mentioned.[52,91]

The Periodic Lateralized Epileptiform Discharges Pattern (PLEDS)

As the term implies, this pattern consists of stereotyped, repetitive, paroxysmal complexes occurring at around 1 Hz, lasting at least 10 min but often much longer, even for days[75,92] (Figure 8–4). To fit a PLEDS definition, these discharges ought to exhibit no evolution in morphology, frequency, or field, and should not be associated with ictal manifestations. Thus most criteria for PLEDS in neonates are similar to those previously described in children and adults.[93–96]

Scher and Beggarly[92] suggested that "periodic discharges" (presumably similar to what we call LFD) are distinguishable from PLEDS on the basis of lack of evolution and longer persistence of PLEDS, as well as lack of association with clinical seizure manifestations. In a review of 1,114 EEGs of 592 neonates, Scher and Beggarly found periodic discharges in 57 (5%) of the recordings performed in 34 neonates (26 premature and 8 full-term, similar to the incidence we have found for LFD). PLEDS were present in 4 of the recordings. Of the 34 neonates, 15 (44%) died, and of the 19 survivors, 11 (58%) had abnormal neurodevelopmental outcomes. Hence, the prognosis was poor for about 75% of this cohort. This incidence of poor outcomes found by Scher and Beggarly[92] is similar to that observed in neonates with seizures who had LFD ictal pattern.[56,85] Scher and Beggarly[92] found that stroke was the most common brain lesion (53%). They concluded that in neonates focal periodic discharges, including PLEDS, have the same ominous prognosis as in older patients. McCutchen et al.[75] recorded seizures in 13 of 16 asphyxiated neonates. Five of these had PLEDS and the authors stated that "electrographic seizures may consist of a run of PLEDS." They also concluded that "distinction between PLEDS and EEG seizures with similar wave forms may be difficult."

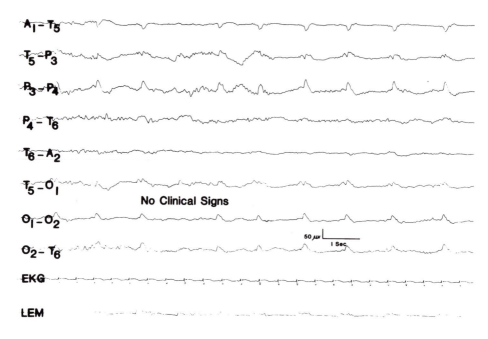

FIGURE 8–4.   PLEDS in term infant with hypoxic-ischemic encephalopathy.

Further problems in trying to clearly separate PLEDS from LFD can be found in the literature. Hughes and Schlaugenhauff[97] used interchangeably terms such as "atypical PLEDS" and "pseudo-periodic discharges;" Schwartz et al.[98] spoke of the evolution of PLEDS; Sainio et al.[99] in describing the EEG in neonatal herpes simplex encephalitis used interchangeably terms of "electrical seizures" and "pseudo-periodic discharges." There is some question regarding another criterion for PLEDS, namely their prolonged duration, because some of these papers refer to PLEDS runs that last only a few minutes.

PLEDS may represent a continuum of a similar pathophysiological substratum appearing in generally brain-damaged infants who may or may not exhibit clinically detectable seizure and who usually display other EEG background abnormalities and disorganized states. Prognosis appears similarly poor whether their EEGs show the LFD or PLED pattern. Clues for a less ominous outcome come primarily from determining the underlying etiology. The EEG—if it exhibits less abnormal background, is reactive to stimulation, and still shows some changes appropriate for various states—may indicate a better prognosis. This is reinforced if these patterns subside in repeated recordings.

Multifocal Ictal Discharge

The main characteristic of this pattern is the appearance of discharges erupting independently from two or more locations (Figure 8–5). The frequencies

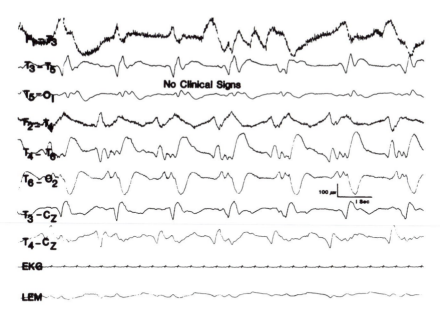

FIGURE 8–5. Multifocal discharges in term infant with hypoxic-ischemic encephalopathy.

of these discharges may vary considerably between the different foci and may change within the same location from moment to moment. The discharges may be sustained or wax and wane, assuming variable morphologies during the same event. They may occur in the context of an otherwise normal background but more frequently are seen in EEGs whose background is moderately to severely abnormal and in neonates whose state organization is disrupted, from invariance to excessive lability. The corresponding clinical expressions also vary from focal clonic or tonic seizures, often to those of the fragmentary anarchic type or those with subtle expression. In general, in the presence of interictal abnormal backgrounds the clinical concomitants are more likely to fall within the subtle or fragmentary types, while in the presence of more normal backgrounds, the clinical concomitants tend to be more organized and sustained, with clonic or, less often, with tonic components.

In this pattern, the EEG exhibits polymorphic discharges varying in morphology, periodicity, and location. Background patterns are invariably abnormal. It is a pattern similar to the hypsarrhythymic pattern seen in infancy, not to be confused with the invariant burst-suppression pattern that is seen in neonates with the proposed syndromes of Early Myoclonic Epileptic Encephalopathy (EMEE) and Early Infantile Epileptic Encephalopathy (EIEE).[100–103]

If the multifocal discharges occur within the context of relatively normal backgrounds and of still-differentiated states, the outcomes are better when the backgrounds and state organizations are abnormal.

Serial Recording for Prognosis

Repeated recordings at appropriate intervals will provide the clinician with greater predictive information than can be derived from a single EEG. There are, however, some EEGs so severely abnormal that they are thought to be valid for the formation of prognosis, without the need for serial tests. Thus some authors feel that predictions can accurately be advanced when the initial EEG shows electrocerebral inactivity, a low-voltage undifferentiated, unreactive pattern, or a burst-suppression pattern, even if the test is obtained shortly after birth.[7,32,51,56, 68,77,80,104] The EEG can show valid prognostic and diagnostic clues, detect unsuspected ictal events, and reveal catastrophic brain pathologies that may not be clinically evident. This may occur in infants with migrational abnormalities, severe hypoxic-ischemic insults, or prenatally acquired insults. For example, an intrauterine brain infarction is often unsuspected clinically and may be suspected by an abnormal EEG obtained soon after birth, confirmed later by neuroimaging.[57,105–107] Conversely, there are situations in which a single test result, while containing abnormal features, is not sufficient to reliably determine prognosis.[108]

The electroencephalographer has little control over the many variables that transiently alter the neonate's organization of states and thus alter the EEG. This is particularly true for very ill infants subjected to the many interventions and stimulations of an intensive care nursery. Recordings are often requested on infants who are systemically ill or have already received drugs known to affect both states and EEG background. There are infants who have on-going CNS problems, such as infections, or in whom hypoxic-ischemic encephalopathy develops after birth. For these and other neonates the disappearance, persistence, or emergence of abnormal EEG patterns evidently will affect the prognostic correlations. This is quite cogent for those infants whose EEGs exhibit mainly "dysmaturity" features and for whom only serial recordings will separate "transient" from "persistent" dysmaturities to allow a favorable or an alarming predictive statement to be reached.[109,110] There are also situations in which the EEG shows persistent or worsening features while clinical observations suggest improvement; this evaluation indicates a worse outcome than otherwise suggested by the clinical course. In a prospective study of 82 neonates, Tharp et al.[104] found that 41% of those infants who had an initial normal EEG, which became abnormal in a subsequent recording, were left with major neurological sequelae in contrast to only 3% with normal outcome and 15% with minor sequelae.

In performing serial EEG tests, it is important to remember that the EEG continues to evolve. As demonstrated by Takeuchi and Watanabe,[31] prognosis may depend on the time when the recording occurs. They analyzed the evolutionary changes of the EEG background in 173 neonates with perinatal hypoxic encephalopathy. Infants who had only mildly depressed background on the first day of life developed normally, while infants with similarly depressed background activity in the EEG recorded after day 7 or day 12 developed neurological deficits. Hence, similar degrees of EEG abnormalities had a different prognostic significance according to the number of days after the insults before the test was first performed. Our observations are in full agreement; hence, to extract valid prognostications from an analysis of EEG background patterns in neonates with acquired pathologies, one needs to take into account the time elapsed since the insult. It is also important to be aware that whereas serial EEGs may significantly assist predictions of outcome, this is true generally only when the tests are obtained during the neonatal period. It is not unusual that prognostically unfavorable EEG patterns obtained in this epoch of brain ontogenesis may at times appear to normalize as the newborn enters into the cryptic period of early and late infancies. Yet the long-term prognosis generally correlates best with the EEG recorded during the newborn period.

Summary

Neonatal seizures are one of the most common, yet ominous, conditions occurring in neonates. The EEG, when appropriately used, is very useful in both diagnosis[111] and treatment.[112]

REFERENCES

1. Blanc JF, Langue J, Bochu M, Dutruge J, Salle B. Intracranial hemorrhage in infants born at term. *Arch Fr Pediatr* 1982;39:251–253.
2. Cukier F, Andre M, Monod N, Dreyfus-Brisac C. Apport de l'E.E.G au diagnostic des hemorragies intra-ventriculaires du premature. *Rev Electroencephalogr Neurophysiol Clin* 1972;2:318–322.
3. Greisen G, Hellstrom Westas L, Lou H, Rosen I, Svenningsen NW. EEG depression and germinal layer haemorrhage in the newborn. *Acta Pediatr Scand* 1987;76:519–525.
4. Lacey DJ, Topper WH, Buckwald S, Zorn WA, Berger PE. Preterm very-low-birth-weight neonates: Relationship of EEG to intracranial hemorrhage, perinatal complications and developmental outcome. *Neurology* 1986;36:1084–1087.
5. Navelet Y, Dallest AM, Ropert JC. Aspects EEG observes chez quarante nouveau-nes decedes avec une hemorragie intra-ventriculaire. *Rev Electroencephalogr Neurophysiol Clin* 1980;10:19–20.
6. Staudt F, Howieson J, Benda GJ, Engel RC. EEG in newborn infants with intracranial hemorrhages: A comparison with clinical findings and CT scan. *EEG. EMG* 1982;13:143–147.
7. Watanabe K, Hakamada S, Kuroyanagi M, Yamazaki T, Takeuchi T. Electroencephalographic study of intraventricular hemorrhage in the preterm infant. *Neuropediatrics* 1983;14:225–230.
8. Sternberg B, Mises J, Lerique-Koechlin A. EEG et hydrocephalies neo-natales. *Rev Neurol* 1970;122:491–493.

9. Mises J, Daviet F, Mousalli Salefranque F, Sternberg B, Flandin C, Renier D. Brain abscess in the newborn infant (27 cases: initial electroclinical study, course). *Rev Electroencephalogr Neurophysiol Clin* 1987;17:301–308.

10. De Giorgis GF, Antonozzi I, Del Castello PG, Rosano M, Loizzo A. EEG as a possible prognostic tool in phenylketonuria. *Electroenceph Clin Neurophysiol* 1985;55:60–68.

11. Mises J, Moussali Salefranque F, Hagenmuller MP, Plouin P. Fast rhythms in metabolic diseases in children. *Rev Electroencephalogr Neurophysiol Clin* 1983;13:61–67.

12. Mises J, Moussalli Salefranque F, Plouin P, Saudubray JM. The EEG in methylmalonic acidaemia (author's trans). *Rev Electroencephalogr Neurophysiol Clin* 1978;8:71–77.

13. Parain D, Samson-Dollfus D. Etude electrophysiologique d'une hypoglycemie neo-natale prolongee par hyperinsulinisme. *Rev EEG Neurophysiol Clin* 1983;12:157–161.

14. Clancy RR, Chung HJ. EEG changes during recovery from acute severe neonatal citrullinema. *Electroenceph Clin Neurophysiol* 1991;78:222–227.

15. Verma NP, Hart ZH, Kooi KA. Electroencephalographic findings in urea-cycle disorders. *Electroenceph Clin Neurophyiosl* 1984;57:105–112.

16. Matalon R, Naidu S, Hughes JR, and Michals K. Nonketotic hyperglycinemia: Treatment wtih diazepam—a competitor for glycine receptors. *Pediatrics* 1983;71:581–584.

17. Melancon SB, Dallaire L, Vincelette P, Potier M, Geoffroy G. Early treatment of severe infantile glycine encephalopathy (nonketotic hyperglycinemia) with strychnine and sodium benzoate. *Prog Clinc Biol Res* 1979;34:217–229.

18. Moura Ribeiro MV, Ferlin ML, Gallina RA, Funayama CA, Fernandes RM. Nonketotic hyperglycinemia. Study of a case. *Arq Neuropsiquiatr* 1987;45:67–71.

19. Ohya Y, Ochi N, Mizutani N, Hayakawa C, Watanabe K. Nonketotic hyperglycinemia: Treatment with NMDA antagonist and consideration of neuropathogenesis. *Pediatr Neurol* 1991;7:65–68.

20. Scher MS, Bergman I, Ahdab-Barmada M, Fria T. Neurophysiological and anatomical correlations in neonatal nonketotic hyperglycinemia. *Neuropediatrics* 1986;17:137–143.

21. Holmes GL, Rowe J, Hafford J, Schmidt R, Testa M, Zimmerman A. Prognostic value of the electroencephalogram in neonatal asphyxia. *Electroenceph Clin Neurophysiol* 1982;53:60–72

22. Andre M, Vert P, Debruille C. Diagnosis and outcome of cerebral distress in newborn infants who presented signs of fetal hypoxia. Prospective study. *Arch Fr Pediatric* 1978;35:23–36.

23. Greiser G, Pryds O. Low CBF, discontinuous EEG activity, and periventricular brain injury in ill, preterm neonates. *Brain Dev* 1989;11:164–168.

24. Greisen G, Pryds O, Rosen I, Lou H. Poor reversibility of EEG abnormality in hypotensive, preterm neonates. *Acta Paediatr Scan* 1988;77:785–790.

25. Gyorgy I. Prognostic value of sleep analysis in newborns with perinatal hypoxic brain injury. *Acta Paediatr Acad Sci Hung* 1983;24:1–6.

26. Karch D, Kastl E, Sprock I, von Bernuth H. Perinatal hypoxia and bioelectric brain maturation of the newborn infant. *Neuropadiatrie* 1977;8:253–262.

27. Karch D, Kinderman E, Arnold G. The prognostic significance of determining bioelectric brain maturity in newborn infants with perinatal complication. *Klin Padiat* 1981;193:301–304

28. Karch D, Sprock I, Lemburg P. Early diagnosis of severe brain damage of premature and newborn infants under intensive care. A polygraphic study. *Monatsschr Kinderheilkd* 1977;125:923–928.
29. Lombroso CT. Normal and abnormal EEG's in neonates. In Henry CE (ed.), *Current clinical neurophysiology: Update on EEG and evoked potentials.* North-Holland, Amsterdam: Elsevier, 1980, pp. 83–150.
30. Monod N, Pajot N. Methods of assessing neonatal anoxia with EEG studies. *Electroenceph Clinc Neurophysiol* 1967;23:383.
31. Takeuchi T, Watanabe K. The EEG evolution and neurological prognosis of neonates with perinatal hypoxia. *Brain Dev* 1989;11:115–120.
32. Watanabe K, Hara K, Miyazaki S, Hakamda S. The role of perinatal brain injury in the genesis of childhood epilepsy. *Folia Psychiatr Neurol Jpn* 1980;34:227–232.
33. Watanabe K, Kuroyanagi M, Hara K, Miyazaki S. Neonatal seizures and subsequent epilepsy. *Brain Dev* 1982;4:341–346.
34. Watanabe K, Miyazaki S, Hara K, Hakamada S. Behavioral state cycles, background EEGs and prognosis of newborns with perinatal hypoxia. *Electroenceph Clinc Neurophysiol* 1980;49; 618–625.
35. Tharp BR, Laboyrie PM. The incidence of EEG abnormalities and outcome of infants paralyzed with neuromuscular blocking agents. *Crit Care Med* 1983; 11:926–929.
36. Staudt F, Roth JG, Engel RC. The usefulness of electroencephalography in curarized newborns. *Electroenceph Clin Neurophysiol* 1981;51:205–208.
37. Goldberg RN, Goldman SL, Ramsay RE, Feller R. Detection of seizure activity in the paralyzed neonate using continuous monitoring. *Pediatrics* 1982;69: 583–586.
38. Eyre JA, Oozeer RC, Wilkinson AR. Diagnosis of neonatal seizure by continuous recording and rapid analysis of the electroencephalogram. *Arch Dis Child* 1983;58:785–790.
39. Hakeem VF, Wallace SJ. EEG monitoring of therapy for neonatal seizures. *Dev Med Child Neurol* 1990;32:858–864.
40. Brod SA, Ment LR, Ehrenkranz RA, Bridgers S. Predictors of success for drug discontinuation following neonatal seizures. *Pediatr Neurol* 1988;4:13–17.
41. Clancy RR, Legido A. Postnatal epilepsy after EEG-confirmed neonatal seizures. *Epilepsia* 1991;32:69–76.
42. Lombroso CT. Seizures in the newborn period. In Vinken PJ, Bruyn GW (eds.), *Handbook of clinical neurology,* Vol. 15. North-Holland, Amsterdam: The Epilepsies, 1974, pp. 189–218.
43. Aicardi J. *Epilepsy in children.* New York: Raven Press, 1986.
44. Dennis J. Neonatal convulsions. Aetiology, late neonatal status and long-term outcome. *Dev Med Child Neurol* 1981;23:389–403.
45. Estivill E, Monod N, Amiel-Tison C. Etude electroencephalographique d'un cas d'encephalite herpetique-neo-natal. *Rev EEG Neurophysiol Clin* 1977;7: 380–385.
46. Fenichel GM. Convulsions. In *Neonatal neurology.* London: Churchill Livingstone, 1985, pp. 25–52.
47. Holden KR, Mellitis ED, Freeman JM. Neonatal seizures: I, Correlation of prenatal and perinatal event with outcomes. *Pediatrics* 1982;70:165–176.
48. Lombroso CT. Prognosis in neonatal seizures. In Delgada-Escueta AV, Waterlain DM, Treman DM, Porter RJ (eds.), *Advances in neurology,* Vol. 34, *Status epilepticus.* New York: Raven Press, 1983, pp. 101–113.

49. Watanabe K, Miyazaki S, Hara K, Hakamada S. Behavioral state cycles, background EEGs and prognosis of newborns with perinatal hypoxia. *Electroencephalogr Clinc Neurophysiol* 1980;49:618–625.
50. Lombroso CT. Neonatal seizure states. In *XI International congress of pediatrics proceedings.* Tokyo: University of Tokyo Press, 1965, pp. 38–49.
51. Rose AL, Lombroso CT. Neonatal seizures stats. A study of clinical, pathological, and electroencephalographic features in 137 full-term babies with a long-term follow-up. *Pediatrics* 1970;45:404–425.
52. Monod N, Pajot N, Guidasci S. The neonatal EEG: Statistical studies and prognostic value in full-term and preterm babies. *Electroencepha Clinc Neurophysiol* 1972;32:529–544.
53. Rowe JC, Holmes GL, Hafford J, Baboval D, Robinson S, Philipps A, Rosenkrantz T, Raye J. Prognostic value of the electroencephalogram in term and preterm infants following neonatal siezures. *Electroencephalogr Clin Neurophysiol* 1985;60:183–196.
54. Scher MS, Painter MJ, Bergman I, Barmada MA, Brunberg J. EEG diagnoses of neonatal seizures: Clinical correlations and outcome. *Pediatr Neurol* 1989; 5:17–24.
55. Hrachovy RA, Mizrahi EM, Kellaway P. Electroencephalography of the newborn. In Daly DD, Pedley TA (eds.), *Current practice of clinical electroencephalography.* New York: Raven Press, 1990, pp. 201–252.
56. Lombroso CT. Some aspects of EEG polygraphy in newborns at risk from neurological disorders. *Electroencephalogr Clinc Neurophysiol Suppl* 1982;36: 652–663.
57. Lombroso CT. Neonatal polygraphy in full-term and premature infants. A review of normal and abnormal findings. *J Clinc Neurophysiol* 1985;2:105–153.
58. Dreyfus-Brisca C, Curzi-Dascalova L. The EEG during the first year of life. In Leiry G (ed.), *Handbook of electroencephalography and clinical neurophysiology,* Vol. 6B. Amsterdam: Elsevier, 1975, pp. 24–30.
59. Rung GW, Wickey GS, Myers JL, Salus JE, Hensley FA, Martin DE. Thiopental as an adjunct to hypothermia for EEG suppression in infants prior to circulatory arrest. *J Cardiothoracic Vasc Anesth* 1991;5:337–342.
60. Thoman EB, Davis DH, Raye JR, Philipps AF, Rowe JC, Denenberg VH. Theophylline affects sleep-wake state development in premature infants. *Neuropediatrics* 1985;16:13–18.
61. Denenberg VH, Zeidner LP, Thoman EB, Kramer P, Rowe JW, Phillips AF, Raye JR. Effects of theophylline on behavioral state development in the newborn rabbit. *J Pharmacol Exp Ther* 1982;221:604–608.
62. Watanabe K, Hara K, Miyazaki S, Hakamada S. Neurophysiological study of newborns with hypocalcemia. *Neuropediatrics* 1982;13:34–38.
63. Radvanyi-Bouvet MF, Monset-Couchard M, Morel-Kahn F, Vicente G, Dreyfus-Brisac C. Expiratory patterns during sleep in normal full-term and premature neonates. *Biol Neonate* 1982;41:74–84.
64. Staudt F, Scholl ML, Coen RW, Bickford RB. Phenobarbital therapy in neonatal seizures and the prognostic value of the EEG. *Neuropediatrics* 1982;13:24–33.
65. Benda GI, Engel RC, Zhang YP. Prolonged inactive phases during the discontinous pattern of prematurity in the electroencephalogram of very-low-birthweight infants. *Electroenceph Clinc Neurophysiol* 1989;72:189–197.
66. Ashwal S. Brain death in the newborn. *Clin Perinatol* 1989;16:501–518.

67. Ashwal S, Schneider S. Brain death in the newborn. *Pediatrics* 1989;84:429–437.
68. Pezzani C, Radvanyi Bouvet MF, Relier JP, Monod N. Neonatal electroencephalography during the first twenty-four hours of life in full-term newborn infants. *Neuropediatrics* 1986;17:11–18.
69. Abroms IF. EEG and prognosis in neonatal seizures. *Proc Royal Soc Med* 1971;64:471–472.
70. Scher MS, Richardson GA, Coble PA, Day NL, Stoffer DS. The effects of prenatal alcohol and marijuana exposure: Disturbances in neonatal sleep cycling and arousal. *Pediatr Res* 1988;24:101–105.
71. Loffe S, Childiaeva R, Chernick V. Prolonged effects of maternal alcohol ingestion on the neonatal electroencephalogram. *Pediatrics* 1984;74:330–335.
72. Clancy RR, Legido A. The exact ictal and interictal duration of electroencephalographic neonatal seizures. *Epilepsia* 1987;28:537–541.
73. Clancy RR, Legido A, Lewis D. Occult neonatal seizures. *Epilepsia* 1988;29: 256–261.
74. Scher MS, Painter MJ. Electroencephalographic diagnosis of neonatal seizures: Issues of diagnostic accuracy, clinical correlation and survival. In Wasterlain CG, Vert P (eds.), *Neonatal seizures.* New York: Raven Press, 1990, pp. 15–25.
75. McCutchen CB, Coen R, Iragui VJ. Periodic lateralized epileptiform discharges in asphyxiated neonates. *Electroencephalogr Clinc Neurophysiol* 1985;61: 210–217.
76. Aicardi J. *Epilepsy in children.* New York: Raven Press, 1986, pp. 1–413.
77. Dreyfus-Brisac C, Monod N. Neonatal status epilepticus. In Remond A (ed.), *Handbook of electroencephalography and clinical neurophysiology,* Vol. 15. Amsterdam: Elsevier, 1972, pp. 38–52.
78. Dreyfus-Brisac C, Monod N. The EEG of full-term and premature infants. In Leiry G (ed.), *Handbook of electroencephalography and clinical neurophysiology,* Vol. 6–B, Amsterdam: Elsevier, 1975, pp. 6–23.
79. Dulac O, Aubourg P, Plouin P. Other epileptic syndromes in neonates. In Roger J, Dravet C, Bureau M, Dreifuss FE, Wolf P (eds.), *Epileptic syndromes in infants, childhood and adolescence.* London: John Libbey Eurotext Ltd, 1985, pp. 23–29.
80. Engel R. *Abnormal electroencephalogram in the newborn.* Springfield, IL: Charles C. Thomas, 1975.
81. Holmes GL. Neonatal seizures. In Pedley TA, Meldrum BS (eds.), *Recent advances in epilepsy,* Number two. New York: Churchill Livingstone, 1985, pp. 207–237.
82. Stockard-Pope JE, Wernser SS, Bickford RG. *Atlas of neonatal electroencephalography.* New York: Raven Press, 1992, pp. 1–401.
83. Shewmon DA. What is a neonatal seizure? Problems in definition and quantification for investigative and clinical purposes. *J Clinc Neurophysiol* 1990;7: 315–368.
84. Shewmon DA. Brief interictal rhythmic discharges in newborns. *Electroenceph Clin Neurophysiol* 1983;56:24.
85. Lombroso CT. Neonatal electroencephalography. In Neidermeyer E, Lopes da Silva F (eds.), *Electroencephalography: Basic principles, clinical application and related fields.* Baltimore: Urban & Schwarzberg, 1982, pp. 599–637.

86. Mikati MA, Feraru E, Krishnamoorthy K, Lombroso CT. Neonatal herpes simplex meningoencephalitis: EEG investigations and clinical correlates. *Neurology* 1990;40:1433–1437.
87. Kellaway P, Mizrahi EM. Neonatal seizures. In Luders H, Lesser RP (eds.), *Epilepsy: Electroclinical syndromes.* Amsterdam: Springer-Verlag, 1987, pp. 13–47.
88. Pettay O, Leinikki P, Donner M, Lapinlimer K. Herpes simplex virus infection in the newborn. *Arch Dis Child* 1972;47:97–103.
89. Mizrahi EM, Tharp BR. A characteristic EEG pattern in neonatal herpes simplex encephalitis. *Neurology* 1982;32:1215–1220.
90. Holmes GL, Kull LL. Neonatal seizures. *Am J EEG Technol* 1990;30:281–308.
91. Tharp BR. Pediatric electroencephalography. In Aminoff M (ed.), *Electrodiagnosis in clinical neurology.* New York: Churchill Livingstone, 1980, pp. 83–150.
92. Scher MS, Beggarly M. Clinical significance of focal periodic discharges in neonates. *J Child Neurol* 1989;4:175–185.
93. Chatrian GE, Shaw CM, Leffman H. The significance of periodic lateralized epileptiform discharges in EEG: An electrographic, clinical and pathological study. *Electroenceph Clin Neurophysiol* 1964;17:177–193.
94. Kuroiwa Y, Celesia GG. Clinical significance of periodic EEG patterns. *Arch Neurol* 1980;37:15–20.
95. PeBenito R, Cracco JB. Periodic lateralized epileptiform discharges in infants and children. *Ann Neurol* 1979;6:47–50.
96. Westmoreland BF, Klass DW. A distinctive rhythmic EEG discharge of adults. *Electroenceph Clin Neurophysiol* 1981;51:186–191.
97. Hughes JR, Schlaugenhauff RE. The periodically recurring focal discharges. *Epilepsia* 1965;6:156–166.
98. Schwartz MS, Prior PF, Scott DF. The occurrence and evolution in the EEG of a lateralized periodic phenomenon. *Brain* 1973;96:613–622.
99. Saino K, Granstrom ML, Pettay O, Donner M. EEG in neonatal herpes simplex encephalitis. *Electroenceph Clinc Neurophysiol* 1983;56:556–561.
100. Aicardi J. Early myoclonic encephalopathy. In Roger J, Dravet C, Bureau M, Dreifuss FE, Wolf P (eds.), *Epileptic syndromes in infancy, childhood and adolescence.* London: John Libbey Eurotext Ltd, 1985, pp. 12–22.
101. Lombroso CT. Early myoclonic encephalopathy, early infantile epileptic encephalopathy and benign and severe infantile myoclonic epilepsies. A critical review and personal contributions. *J Clinc Neurophysiol* 1990;7:380–403.
102. Ohtahara S, Ishida T, Oka E. On the specific age dependent epileptic syndrome. The early infantile epileptic encephalopathy with suppression-burst. *No To Hattatsu* 1976;8:270–280.
103. Ohtahara S, Ohtuska Y, Yamatogi Y, Oka E. The early-infantile epileptic encephalopathy with suppression-burst: Developmental aspects. *Brain Dev* 1987;9:371–376.
104. Tharp B, Cukier F, Monod M. The prognostic value of the EEG in premature infants (author's trans). *Rev Electroencephalogr Neurophysiol Clin* 1977;7:386–391.
105. Aso K, Scher MS, Barmada MA. Neonatal electroencephalography and neuropathology. *J Clin Neurophysiol* 1989;6:103–123.
106. Levy S, Abroms I. Seizures and cerebral infarctions in the full-term newborn. *Ann Neurol* 1985;17:366–372.

107. Ment LR, Duncan CC, Ehrenkranz RA. Prenatal cerebral infarction. *Ann Neurol* 1984;16:559–568.
108. Plouin P, Moussalli F, Lerique A, Mises J, Lavoisy P, Navelet Y. Clinical course following a neonatal EEG recording reported as severely abnormal. *Rev Electroencephalogr Neurophysiol Clin* 1977;7:410–415.
109. Lombroso CT. Neurophysiological observations in diseased newborns. *Biol Psychiat* 1975;10:527–558.
110. Tharp BR. Electrophysiological brain maturation in premature infants: An historical perspective. *J Clin Neurophysiol* 1990;7:302–314.
111. Lombroso CT, Holmes GL. Value of the EEG in neonatal seizures. *J Epilepsy* 1993;6:39–70.
112. Holmes GL, Lombroso CT. Prognostic value of background patterns in the neonatal EEG. *J Clin Neurophysiol* 1993;10:323–352.

CHAPTER 9

Transcranial Doppler Technology: The Noninvasive Monitoring of Cerebral Perfusion During Cardiopulmonary Bypass

Frederick A. Burrows

Introduction

Transcranial Doppler (TCD) sonography is a noninvasive technique which allows instantaneous measurements of cerebral blood flow velocity (CBFV) in cerebral vessels in real time. This technique can be used to monitor cerebral perfusion and to detect cerebral emboli during cardiopulmonary bypass (CPB).

The two major support techniques used in repair of complex congenital heart lesions are deep hypothermic circulatory arrest (DHCA) and deep hypothermia with continuous low-flow cardiopulmonary bypass (low-flow CPB) during which the patient is cooled as during DHCA (nasopharyngeal or tympanic temperature <20°C). The use of DHCA for open heart surgery assumes that there is a safe duration of total DHCA, which is inversely related to body temperature and is characterized by the absence of detectable structural or functional organ derangement in the early or late postoperative period.[1] The organ with the shortest safe circulatory arrest time is the brain. Conflicting reports of transient cerebral dysfunction and late neurologic and developmental adverse effects after DHCA[2,3] have generated controversy about its use. The alternative support method, low-flow bypass, maintains continuous cerebral circulation during repair and has been advocated as preferable to DHCA with respect to neurologic outcome.[4,5] Both of these techniques are based on the premise that the reduction in brain temperature during cardiopulmonary bypass provides a sufficient margin of safety during the low-flow or circulatory arrest period. At normothermia the mean ratio of CBF to $CMRO_2$ is 20 to 1 and becomes increasingly luxuriant with temperature reduction until at profound hypothermia the ratio increases to 75 to 1.[6] In theory then, low-flow CPB could provide an indefinite period of effective cerebral perfusion during hypothermia if adequate cerebral oxygen delivery is maintained.

The effectiveness of low-flow CPB in providing improved cerebral protection, however, remains controversial. In a study using a dog model, Wantanabe et al.[7] reported that a 60-minute period of circulatory arrest was followed by an irreversible decrease in brain pH and oxygen tension and an increase in brain carbon dioxide tension, whereas 120 minutes of low-flow CPB $(25 \text{ mL/m}^{-2}/\text{m}^{-1})$ demonstrated recovery in brain pH and carbon dioxide tension, suggesting that low-flow CPB may offer more cerebral protection than DHCA. However, Rossi et al.[8] found that creatine kinase brain isoenzyme, a marker of cerebral ischemia, increased equally after both DHCA and low-flow CPB and concluded that there was no benefit to low-flow CPB. The purpose of this chapter is to review the use and the limitations of TCD in assessing cerebral perfusion during cardiopulmonary bypass (CPB) in the pediatric population.

Cerebral Blood Flow Velocity

The transcranial Doppler technique uses a range-gated, pulsed-wave, direction-sensitive Doppler probe (area = 1.5 cm^2), with an emitting power of 100 mW and a resolution of 3 cm/s, to transmit low-frequency sound (1 to 2.5 MHz) through thin areas (windows) of the skull. For the purposes of monitoring cerebral perfusion during CPB, the CBFV is measured via the temporal window in the M1 segment of the middle cerebral artery (MCA), the largest of the basal cerebral arteries and the dominant one with regard to perfusion (70% of the ipsilateral hemispheric flow). The MCA is a direct continuation and the main branch of the internal carotid artery (ICA), coursing in a horizontal plane laterally and slightly anteriorly. The initial or precommunicating portion of the MCA is referred to as the M1 segment and gives rise to numerous lenticulostriate perforators. In adults the M1 segment has a mean length of 16.2 mm. To ensure a reproducible window for monitoring, the transducer probe is adjusted so that the M1 segment flow velocity is accompanied with retrograde anterior cerebral artery flow velocity (Figure 9–1). The frequency spectrum of Doppler signals is displayed on a frequency analyzer in real time and can be stored, digitized, and analyzed at a later date for research or archiving purposes.

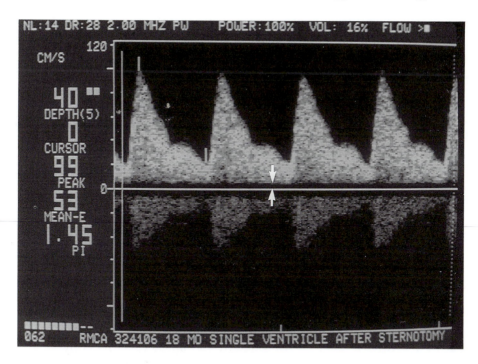

FIGURE 9–1. Example of a typical transcranial Doppler spectral display when the sample volume is centered on the M1 segment of the middle cerebral artery. Positive deflections represent flow towards the Doppler probe in the M1 segment. Retrograde anterior cerebral artery flow is represented by the negative deflections. The threshold of resolution of the TCD is apparent as the acoustically silent area (arrow) between 0 and approximately 3 cm/s velocity.

Limitations

The use of CBFV as an index of cerebral perfusion depends on the ability of the TCD to correlate with cerebral blood flow (CBF) and this, among other considerations, depends on the cross-sectional area of the M1 segment of the MCA remaining constant. The diameter of the M1 segment is believed to be rigidly fixed by bone such that alterations in vessel diameter producing changes in CBFV cannot occur.[9] As such, any changes in CBFV in the M1 segment must reflect changes in CBF. However, such consistency of the diameter of the M1 segment is controversial.[10] Other potential problems in the measurement of CBFV are based both on errors due to the physics of sound waves and errors due to limitations of the Doppler instruments. Among these potential errors, the most important are attributable to the angle of insonation of the Doppler beam and to the resolution of the TCD. Cadaveric studies have shown that the angle of insonation between the temporal window and the M1 segment of the MCA is less than 20°. The Doppler shift is proportional to the cosine of this angle, and the maximum error generated by this variation in the angle is 7%. Doppler resolution is determined by the frequency of the transducer (carrier frequency) and the angle of the Doppler beam. The angle of insonation, as discussed above, is minimal, and the filters are active from 100 to 150 Hz. This translates into a minimal display velocity of approximately 3 to 4 cm/s (see Figure 9–1). When CBF and CBFV are severely reduced with the institution of low-flow CPB, the resolution of the TCD can become problematic. With a resolution of 3 to 4 cm/s, a blind spot exists in TCD assessment of cerebral perfusion when perfusion may be present but below the threshold of resolution of the TCD and therefore is not detected.[11]

Absolute flow velocities measured with TCD vary with many factors including age, $PaCO_2$, and regional cerebral metabolic activity.[12] Recently it has been demonstrated, *in vitro*, that changes in temperature and in hematocrit have no effect on flow velocity when constant flow is maintained in a carrier vessel of constant diameter.[13] Whether TCD, as currently configured, is an appropriate substitute for other clinical methodologies for quantification of cerebral perfusion is unclear. The relationship between CBFV and CBF is inconsistent. Although changes in MCA velocity correlate well with CBF changes, the velocities do not necessarily correlate directly with CBF,[10,14] due in part to interindividual variation in the caliber of cerebral vessel being insonated.[15] In addition, increases in TCD flow velocity correlate inversely with vessel diameter in the presence of cerebral vasospasm but may be directly proportional to vessel diameter in the face of distal peripheral vasodilatation. As such, it can be difficult to ascertain if increased flow velocity represents an increase or a reduction in CBF. Similarly, when TCD data are employed to calculate cerebrovascular resistance,[16] it must be recognized that currently there is no TCD literature quantifying the level to which resistance must be increased before a change in CBFV is observed. The ability to use TCD as a monitor of cerebral perfusion requires the premise that only one variable is changing at any given time to effect the observed change in CBFV.

Validity Studies

The combined measurement of flow velocity and diameter of a cerebral artery provides data that agree well with what is obtained with the microsphere technique.[17] Only marginal changes in the mean diameter of the MCA are assumed to take place,[18] leading to the suggestion that changes in CBFV can be used to estimate changes in CBF. This concept has been supported by experimental and clinical studies performed in normal subjects and in patients at normothermia or moderate hypothermia.[14,19] Bishop and coworkers found a correlation coefficient of 0.85 between changes in MCA flow velocity and xenon washout measurements of cerebral blood flow.[14]

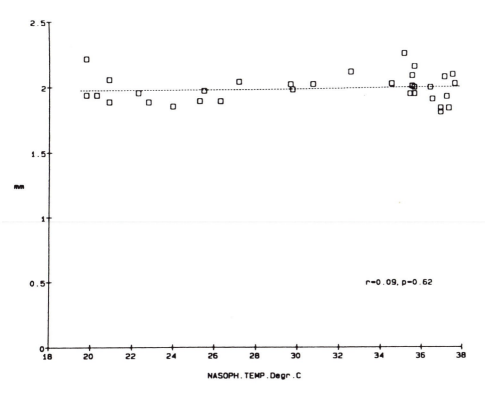

FIGURE 9-2. Nasopharyngeal temperature versus mean diameter of the middle cerebral artery in a single patient. (Reprinted with permission from van der Linden J, Priddy R, Ekroth R, et al. Cerebral perfusion and metabolism during profound hypothermia in children: A study of middle cerebral artery ultrasonic variables and cerebral extraction of oxygen. *J Thorac Cardiovasc Surg* 1991;102:103–114.)

Lindegaard and coworkers observed a correlation coefficient of 0.95 between changes in MCA flow velocity and electromagnetically measured flow in the ipsilateral internal carotid artery.[19] Recent studies by van der Linden and coworkers, using computerized echocardiographic tracking to monitor MCA diameter during profound hypothermic cardiac operations in small children, indicated that this artery did not change its mean diameter significantly during changes in temperature (Figure 9–2), PaCO$_2$, mean arterial pressure, or pump flow rate.[20] Other work demonstrated a close correlation between MCA flow velocity and CBF at similar temperature (Figure 9–3) supporting the Doppler technique as useful at deep hypothermic conditions.[20] The intra-observer, between-observer, and long-term repeatability of TCD measurements have been investigated and determined to be accurate.[21]

The use of relative units facilitates the comparison of CBFV values to CBF. This method of displaying the TCD measurements examines changes in CBFV in comparison to a baseline or control value obtained under stable

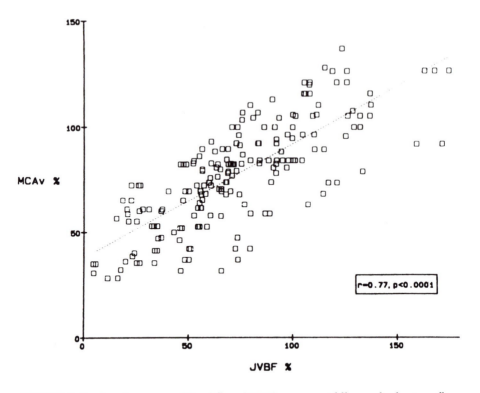

FIGURE 9–3. Jugular venous blood flow (JVBF) versus middle cerebral artery flow velocity (MCAv), expressed in percent of individual awake values. Combined data from 7 patients. (Reprinted with permission from van der Linden J, Wesslen O, Ekroth R, Tyden H, von Ahn H. Transcranial Doppler-estimated versus thermodilution-estimated cerebral blood flow during cardiac operations: Influence of temperature and arterial carbon dioxide tension. *J Thorac Cardiovasc Surg* 1991;102: 95–102.)

conditions such as awake values[22] or values obtained when stable on CPB.[16] The use of such proportional changes have been demonstrated to correlate well (see Figure 9–3) with observed proportional changes in CBF.[22]

Clinical Studies

The introduction of TCD sonography enabled noninvasive investigation of the effects of DHCA and of low-flow CPB on cerebral perfusion and hemodynamics. Studies performed by Hillier, et al.[16] have demonstrated that the changes in CBFV induced by CPB with DHCA (Figure 9–4) paralleled those changes demonstrated by Greeley and coworkers[23] using more invasive techniques. Van der Linden and coworkers have demonstrated that, when compared with normalized jugular venous blood flow, changes in MCA flow velocity accurately reflect changes in jugular venous blood flow to levels as

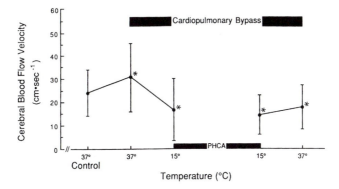

FIGURE 9-4. Changes in cerebral blood flow velocity before cardiopulmonary bypass and before and after profound hypothermic circulatory arrest at normothermia and deep hypothermia. Values represent mean (+ SD). *p<.05 compared with control. (Reprinted with permission from Hillier SC, Burrows FA, Bissonnette B, Taylor RH. Cerebral hemodynamics in neonates and infants undergoing cardiopulmonary bypass and profound hypothermic circulatory arrest: Assessment by transcranial Doppler sonography. *Anesth Analg* 1991;72:723-728.)

low as 10% of normal (see Figure 9-3).[22] These studies demonstrate the ability of TCD sonography to detect cerebral perfusion and changes in cerebral perfusion when directly measured values have decreased to very low levels. The presence and adequacy of cerebral perfusion during periods of low-flow CPB are important if it is to be considered an advantage over DHCA. Greeley, et al. have demonstrated an increase in the margin of safety with the introduction of hypothermia[6] and pump flows as low as 0.5 L/min/m[2 20] and 5 to 10 mL/kg/min[2 24] have been suggested to be adequate. However, reports and studies by Taylor et al.[11,25] suggest that cerebral perfusion may become limited or absent when CPP decreases below 7 to 12 mm Hg (Figures 9-5 and 9-6). These results have been questioned by others who have not been able to reproduce these results in their own clinical setting.[26] It is possible that the threshold of resolution of the TCD has produced these results in that cerebral perfusion may still be present but not detectable by the TCD. Alternatively, it is equally possible that different clinical settings produce different responses to low-flow CPB. Further studies support the contention that cerebral perfusion may become absent during low-flow CPB. Distinctive patterns of recovery of CBFV have been demonstrated during increasing pump flow after low-flow CPB with continued cerebral perfusion and after DHCA (Figure 9-7). In patients undergoing low-flow CPB in whom CBFV became nondetectable, two subgroups were identified: those in whom the pattern of recovery was the same as those undergoing low-flow CPB but in

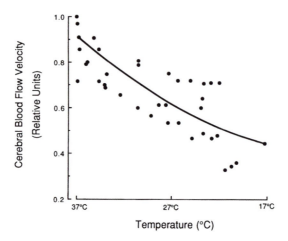

FIGURE 9–5. The exponential relationship between nasopharyngeal temperature and cerebral
blood flow velocity during cooling and before
deep hypothermic circulatory arrest (r=.78).
(Reprinted with permission from Hillier SC, Burrows FA, Bissonnette B, Taylor RH. Cerebral hemodynamics in neonates and infants undergoing
cardiopulmonary bypass and profound hypothermic circulatory arrest: Assessment by transcranial Doppler sonography. *Anesth Analg* 1991;72:
723–728.)

whom detectable perfusion was present during the procedure and those in
whom the pattern of recovery was the same as those undergoing DHCA.[27]
Other work has demonstrated an increase in cerebral production of lactate
in some patients who are undergoing low-flow CPB.[28] This implies that cerebral perfusion may not necessarily cease but instead may become undetectable because it is below the threshold of resolution of the TCD. Such
limited perfusion may be too low to provide sufficient substrate to the
brain.[29,30] Clinical work comparing pH management during low-flow CPB
and DHCA has suggested that a more alkaline pH strategy, such as alpha-
stat, may result in less effective cerebral protection in neonates and infants
who have received such support techniques.[31] Recently, studies have been
undertaken to compare the effects of alpha-stat versus pH-stat pH management on CBFV during hypothermic cardiopulmonary bypass. The results of
this study are preliminary, but early trends suggest that the reduction of
CBFV during the induction of hypothermia and during low-flow CPB is less
and recovery after DHCA is more rapid when pH-stat management is
employed. This is in partial agreement with microsphere studies performed
in rabbits, in which a greater global cerebral blood flow was demonstrated

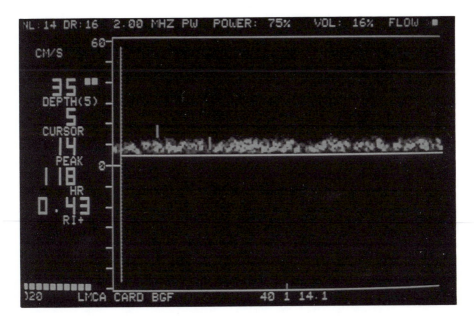

FIGURE 9–6A.   Transcranial Doppler display spectral during full (2.4 L/min/m²) continuous cardiopulmonary bypass flow. Nasopharyngeal temperature is 14.1°C. Left middle cerebral artery (LMCA). (Reprinted with permission from Taylor RH, Burrows FA, Bissonnette B. No flow during low-flow cardiopulmonary bypass (Letter). *J Thorac Cardiovasc Surg* 1991;101:363–365.)

during pH-stat acid-base management at normal pump flow rates (100 to 150 mL/kg/m).[32] The implications of these trends to cerebral injury during pediatric cardiac surgery are also under investigation.

Cerebral Emboli

Transcranial Doppler detection of gaseous and solid (thrombi and platelet aggregates) emboli has been demonstrated (Figure 9–8), and a relationship has been demonstrated between the number of emboli detected by TCD and a decline in neuropsychological function after cardiopulmonary bypass.[33] The emboli appear as short-duration, high-intensity signals in the Doppler spectrum. The intensity of the Doppler signal from an artery containing an embolus depends on the density difference between the embolic material and blood. This difference is greatest for gaseous emboli, which are therefore the easiest to detect; solid emboli, such as thrombi and platelet aggregates, result in less intense signals. Studies in *in vitro* and *in vivo* models demonstrate that this technique provides information on the size and type of emboli. Larger emboli produce signals of greater intensity and duration.[34]

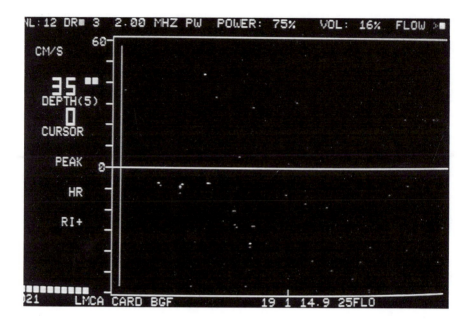

FIGURE 9–6B. Transcranial Doppler display during 25% of full flow (0.6 L/min/m²) in the same infant, no perfusion is detected in the left middle cerebral artery. (Reprinted with permission from Taylor RH, Burrows FA, Bissonnette B. No flow during low-flow cardiopulmonary bypass (Letter). *J Thorac Cardiovasc Surg* 1991;101:363–365.

Practical patient monitoring will require automatic emboli detectors incorporated into the Doppler machine; such programs are being developed. The prognostic significance of such emboli in children remains to be determined.

Summary

Transcranial Doppler sonography (TCD) has enabled noninvasive study of cerebral perfusion. This modality has proven useful in the management and study of patients undergoing repair of complex congenital heart lesions (CHD). Deep hypothermic circulatory arrest (DHCA) and deep hypothermia with continuous low-flow cardiopulmonary bypass (low-flow CPB) are two support techniques used to facilitate the repair of such lesions. Extended periods of DHCA may impair cerebral function and metabolism and produce ischemic brain injury. Low-flow CPB has been advocated as preferable to DHCA with respect to neurologic outcome because it maintains continuous cerebral circulation during repair of CHD. Several studies have suggested that low-flow CPB produces equal degrees of cerebral injury to correspond-

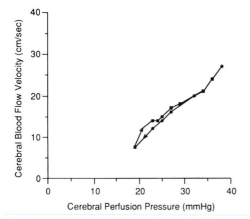

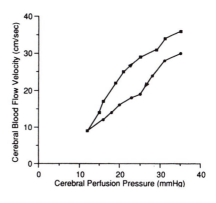

FIGURE 9–7A. Interpolated values of cerebral blood flow velocity (CBFV) changes representing one patient during decreasing and increasing cerebral perfusion pressure (CPP), induced by alterations in pump flow within the normal range. The slope of the CBFV-to-CPP relationship during decreasing (0.95 cm/s/mm Hg) and increasing (0.86 cm/s/mm Hg) pump flow respectively were determined by linear regression analysis. There was no statistical difference between the dV/dP (p=.42) or the y intercept (p=.29) of the lines. (Reprinted with permission from Burrows FA, Bissonnette B. Cerebral blood flow velocity patterns during cardiac surgery utilizing profound hypothermia with low-flow cardiopulmonary bypass or circulatory arrest in neonates and infants. *Can J Anaesth* 1993;40:1–10.)

FIGURE 9–7B. Interpolated values of cerebral blood flow velocity (CBFV) changes representing one patient during decreasing and increasing cerebral perfusion pressure (CPP), induced by alterations in pump flow to establish low-flow cardiopulmonary bypass (CPB). The slope of the CBFV-to-CPP relationship during decreasing (0.95 cm/s/mm Hg) and increasing (1.15 cm/s/mm Hg) pump flow respectively were determined by linear regression analysis. The dV/dP during decreasing pump flows and CPP was significantly less than during increasing pump flows and CPP after low-flow CPB (p=.04). (Reprinted with permission from Burrows FA, Bissonnette B. Cerebral blood flow velocity patterns during cardiac surgery utilizing profound hypothermia with low-flow cardiopulmonary bypass or circulatory arrest in neonates and infants. *Can J Anaesth* 1993;40:1–10.)

ing periods of DHCA. Transcranial Doppler sonography has enabled the noninvasive study of cerebral perfusion during operations utilizing either DHCA or low-flow CPB. Although these studies have demonstrated the presence of cerebral perfusion at low perfusion pressures, it has been suggested that cerebral perfusion may be limited or cease at low cerebral perfusion pressures and at extremely low pump flow rates. Transcranial Doppler sonography is a useful tool for monitoring cerebral perfusion during low-flow CPB. Studies with this modality may help to define and develop improved modes of cerebral protection during repair of CHD.

FIGURE 9–7C. Interpolated values of cerebral blood flow velocity (CBFV) changes representing one patient during decreasing and increasing cerebral perfusion pressure (CPP), induced by alterations in pump flow to establish low-flow cardiopulmonary bypass (CPB). The slope of the CBFV-to-CPP relationship during decreasing (0.92 cm/s/mm Hg) and increasing (0.57 cm/s/mm Hg) pump flow respectively were determined by linear regression analysis. The dV/dP during decreasing pump flows and CPP was significantly greater than during increasing pump flows and CPP after

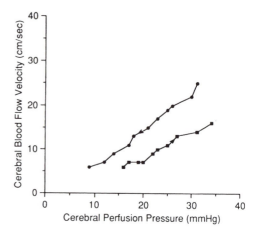

DHCA (p=.03). (Reprinted with permission from Burrows FA, Bissonnette B. Cerebral blood flow velocity patterns during cardiac surgery utilizing profound hypothermia with low-flow cardiopulmonary bypass or circulatory arrest in neonates and infants. *Can J Anaesth* 1993;40:1–10.)

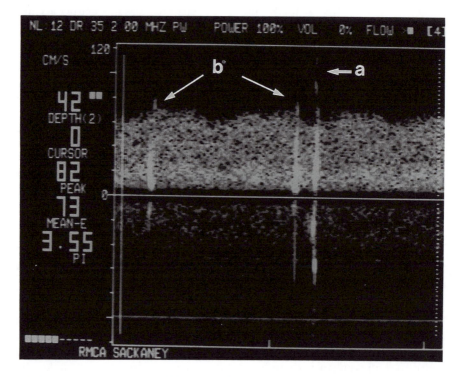

FIGURE 9–8. Transcranial Doppler display during cardiopulmonary bypass. The signal identified as "a" is suggestive of air while the signals identified as "b" are suggestive of particulate emboli.

References

1. Kirklin JW, Barratt-Boyes BG (eds.), *Cardiac surgery*. New York: John Wiley and Sons, 1986: pp. 30–74.
2. Ferry PC. Neurological sequelae of cardiac surgery in children. *Am J Dis Child* 1987;141:309–312.
3. Ferry PC. Neurological sequelae of open-heart surgery in children. An "irritating question." *Am J Dis Child* 1990;144:369–373.
4. Fox LS, Blackstone RH, Kirklin JW. Relationship of brain blood flow and oxygen consumption to perfusion flow rate during profoundly hypothermic cardiopulmonary bypass. *J Thorac Cardiovasc Surg* 1984;87:658–64.
5. Rebeyka IM, Coles JG, Wilson GJ, et al. The effect of low-flow cardiopulmonary bypass on cerebral function: An experimental and clinical study. *Ann Thorac Surg* 1987;43:391–396.
6. Greeley WJ, Kern FH, Ungerleider RM, et al. The effect of hypothermic cardiopulmonary bypass and total circulatory arrest on cerebral metabolism in neonates, infants, and children. *J Thorac Cardiovasc Surg* 1991;101: 783–794.
7. Watanabe T, Orita H, Kobayashi M, Washio M. Brain tissue pH, oxygen tension, and carbon dioxide tension in profoundly hypothermic cardiopulmonary bypass. *J Thorac Cardiovasc Surg* 1989;97:396–401.
8. Rossi R, Ekroth R, Thompson RJ. No flow or low flow? A study of the ischaemic marker creatine kinase BB after deep hypothermic procedures. *J Thorac Cardiovasc Surg* 1989;98:193–199.
9. Carpenter MB, Sutin J. *Human neuroanatomy*, 8th ed. Baltimore: Williams & Wilkins, 1983:872.
10. Kontos HA. Validity of cerebral arterial blood flow calculations from velocity measurements. *Stroke* 1989;20:1–3.
11. Taylor RH, Burrows FA, Bissonnette B. Cerebral pressure-flow velocity relationship during hypothermic cardiopulmonary bypass in neonates and infants. *Anesth Analg* 1992;74:636–642.
12. Caplan L, Brass LM, DeWitt LD, et al. Transcranial Doppler ultrasound: Present status. *Neurology* 1990;40:696–700.
13. Reimer H, Bissonnette B. Temperature and hematocrit do not affect the relationship between blood flow velocity and blood flow. *Anesth Analg* 1993;76:S345.
14. Bishop CCR, Powell S, Rutt D, Browse NL. Transcranial Doppler measurement of middle cerebral artery flow velocity: A validation study. *Stroke* 1986;17:913–915.
15. Gabrielson TO, Greitz T. Normal size of the internal carotid, middle cerebral and anterior cerebral arteries. *Acta Radiol* 1970;10:1–10.
16. Hillier SC, Burrows FA, Bissonnette B, Taylor RH. Cerebral hemodynamics in neonates and infants undergoing cardiopulmonary bypass and profound hypothermic circulatory arrest: Assessment by transcranial Doppler sonography. *Anesth Analg* 1991;72:723–728.
17. Buijs J, Van Bel F, Nandorff A, Hardjowijono R, Steijnen T, Ottenkamp J. Cerebral blood flow pattern and autoregulation during open-heart surgery in infants and young children: A transcranial, Doppler ultrasound study. *Crit Care Med* 1992;20:771–777.

18. Huber P, Handa J. Effect of contrast material, hypercapnea, hyperventilation, hypertonic glucose and papaverine in the diameter of cerebral arteries: Angiographic determination in man. *Invest Radiol* 1967;2:17–32.
19. Lindegaard KF, Lundar T, Wiberg J, Sjöberg D, Aaslid R, Nornes H. Variations in middle cerebral artery blood flow investigated with noninvasive transcranial blood velocity measurements. *Stroke* 1987;18:1025–1030.
20. van der Linden J, Priddy R, Ekroth R, et al. Cerebral perfusion and metabolism during profound hypothermia in children: A study of middle cerebral artery ultrasonic variables and cerebral extraction of oxygen. *J Thorac Cardiovasc Surg* 1991;102:103–114.
21. Demolis P, Chalon S, Giudicelli J-F. Repeatability of transcranial Doppler measurements of arterial blood flow velocities in healthy subjects. *Clin Sci* 1993;84:599–604.
22. van der Linden J, Wesslén Ö, Ekroth R, Tydén H, von Ahn H. Transcranial Doppler-estimated versus thermodilution-estimated cerebral blood flow during cardiac operations: Influence of temperature and arterial carbon dioxide tension. *J Thorac Cardiovasc Surg* 1991;102:95–102.
23. Greeley WJ, Ungerleider RM, Kern FH, Brusino FG, Smith LR, Reves JG. Effects of cardiopulmonary bypass on cerebral blood flow in neonates, infants, and children. *Circulation* 1989;80(suppl I):209–215.
24. Mault JR, Ohtake S, Klingensmith M, Heinle JS, Greeley WJ, Ungerleider RM. Cerebral metabolism and circulatory arrest: Effects of duration and strategies for protection. *Ann Thorac Surg* 1993;55:57–64.
25. Taylor RH, Burrows FA, Bissonnette B. No flow during low-flow cardiopulmonary bypass (Letter). *J Thorac Cardiovasc Surg* 1991;101:363–365.
26. Jonas RA, Hickey P. Invited letter concerning: No flow during low flow cardiopulmonary bypass. *J Thorac Cardiovasc Surg* 1991;101:364–365.
27. Burrows FA, Bissonnette B. Cerebral blood flow velocity patterns during cardiac surgery utilizing profound hypothermia with low-flow cardiopulmonary bypass or circulatory arrest in neonates and infants. *Can J Anaesth* 1993;40:1–10.
28. Reimer H, Burrows FA, Bissonnette B. Cerebral metabolism during low-flow cardiopulmonary bypass and profound hypothermic circulatory arrest. *Anesthesiology* 1992;77:A1135.
29. Miyamoto K, Kawashima Y, Matsuda H, et al. Optimal perfusion flow rate for the brain during deep hypothermic cardiopulmonary bypass at 20°C. *J Thorac Cardiovasc Surg* 1986;92:1065–1070.
30. Swain JA, McDonald TJ, Jr., Griffith PK, Balaban RS, Clark RE, Ceckler T. Low-flow hypothermic cardiopulmonary bypass protects the brain. *J Thorac Cardiovasc Surg* 1991;102:76–84.
31. Jonas RA, Bellinger DC, Rappaport LA, et al. Relation of pH strategy and developmental outcome after hypothermic circulatory arrest. *J Thorac Cardiovasc Surg* 1993;106:362–368.
32. Hindman BJ, Funatsu N, Harrington J, et al. Differences in cerebral blood flow between alpha-stat and pH-stat management are eliminated during periods of decreased systemic flow and pressure. *Anesthesiology* 1991;71:1096–1102.
33. Stump DA, Tegler CH, Rogers AT, et al. Neuropsychological deficits are associated with the number of emboli detected during cardiac surgery. *Stroke* 1993;24:A509.
34. Markus H. Transcranial Doppler detection of circulating emboli: A review. *Stroke* 1993;24:1246–1250.

CHAPTER 10

PET and SPECT in the Assessment of Cerebral Function

Adre J. du Plessis
S. Ted Treves

Cerebral injury during pediatric cardiac surgery may result from several different mechanisms.[1,2] Cerebral ischemia is a leading candidate mechanism either resulting from diffuse hypoperfusion or focal vaso-occlusive events related to bypass pump-related embolic phenomena. Cerebroprotective measures are directed mainly at depressing cerebral metabolism[3] (by hypothermia and drugs) to maintain a positive substrate supply-utilization balance and to prevent the development of ischemia during periods of attenuated blood flow. During cardiopulmonary bypass (CPB), our ability to monitor the adequacy of this balance between supply and demand is limited. At the same time, the brain's normal mechanisms of autoregulating the balance between perfusion pressure, CBF, and metabolism may be disrupted.[4,5] Thus, this complex scenario demands that the investigation of ischemic mechanisms of brain injury during cardiac surgery address cerebral metabolism and perfusion simultaneously.

Two functional brain imaging techniques, positron emission tomography (PET) and single photon emission computed tomography (SPECT), allow the *in vivo* study of regional cerebral biochemical and hemodynamic processes. The advantages and constraints of these techniques, as well as their applicability to the questions of brain injury during cardiac surgery will be discussed.

Positron Emission Tomography (PET)

Over the four decades since the conception of positron imaging, technological and methodological advances have evolved PET into the gold standard of

143

functional brain-scanning techniques.[6] PET is capable of accurately measuring regional concentrations of radiotracer in tissue. Quantitative analysis of numerous regional biological processes in the brain can be made, including regional cerebral blood volume and flow and the regional metabolism of oxygen and glucose, by attaching PET radiopharmaceuticals to substances that distribute according to function.

When positrons (positively charged electrons) collide with electrons, the annihilation event results in two high-energy photons, emitted in opposite directions.[7] PET utilizes this phenomenon by recording photons in diametrically opposed pairs of detectors. These detector pairs are arranged in geometric arrays, connected by coincidence circuits. Photon signals are recorded only if detector pairs register photon pairs virtually simultaneously (Figure 10–1). This coincidence detection system underlies the localizing ability of PET and reduces the signal degradation caused by scattered radiation. Positron-emitting radionuclides (such as ^{15}O, ^{11}C, and ^{13}N) may be incorporated into a variety of biological substrates and drugs. Flow-specific tracers such as $H_2^{15}O$ allow the measurement of regional cerebral blood flow (rCBF); substrate analogs such as ^{18}F-deoxyglucose, the cerebral metabolic rate for glucose (CMRGl); $^{15}O\text{-}O_2$, the cerebral metabolic rate for oxygen (CMRO$_2$); and ^{15}O-carbon monoxide, the cerebral blood volume (CBV). The short physical half-lives of these radionuclides permits repeated measurements of rapid metabolic processes but also necessitates an on-site cyclotron for isotope generation. Specific biological questions can be investigated by applying tracer kinetic models to the PET data. Finally, computerized tomographic reconstruction of data from the coincidence detector pairs yields a three-dimensional representation of the data.

Numerous questions of normal and abnormal cerebral function have been addressed by PET. Major clinical applications (largely in adults) have been epilepsy,[8,9] cerebrovascular disease,[10,11] dementia,[12] brain tumors,[13,14] and movement disorders.[15–17] This discussion will focus on studies of cerebral ischemia.

In adults suffering cerebrovascular accidents, several PET studies have addressed the complex relationship between regional CBF, CBV, CMRO$_2$, and CMRGl.[10,11] When compared to lesions detected by structural imaging (CT/MRI), abnormalities detected by PET occur earlier and are often more extensive. In addition, PET studies of cerebral infarction have demonstrated areas of hypoperfusion remote from the CT/MRI delineated area of infarction.[18,19] This phenomenon is believed to result from depression of cerebral function in remote projection areas, due to deafferentation (diaschisis) of projection pathways involved in the primary area of infarction. During evolving ischemia, PET has delineated the temporal and spatial relationships among cerebral metabolism (oxygen and glucose), cerebral oxygen extraction (COE), and CBF.[10] With decreasing cerebral perfusion pressure, CMRO$_2$ is initially maintained by an increase in CBV (due to vasodilation) and subsequently is maintained by increasing cerebral oxygen extraction (COE).[20] As perfusion

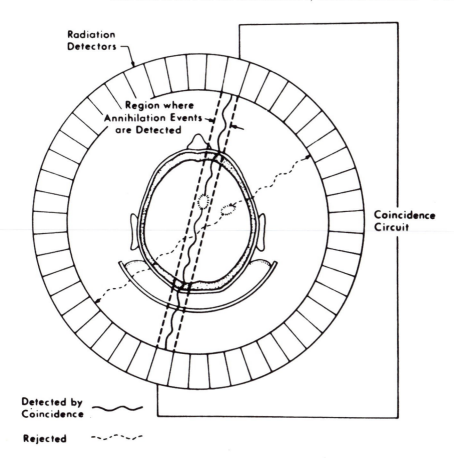

FIGURE 10–1.   Positron emission tomography: the basic principles underlying the coincidence detection of photon emission resulting from the annihilation collision of positrons and electrons (Reprinted with permission from Volpe J, Herscovitch P, Perlmann J, Raichle M. Positron emission tomography in the newborn: Extensive impairment of regional cerebral blood flow with intraventricular hemorrhage and hemorrhagic intracerebral involvement. *Pediatrics* 1983;72(5):589–601.)

decreases further, these compensatory mechanisms fail and $CMRO_2$ falls; a persistent depression of $CMRO_2$ results in infarction.

Although the number of PET studies in young infants and children is limited, several important studies of normal and abnormal cerebral hemodynamics and metabolism in this age group have been reported. Using [18]FDG to study CMRGl, normal patterns for the metabolic maturation of the infant brain have been described.[21,22] Distinct maturational differences in cerebral blood flow and oxygen metabolism have also been demonstrated. Altman, et al. demonstrated that in the newborn, CBF well below the adult threshold for cerebral infarction (i.e., less than 10mL/100gm/min) is compatible with a normal neurological and cognitive outcome.[23] In a later study, these authors demonstrated similar maturational differences for cerebral oxygen metabolism.[24] In the newborn, $CMRO_2$ values significantly lower than that required to maintain neuronal viability in the adult were seen without subsequent evidence of neurologic injury. In some preterm infants oxygen metabolism appeared to be virtually absent. These findings suggested that cerebral energy requirements in the human newborn were either minimal and/or were met by nonoxidative metabolism.[24] In the preterm infant with intraventricular-intraparenchymal hemorrhage, PET has demonstrated dramatic disturbances in CBF extending well beyond the regions of parenchymal injury as depicted by cranial ultrasound.[25] At autopsy these regions of hypoperfusion correlated with extensive infarction suggesting that the mechanism of parenchymal hemorrhage in these infants was ischemic in origin. A PET study of rCBF using $^{15}O\text{-}H_2O$ in 17 birth-asphyxiated term infants[26] demonstrated symmetric impairment of CBF to the parasagittal regions of the cerebral hemispheres, suggesting ischemic injury to the "watershed" regions between the end zones of major cerebral arterial supply territories, presumably due to global cerebral hypoperfusion. This finding was again supported by neuropathological and experimental data. Positron emission tomography has also been used to study the rCBF in infant survivors of ECMO.[27] These studies showed symmetric hemispheric rCBF regardless of the state of the carotid arteries (i.e., ligated or reanastomosed). Other than an isolated case report, there are currently no available PET data on cerebral metabolism or blood flow following cardiopulmonary bypass or cardiac surgery. An ^{18}FDG PET study of CMRGl in a case of postpump chorea following cardiac surgery showed focal regions of impaired cerebral metabolism despite the lack of structural defects on MRI scan.[28]

Single Photon Emission Computed Tomography (SPECT)

The value of SPECT as a functional brain-scanning technique is based on the usual tight coupling of cerebral blood flow to metabolism.[29,30] Unlike PET, no specific metabolic tracers are currently available. Lipophilic perfusion tracers, which diffuse freely and rapidly through the intact blood brain barrier (BBB), are utilized to reflect regional perfusion and thus usually local cerebral metabolism.[31] Beyond the BBB, these tracers undergo hydrophilic transformation, which delays their washout, thereby effectively trapping them in the brain for up to several hours. Tracers are now available which can be stored at the bedside. At the time of a spontaneous clinical event of interest (e.g., a seizure), the tracer can be injected allowing the stable CBF pattern to be imaged later. With newer tracers such as technetium-99m hexamethyl-prolene amine oxime ($^{99m}Tc\text{-}HMPAO$), stable images can be recorded 10 minutes after the injection and for longer than 4 hours thereafter. These features allow the rCBF related to specific clinical events to be "freeze-framed" at the time of injection of the tracer for later imaging.

Brain SPECT has been applied to a broad spectrum of clinical questions including epilepsy,[32–34] cerebrovascular disease,[35–38] dementia,[39] brain tumors,[40] and movement disorders.[41–44] As with PET, SPECT perfusion defects tend to precede and exceed the lesions noted on CT or MRI scan and often correlate more closely with the clinical picture.[35] Perfusion SPECT has been used to address pediatric cerebrovascular disease. Shahar, et al. described SPECT findings in 15 infants and children presenting with hemiparesis.[37] Perfusion SPECT in the newborn was shown to correlate, in most cases, with abnormalities on head ultrasonography (US); however, in this study SPECT appeared less sensitive than US to defects in the deep white matter and more sensitive to changes in the parasagittal regions.[45] ^{99m}Tc-HMPAO perfusion SPECT studies of CBF patterns in 13 survivors of infant ECMO demonstrated regional CBF defects in 7 cases, while only 2 cases had focal abnormalities on structural imaging studies (US, CT, or MRI).[46] In acute infantile hemiplegia, SPECT perfusion defects were more enduring than EEG abnormalities, suggesting that SPECT was sensitive to reductions in CBF above the threshold for electrical failure.[38]

To date, perfusion SPECT studies of CBF in survivors of congenital heart disease and cardiac surgery are limited.[34,47] We recently used ^{99m}Tc-HMPAO perfusion SPECT to study rCBF patterns in 11 children who developed a movement disorder following cardiac surgery.[47] While none of these cases showed focal structural defects on structural imaging (CT or MRI) scans, perfusion SPECT showed regional cortical and subcortical cerebral hypoperfusion in 9 of 11 cases (Figure 10–2). Perfusion defects were evident in the deep grey matter regions in 6 of 11 and in the cortical regions in 9 of 11 patients. These defects showed a strong unexplained right-sided predilection. Perfusion abnormalities were extensive, involving more than two brain lobes in eight cases. In no case was hypoperfusion confined to the territory of any one major cerebral vessel. These findings suggested functional brain injury in these patients, undetected by conventional cranial CT and MRI.

One further potential application of these techniques also relates to the rare but potentially devastating movement disorders[48] seen in infants undergoing hypothermic cardiac surgery. In adults, PET and SPECT have been utilized in the study of neurotransmitter-receptor systems and their alteration in disease.[16,41,43,44,49] New SPECT neuroreceptor imaging agents, such as dopaminergic, muscarinic, serotinergic, and benzodiazepine compounds, are being developed.[30,50] These new imaging agents may prove valuable in delineating complex neurotransmitter disturbances underlying these movement disorders and may shed light on their etiology as well as facilitate the development of effective therapies currently so lacking.

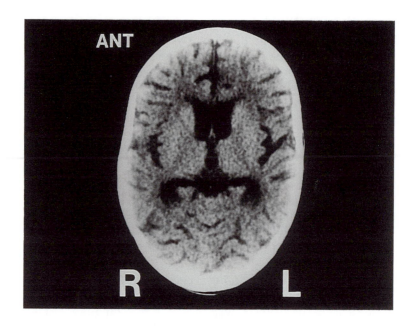

FIGURE 10–2A.   Brain CT scan (transverse view) of a patient with choreoathetosis following deep hypothermic cardiac surgery, showing diffuse cerebral atrophy without focal structural defects.

Emission Tomography: Current Limitations and Future Directions

Although the functional brain imaging techniques of PET and SPECT have advanced our understanding of cerebral metabolism and hemodynamics, these techniques have certain constraints. The major limitation of PET relates to its cost and complexity, factors which have restricted the widespread application of the technique. The short half-life of PET isotopes necessitates an on-site cyclotron, and the complexities of radiotracer synthesis require a radiochemist. Single photon emission tomography is a less costly, less cumbersome, and more accessible alternative, which in many circumstances is able to demonstrate the same information as PET.[51] However, several limitations restrict the SPECT technique. First, the inability to measure metabolism directly may limit the value of SPECT, particularly in the study of ischemia when the normal coupling of CBF to metabolism may break down. In addition, recent evidence suggests that the fractional fixation of ^{99m}Tc-HMPAO may be altered in certain disease states, including cerebral ischemia.[52] Second, SPECT is currently semiquantitative. Ongoing efforts are aimed at quantitative validation.[33]

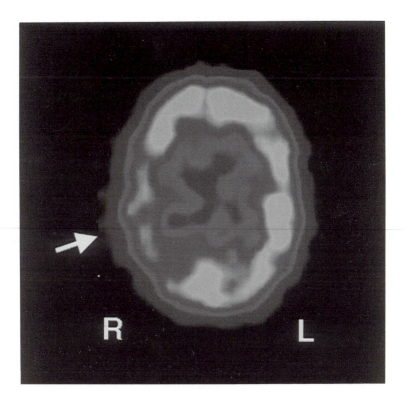

FIGURE 10–2B. ^{99m}Tc-HMPAO Brain SPECT of the same patient (Figure 10–2A) at the equivalent horizontal level, showing regional cerebral hypoperfusion in the right (R) temporoparietal region (arrow) and right deep gray matter.

The area of functional brain imaging using emission tomography is a rapidly evolving field, and a number of exciting developments are on the horizon. Technological advances, such as the development of automated radionuclide generators and smaller cameras, may reduce the cost and technical complexity, thereby expanding the future clinical role of emission tomography.[7] The spatial resolution of PET has improved dramatically over the past ten years, increasing from 30 mm to 3.5 mm, and is currently approaching its theoretical limit. Spatial resolution with SPECT is also improving as older, single-headed rotating SPECT cameras are being replaced by multidetector units. These technological advances in SPECT instrumentation have also decreased the imaging times required. Together with progress in the area of quantitation[33] and radiotracer development, these advances will continue to expand the clinical applications of SPECT.[30] A further exciting feature unique to both these techniques is the potential for custom designing new radiopharmaceuticals to address new questions;

already over 500 substrates and drugs have been labeled for use in PET. The potential for SPECT radiopharmaceutical development is immense. Finally, image fusion techniques have been designed that combine the anatomical detail of MRI with functional data from PET and SPECT.

In summary, these functional imaging techniques represent exciting new ways to measure cerebral function *in vivo.* In addition, the research trajectory in this area would predict the resolution of many of the current limitations of these techniques. While logistic constraints prevent the intraoperative study of cerebral changes during cardiac surgery, the potential application of these techniques to the perioperative period, as well as to experimental questions, remains to be explored.

References

1. Aberg T, Ronquist G, Tyden H, et al. Adverse effects in the brain in cardiac operations as assessed by biochemical, psychometric, and radiologic methods. *J Thorac Cardiovasc Surg* 1984;87:99–105.
2. Henricksen L. Evidence suggestive of diffuse brain damage following cardiac operations. *Lancet* 1984;1:816–820.
3. Gisvold S, Steen P. Drug therapy in cerebral ischemia. *Br J Anaesth* 1985;57: 96–109.
4. Murkin J, Farrar J, Tweed W, et al. Cerebral autoregulation and flow/metabolism coupling during cardiopulmonary bypass: The influence of $PaCO_2$. *Anesth Analg* 1987;66:825–832.
5. Henricksen L, Hjelms E, Lindeberg T. Brain hyperperfusion during cardiac operations. *J Thorac Cardiovasc Surg* 1983;86:202–208.
6. Hoffman J, Hansom M, Coleman R. Clinical positron emission tomography imaging. *Radiol Clin North Amer* 1993;31(4):935–959.
7. Phelps M. PET: A biological imaging technique. *Neurochem Res* 1991;16(9): 929–940.
8. Engel J, Kuhl D, Phelps M, et al. Comparative localization of epileptic foci in partial epilepsy by PET and EEG. *Ann Neurol* 1982;12:529.
9. Kuhl D, Engel J, Phelps M, et al. Epileptic patterns of local cerebral metabolism and perfusion in humans determined by emission computed tomography of 13F-FDG and 3NH3. *Ann Neurol* 1980;8:348.
10. Wise R, Bernardi S, Frackowiak R, et. al. Serial observations on the pathophysiology of acute stroke. *Brain* 1983;106:197–222.
11. Frackowiac R, Wise R. Positron tomography in ischemic cerebrovascular disease. *Neurol Clin* 1983;1:183–201.
12. Alavi A, Ferris S, Wolf A, et al. Determination of cerebral metabolism in senile dementia using F-1 8-deoxyglucose and positron emission tomography. *J Nuc Med* 1980;21:21.
13. DiChiro G, Brooks R, Patronas N, et. al. Issues in the in vivo measurement of glucose metabolism of human CNS tumors. *Ann Neurol* 1984;15 (Suppl l):S137.
14. Patronas N, DiChiro G, Kufta C, et al. Predictions of survival in glioma patients by means of positron emission tomography. *J Neurosurg* 1985;62:816.

15. Kuhl D, Phelps M, Markham C, et al. Cerebral metabolism and atrophy in Huntington's disease determined by 1 ~ FDG and computed tomographic scan. *Ann Neurol* 1982;12:425.

16. Leenders K, Frackowiac R, Quinn N, et al. Brain energy metabolism and dopaminergic function in Huntington's disease measured in vivo using positron emission tomography. *Mov Disord* 1986;1:69–77.

17. Holthoff V, Koeppe R, Frey K, et al. Positron emission tomography measures of benzodiazepine receptors in Huntington's disease. *Ann Neurol* 1993;34: 76–81.

18. Kushner M, Alavi A, Reivich M, et al. Contralateral cerebellar hypometabolism following cerebral insult: A positron emission tomographic study. *Ann Neurol* 1984;15:425–434.

19. Martin W, Raichle M. Cerebral blood flow and metabolism in cerebral hemisphere infarction. *Ann Neurol* 1983;14:168–176.

20. Powers W, Raichle M. Positron emission tomography and its application to the study of cerebrovascular disease in man. *Stroke* 1985;16(3):361–376.

21. Chugani H, Phelps M, Mazziotta J. Positron emission tomography study of human brain functional development. *Ann Neurol* 1987;22:487–497.

22. Chugani H, Phelps M, Barnes D. PET in normal and abnormal brain development. In Swann JW, Messer A (ed.), *Disorders of the developing nervous system: Changing views on their origins, diagnoses, and treatments.* New York: Alan R. Liss, Inc., 1988, pp. 51–67.

23. Altman D, Powers W, Perlman J, et al. Cerebral blood flow requirement for brain viability in newborn infants is lower than in adults. *Ann Neurol* 1988;24: 218–226.

24. Altman D, Perlman J, Volpe J, Powers W. Cerebral oxygen metabolism in newborns. *Pediatrics* 1993;92(1):99–104.

25. Volpe J, Herscovitch P, Perlmann J, Raichle M. Positron emission tomography in the newborn: Extensive impairment of regional cerebral blood flow with intraventricular hemorrhage and hemorrhagic intracerebral involvement. *Pediatrics* 1983;72(5):589–601.

26. Volpe J, Herscovitch P, Perlman J, et al. Positron emission tomography in the asphyxiated term newborn: Parasagittal impairment of cerebral blood flow. *Ann Neurol* 1985;17:287–296.

27. Perlman J, Altman D. Symmetric cerebral blood flow in newborns who have undergone successful extracorporeal membrane oxygenation. *Pediatrics* 1992; 89:235–239.

28. Medlock M, Cruse R, Winek S, et al. A 10-year experience with postpump chorea. *Ann Neurol* 1993;34:820–826.

29. Sokoloff L. Relationship among local functional activity, energy metabolism and blood flow in central nervous system. *Fed Proc* 1981;40:2311–2316.

30. Van Heertum R, Miller S, Mosesson R. SPECT brain imaging neurologic disease. *Radiol Clin North Amer* 1993;31(4):881–907.

31. Kung H, Ohmomo Y, Kung M-P. Current and future radiopharmaceuticals for brain imaging with single photon emission tomography. *Semin Nuc Med* 1990; 20(4):290–302.

32. Rowe C, Berkovic S, Austin M, et al. Patterns of postictal blood cerebral flow in temporal lobe epilepsy: Qualitative and quantitative analysis. *Neurology* 1991; 41:1096–1103.

33. Cordes M, Christe W, Henkes H, et al. Focal epilepsies: HM-PAO SPECT compared with CT, MR, and EEG. *J Comput Assist Tomog* 1990;14(3):402–409.

34. Uvebrandt P, Bjure J, Ekholm S. Brain single photon emission computed tomography (SPECT) in neuropediatrics. *Neuropediatrics* 1991;22:3–9.

35. Bogousslavsky J, Delaloye-Bischof A, Regli F, et al. Prolonged hypoperfusion and early stroke after transient ischemic attack. *Stroke* 1990;21:40.

36. Kanazawa O, Shirasaka Y, Hattori H, et al. Ictal 99mTc-HMPAo SPECT in alternating hemiplegia. *Pediatr Neurol* 1991;7:121–124.

37. Shahar E, Gilday D, Hwang P, et al. Pediatric cerebrovascular disease. Alterations of regional cerebral blood flow detected by TC 99m-HMPAO SPECT. *Arch Neurol* 1990;47:578–584.

38. Shirasaka Y, Ito M, Okuno T, et al. Sequential 123I-IMP-SPECT in acute infantile hemiplegia. *Pediatr Neurol* 1989;5:306–310.

39. Jagust W, Budinger T, Reed B. The diagnosis of dementia with single photon emission computed tomography. *Arch Neurol* 1987;44:258–262.

40. Black K, Hawkins R, Kim K, et al. Use of thallium-201 SPECT to quantitate malignancy grade of gliomas. *J Neurosurg* 1989;71:342–346.

41. Smith F, Gemmel H, Sharp P, et al. Technetium-99m HMPAO imaging in patients with basal ganglia disease. *Br J Radiol* 1988;61:914–920.

42. Nagel J, Ichise M, Holman B. The scintigraphic evaluation of Huntington's disease and other movement disorders using single photon emission tomography perfusion brain scans. *Semin Nuc Med* 1991;21:11–23.

43. Oertel W, Tatsch K, Schwartz J, et al. Decrease of D2 receptors indicated by 123I iodobenzamide single-photon emission tomography relates to neurological deficit in treated Wilson's disease. *Ann Neurol* 1992;32:743–748.

44. Brucke T, Podreka I, Angelberger P, et al. Imaging of dopamine D2 receptors with SPECT. Studies in patients with extrapyramidal disorders and under neuroleptic treatment. *J Cereb Blood Flow Metab* 1991;11:220–228.

45. Denays R, Van Pachterbeke T, Tondeur M, et al. Brain single photon emission computed tomography in neonates. *J Nuc Med* 1989;30(8):1337–1341.

46. Park C, Spitzer A, Desai H, et al. Brain SPECT in neonates following extracorporeal membrane oxygenation: Evaluation of technique and preliminary results. *J Nuc Med* 1992;33:1943–1948.

47. du Plessis A, Treves S, Hickey P, et al. Regional cerebral perfusion abnormalities after cardiac operations. *J Thorac Cardiovasc Surg* 1994;107:1036–1043.

48. Wong P, Barlow C, Hickey P, et al. Factors associated with choreoathetosis after cardiopulmonary bypass in children with congenital heart disease. *Circulation* 1992; 86 (suppl II):118–126.

49. Hagglund J, Aquilonius S, Eckernas S, et al. Dopamine receptor properties in Parkinson's disease and Huntington's chorea evaluated by positron emissions tomography using 11 C-methyl-spiperone. *Acta Neurol Scand* 1987; 85:87–94.

50. Eckelman W, Reba R, Rzeszotarski W, et al. External imaging of cerebral muscarinic acetylcholine receptors. *Science* 1984; 223:291–293.

51. Gemmel H, Evans N, Besson J, et al. Regional cerebral blood flow imaging: A quantitative comparison of technetium-99m-HMPAO SPECT with C1502 PET. *J Nuc Med* 1990; 31:1595–1600.

52. Sperling B, Lassen N. Hyperfixation of HMPAO in subacute ischemic stroke leading to spuriously high estimates of cerebral blood flow by SPECT. *Stroke* 1993; 24:192–194.

CHAPTER 11

Brain Monitoring Using Optical Imaging and Optical Spectroscopy

David A. Benaron

Introduction

Medical optical imaging (MOI) and spectroscopy (MOS) use light emitted into opaque tissues to determine the interior structure and chemical content.[1] These optical techniques have been developed in an attempt to prospectively identify impending brain injuries before they become irreversible, thus allowing injury to be avoided or minimized. Optical imaging and spectroscopy center around the simple idea that light passes through the body in small amounts and emerges bearing clues about tissues through which it passes. Images can be reconstructed from such data, and this is the basis of optical tomography. This chapter aims to explore state-of-the-art methods, hardware, and applications, beginning with an overview of the needs addressed by such optical techniques. For those readers with an interest in the physics of medical optics, this chapter contains an exploration of the technical basis of MOI and MOS; for those readers with a primary interest in clinical applications, this chapter concludes with sections on medical applications and a set of recently collected optical images. It is hoped that the reader will gain an appreciation of the power and breadth of optical tomography, as well as an understanding of the fundamental limitations and unsolved problems that need study as optical imaging crosses the threshold from laboratory curiosity to clinical tool.

Why Optical Imaging?

Current Imaging Methods Are Limited

Infants undergoing cardiac surgery, particularly those that must undergo prolonged bypass, face a not insignificant risk for perioperative brain injury. In addition, such injury is not predictable because two nearly identical infants may undergo similar corrective procedures, yet one infant may emerge with normal brain function, while the other emerges with major brain injuries leading to the development of cerebral palsy. How one avoids such injuries becomes a question, in part, of detection. In order to prevent death and minimize long-term injury, early diagnosis is essential for the detection of such problems *before* these injuries become irreversible.

Currently, no bedside imaging or monitoring methods excel at either detecting incipient injury or predicting neurologic outcome. Despite recent advances in noninvasive monitoring, such as in the development of chemically-weighted MRI,[2] most imaging techniques remain limited in at least one of four fundamental ways:

Invasive

Imaging techniques often require exposure to potentially noxious substances and thus involve a degree of risk that increases with exposure. CT scanners, which emit carcinogenic ionizing radiation, cannot be used in a continuous fashion, thus preventing their use as operating room or ICU monitors; Positron Emission Tomography (PET) scans require intravenous injection of radiation emitters; prolonged ultrasound exposure is suspected of causing at least some degree of thermal or structural cellular injury, particularly in developing tissues. Other monitoring methods require indwelling catheters that are ports of entry for debilitating or lethal infections or require the taking of blood, which is not only painful but can be dangerous to some, such as premature infants who may have a total circulating blood volume as small as 40 to 160 mL and can be placed into shock by the loss of as little as 10 mL of blood.

Not portable

Children undergoing or recovering from surgery, as any critically ill patients, cannot be easily transported because such movement may adversely affect their care. Many established techniques, such as MRI, CT, and PET, on the other hand, are not portable and thus may not be available in the very clinical situations for which such imaging information is crucial. Further, the more likely a patient is to require a scan, the more likely it is that the patient will be unable to tolerate transport to an imaging facility.

Noncontinuous

Critically ill people tend to have illnesses that are actively changing processes. Thus, an intermittent test (e.g., ultrasound exam or blood test) may miss the early signs of physiologic changes that herald disaster, preventing intervention that could interrupt the process and prevent the problem from becoming more serious or prevent an injury from becoming irreversible. This is particularly important in the intensive care unit and the operating room, places in which dramatic changes can be expected in patient stability, such that monitoring information and images are vitally needed. However, such instability and the need for ongoing care may preclude transfer of the patient to an imaging facility.

Function not measured

Patient death or brain injury often occurs due to problems that have to do with tissue *function*, such as a lack of oxygen to a portion of the brain, rather than with a physical problem that would be more likely to show up on an imaging scan. While the long-term results of such injury (e.g., brain atrophy secondary to stroke or brain hemorrhage secondary to bleeding from injured blood vessels) can be relatively easy to detect using conventional tests, which often image these structural changes quite well, such information may come too late to prevent the primary injury from occurring in the first place. Most imaging technologies have been designed to measure a static physical structure rather than cellular state so that, while conventional images may reflect what is physically there, these images reveal nothing about the *functioning* of the tissue. Computed x-ray tomography (CT), for example, often does not distinguish between healthy or dying tissues, even though such information may be crucial to accurate diagnosis and effective medical treatment. By the time a brain lesion is visible by CT, the damage is already irreversibly far advanced. The perioperative management of children undergoing surgery, as well as the management of patients with conditions such as stroke, Alzheimer's syndrome, hypoxic brain injury, or myocardial infarction, could thus benefit from the availability of images of such functional information that could allow early intervention.

Optical Imaging May Overcome These Limitations

MOI and MOS use light emitted into scattering media, such as human tissue, to determine interior structure and chemical content; both methods have broad application to the field of medicine. These emerging techniques have application to the continuous, noninvasive bedside or operating room monitoring of tissue structure, oxygenation, blood flow, and metabolite concentration. Optical techniques rely upon the facts that variations in the concentration of light-absorbing oxygen-carrying pigments produce proportional changes in the way these proteins absorb light and that such variations in concentration, as well as variations in tissue structure, affect the path of light through tissue. Near-infrared (NIR) MOS has already been shown to be a relatively safe form of nonionizing radiation that functions well as a medical probe.[3-15] Red and near-infrared light pass easily through structures such as the skull,[4,5] penetrate deeply into many tissues such as the brain and breast,[6–8] and are well tolerated in large doses.[9] Due to the high degree of light scattering in tissue, optical images formed *in vivo* using simple transmission of light have been poor. Similarly, optical concentration estimates have been rendered nonquantitative by long, irregular photon paths. However, using NIR light, variations in light absorbance and scattering at different wavelengths can be used to deduce the concentration of physiologic intermediates of deep tissues such as the brain (provided that the distance light has traveled though the tissue between emission and detection is known) and to deduce tissue structure (provided that the path of the light through the tissue is known).

The application of continuous-wave radiation to the imaging of human heart using light in 1971 and transcerebral spectroscopic quantification was first reported by Jöbsis in 1977.[3] In a period of time less than twenty years since this report, the measurement of human brain blood flow and oxygenation by Edwards, Delpy et al.[16] the noninvasive detection and classification of breast tissues and tumors based upon scattering and absorbance properties in an optical biopsy system by Chance et al.,[17] the imaging of animal bodies and human brain by our laboratory,[18,19] and a number of other experiments have suggested that optical imaging and spectroscopy are nearing clinical application. In fact, the commercial availability of several near-infrared cerebral monitors and their use in clinical investigation (e.g., studies of cerebral metabolism during administration of neuroprotective agents such as allopurinol,[20] designed to protect the brain from injury during lack of oxygen, or studies of the effect of vasoactive compounds on brain blood volume),[21,22] demonstrate that, in at least some cases, these technologies are already being applied. Given the potential of light-based technologies to reduce the invasiveness of medical care, to result in better treatments at reduced cost, and to monitor the effectiveness of medical therapies, the potential for the contribution of optical tomography to health care is believed to be great.

The Physics of Optical Monitoring

This section reviews the physics of photon travel through tissue. Those readers with a primary interest in the medical applications of optical imaging and spectroscopy may choose to skip to Medical Optical Spectroscopy (MOS), page 161.

The Problem of Scattering

Photon travel through tissue is not linear due to scattering events caused by interaction with tissue components, most likely the mitochondria. It is these scattering events that cause light passing through tissue to emerge in a diffuse glow, rather than to emerge showing clear outlines of internal structures such as bone. Scattering causes photons to take lengthy, highly irregular paths through tissue, and many photons travel merely a few millimeters into tissue before scattering. Multiple scattering events, therefore, occur for virtually all photons propagating through tissue, producing a wide range in paths taken by photons and in the time required for different photons to traverse tissue. Thus most photons passing through tissue have randomly scattered hundreds or thousands of times before emerging to be detected. In fact, the physical equations that best describe the behavior of photons in tissue are most closely related to equations that describe the diffusion of particles in liquid or the diffusion of heat. As shall be discussed, photon path lengths also are affected by local absorbance and scattering, so that such paths are complex and highly difficult to predict.

Measuring Optical Path

In the 1980s, it was suggested that the path taken by each photon could be measured using the time required for the photon to traverse the tissue and that this information could be used to improve spectroscopic measures or to form an image of the interior of the scattering object. However, to measure the length of the path light travels, called the *optical path length*, emitted light must contain a feature allowing discrimination of path of travel. The two common methods for path measurement, developed more fully over the past decade, are temporal amplitude-modulation (frequency-based) and pulsed source photon counting (time-based). A third method based upon taking samples at multiple points in space (spatial-array methods) may also be effective at achieving the same goals without actually measuring photon path length directly. These methods for measuring optical path are discussed.

Frequency-based methods

Frequency-based devices estimate path length based upon the time-shift between emission and detection of a modulated optical source, as compared to a reference that has not passed though the subject of measurement. Such systems, when using a single frequency, yield a mean path length but not the distribution of all path lengths taken.[18] Use of multiple frequencies of modulation allows significantly more information to be extracted. The first portable frequency-based optical path-measuring device for tissue was developed by Chance[6] at the University of Pennsylvania and used to measure optical path in living infants.[12] Many groups are now using such systems, e.g., Gratton et al. at the University of Illinois, Urbana; Tromberg et al. at the University of California, Irvine, Beckman Laser Center; Ferrari et al. in Italy; and others.

Time-based methods

The second type of path-measuring method is time-resolved photon counting. The initial measurements of path in tissue used a time-based method and were made using large, immobile ultrashort laser systems and detection optics in model systems.[7,23] Early measurements in humans were made shortly thereafter on expired infants.[10] The first portable version of a time-based system, capable of being taken out of the laboratory and placed at the bedside, was developed by our laboratory at Stanford University in 1990.[24] This device, called a TOFAscope, for time-of-flight and absorbance scope, uses pulsed diode lasers as a light source. The TOFA device measures a time delay for each photon detected, in contrast to phase-shift devices that measure ensemble averages. The Stanford device remains the only existing portable time-resolved photon-counting device with IRB approval in the U.S. for clinical imaging testing. Descriptions of the operation of this device have appeared elsewhere.[18,19] Fortunately, due to the decreasing cost of time-resolved optics, other groups are expected to introduce similar devices soon.

Initially, although there was some disagreement as to whether frequency- and time-domain measures were equivalent, elegant theoretical analyses by Arridge et al.[25] and Sevick et al.[26,27] have shown that the methods are indeed comparable. Recent measurements by our laboratory have confirmed that the average path lengths measured by each method are equivalent.[28] Both time-resolved and frequency-resolved techniques have been shown to be useful path-sensitive approaches in image reconstruction and in subsurface object detection, and both approaches yield theoretically equivalent data related by Fourier-transform.[25,29,30]

Spatial-array methods

A third method to help assess the effects of scattering looks at differences in the steady-state diffusion of light to narrowly-separated points in space. This method can be used to measure the absorbance and scattering properties of tissue using optical fibers placed on the surface of the object. So far, this data appears to yield valid measurements but has not yet been successfully used to produce data for imaging.

Optical Path Varies Over Space

Before optical path length measurement was practical, the inherent variability in optical path length was not well appreciated. Once the technology became available to conveniently measure optical path length, we and many other groups commenced study of the range and variability of such path lengths in models, animals, and humans. Disagreement as to the stability and the predictability of these path lengths has lingered for several years. However, it is now becoming clear that path length is in no manner a constant. It has been well documented that there are static variations between tissues, with the only remaining uncertainty being the degree of this variability. To this end, we present data below as to the degree of this variability. Furthermore, it had been known that path can be dynamically variable, and we now present new data to show that such variability can be very large.

We conclude that optical measurements appear to need optical path corrections to be valid.

Several years ago we investigated the magnitude and variability in transcranial optical path length *in vivo*. We studied transcranial optical path length in 34 infants, aged 1 day to 3 years, using phase-modulated spectroscopy at 754 nm and 816 nm.[12] Optical transcranial path lengths (mean ± SE) were 8.58 ± 0.88 cm, 11.13 ± 0.85 cm, and 11.34 ± 0.93 cm at 754 nm; and 8.76 ± 0.90 cm, 11.20 ± 0.79 cm, and 11.13 ± 0.91 cm at 816 nm, using emitter-detector separations of 1.8, 2.5, and 3.0 cm, respectively. Note that the distance light travels through the head is several times the distance that the emitter and detector are separated. Delpy et al. coined the term "differential path length factor" (DPF) to describe this increase in the apparent distance of photon travel compared to the linear separation of the emitter and detector.

Significantly, the ratio of two path lengths at different wavelengths of the light (a measure of wavelength independence) was within 20% of unity for only 2/3 of infants and ranged from 0.5 to 3.2 in the remaining patients, confirming that path is not fully independent of wavelength.[28,31] The dependence of path upon wavelength makes sense because a highly absorbed wavelength of light would have few far-traveling highly scattered photons surviving to reach the detector, while a poorly absorbed wavelength would have many far-traveling photons surviving to be detected. The net effect is that higher absorbance at any wavelength should lead to a shorter net path. In addition, the scattering of light by small particles decreases with increasing wavelength, a process similar to the phenomenon that produces a uniform, highly scattered blue-enriched sky (the blue light being extracted from the sunlight traveling directly from the sun and reaching us after scattering) as well as a horizon at sunset that is depleted of blue light, leaving a red-enriched sunset.

Unfortunately, path length is not accurately predictable. We could not account for all variability in optical path length using the parameters we recorded or by using the error of measurement. The magnitude of the variability in path length has been similar when measured by different groups. Delpy et al. reported brain DPF as 3.85 ± 0.57 (mean) S.D. for the brain of living infants[32] and 4.39 ± 0.28 for the brain of postmortem infants.[10] Cranial DPF for living infants would then be expected to fall between 2.73 and 4.99 for 95% of all living infants tested, and these values are strikingly similar to the DPFs we measured using phase-shift technologies (4.81 at 1.8 cm, 4.47 at 2.5 cm, and 3.75 at 3.0 cm).

It is interesting to speculate on the origins of such variability of path. Possible sources of local variability in optical tissue path length in our study include the known variations in the optical characteristics among the brains of different infants,[33] the local gross topological irregularity of the convoluted brain surface, and the changes in path length that occur during changes in pigment concentration. Delpy and colleagues report that variability in

DPF decreases as emitter-detector spacing increases, particularly over 5 cm, presumably reflecting a lessening of the influence of local irregularities in brain structure at the larger emitter-detector separations. However, persistent variability in DPF was found even at wide emitter-detector separations. Other studies confirm that optical path length L varies over space. Optical path length varies with spatial variation in tissue structure, a fact which can be an advantage when used to form images of phantoms and tissue.[9,18,24,34] Values for this DPF also vary considerably from tissue to tissue (for example, muscle versus brain, infant brain versus adult brain, or tumors versus normal tissue).

Optical Path Varies Over Time

Not only is path length variable between tissues and over space, but path length is also dynamic and varies over time. This conclusion follows logically from consideration that absorption affects photons unequally. Photons that travel the farthest through the tissue are most likely to be extinguished by an absorber. When the concentration of an absorber increases—as occurs when the saturation of hemoglobin with oxygen changes—the longer traveling photons are preferentially absorbed, thus lowering, on average, the length of path of travel of the surviving transmitted photons. This type of analysis led Chance to suggest that path would vary with effective absorbance and thus with the oxygenation state, an observation we later proved in multiple clinical and laboratory studies.[31,35] In fact, a ratio of optical transcranial path lengths taken at different wavelengths of light changed by as much as 10% during the course of experimental variations in cerebral oxygenation.

To more fully study the dynamic variability of path length, we used our TOFAscope to measure the magnitude of dynamic changes in optical path length occurring under several different circumstances.[35] We recorded in subjects the change in path length over time, which occurred both during manipulation and spontaneously. To measure changes in path length induced by changes in position of the body (which primarily alters venous blood volume), the TOFAscope was placed upon an adult foot that was alternately raised and lowered while absorbance and path length were recorded. Mean optical path changed over 30% during these maneuvers, with the primary effect being the loss of far-traveling photons as blood volume increased. Next, cerebral (transcranial) optical path length was monitored during a set of leg lifts that increased cerebral blood volume (CBV). In these experiments, changes in optical path length approached 10%. Finally, we recorded the magnitude of changes in cerebral optical path length occurring spontaneously over time. Over minutes to hours, path length naturally varied by 5% or more. We suspect this variation is secondary to natural fluctuations in CBV and blood oxygenation. These data clearly show that path not only varies from subject to subject, but it also varies over time in a single subject, even in the absence of an intervention.

Medical Optical Spectroscopy (MOS)

Applying Path Correction to Optical Spectroscopy

As with all forms of conventional optical oximetry, quantitative measurement of pigments such as hemoglobin *in vitro* using path-resolved NIRS is based upon the principle that changes in the absorbance of light (DA) are related to changes in concentration (DC). In the simplest, nonscattering conditions, this relationship is given by Beer's Law ($A = eCL$), where L is the distance light has traveled through the medium (called the optical path length) and e is a constant called the extinction coefficient.[10,36] *In vivo*, however, Beer's Law is inaccurate and inappropriate due to additional light losses caused by light scattering, though it serves as a starting point for such discussions. Of note, the inaccuracies from the use of Beer's Law can be reduced when changes in concentration, rather than absolute concentration, are measured.

In theory, near-infrared spectroscopy (NIRS) techniques such as niroscopy[1-12] and regional cerebral spectroscopy[37] allow quantification of changes in concentration of nearly any substance in the body that absorbs light, though current work has focused upon oxygen-carrying pigments, glucose, lipids, and cholesterol. Most current oximetry techniques use changes in absorbance to determine concentration. Temporal variations in absorbance, caused by changes in the optical spectrum of certain proteins (e.g., hemoglobin, myoglobin, mitochondrial cytochrome aa3, cytosolic cytochrome oxidase, and other copper- or iron-containing proteins) as the partial pressure of oxygen varies, have been used to estimate changes in oxygenation in the extremities,[38,39] heart,[40] and brain[3,37,41] as well as to measure local blood volume and flow.[42-44] Estimates can be quantitative when the distance light travels through the tissue is known.[11,31,45]

Oxygen-sensitive NIRS differs from pulse oximetry in that NIRS can be used to independently measure oxygenation in the arteries, veins, and small blood vessels via hemoglobin spectroscopy, to measure oxygen sufficiency within the cell via cytosolic and/or mitochondrial cytochrome spectroscopy, or both. Sensitivity to oxygen-carrying pigments gives NIRS techniques the potential to measure hemoglobin oxygen saturation (HbO$_2$%), cellular and mitochondrial cytochrome aa3 oxygenation state (CytO$_2$), cerebral blood flow (CBF), and cerebral blood volume (CBV). Therefore, NIRS holds promise for early warning and monitoring systems for impending and existing hypoxic injuries, particularly for areas such as the brain.[11,42,43,46-49]

Optical Path in Brain Oxygenation Calculations

The variability of path length has implications for the study of cerebral oxygenation, as optical path would therefore be expected to change radically with changes in blood pressure or during maneuvers such as starting or stopping a bypass pump. This problem could lead to serious errors, either of over- or under-estimation of cerebral oxygenation or blood flow during heart surgery, if the measuring device is not path-corrected. In fact, several optical investigational devices have been found to be very sensitive to such errors during ischemic disease. For example, one will report an apparent rise in oxygenation during severe hypovolemic hypoxia, when the brain is, in reality, acutely hypoxic. Thus, one must use caution in interpreting the results of a device that assumes a constant path. As optical path length varies both among static tissues and dynamically with tissue changes, it is clear that path length cannot be considered a constant. There is both a dynamic and static component to the variability of optical path length. Such variability will necessarily place limits upon the maximum accuracy that can be achieved during deep tissue imaging or spectroscopy, unless an ongoing, dynamic assessment of optical path length is made.

The origins of such errors can be appreciated by review of the equations for optical assessment of oxygenation presented above. While it is well known that light is absorbed by tissue and is a measurable variable, quantitative NIRS techniques have, in the past, been based upon assumptions that the distance light travels through tissue, called the optical path length (L), is constant among subjects and independent of the wavelength of light used. Concentration, or changes in concentration, could then be determined from measurements at several wavelengths by solving multiple equations for multiple unknowns. A constant optical path length cancels out in ratios of concentrations, such as when calculating percentage hemoglobin saturation via pulse oximetry.[36] Similarly, other NIRS methods, such as those used in standard devices available in Europe or the U.S. (Hammamatsu NIR infant monitor or Vander Corporation NIROScope, Somanetics Invios, Critikon NIR monitor), rely upon a predicted value for L, estimated *a priori* from either animal models,[7] human experiment, or the geometry of the emitter and detector.[23] Errors regarding the estimated value of L or the stability of L can result in inaccuracies in estimates of absolute pigment concentration or of changes in pigment concentration.

The following example illustrates the impact that static variability of path has upon the accuracy of oxygenation calculations.[35] Substituting a two-fold difference between optical paths at different wavelengths (a range observed in about 10% of the infants studied) in equations for the determination of saturation from optical measurements could result in an over- or underestimate of the relative concentration of one of the hemoglobin pigments by two-fold. With an estimated venous blood hemoglobin saturation of 66%, a two-fold error could change measured saturation to as low as 50% or as high as 80%. Because these lower- and upper-limit saturations would require different clinical responses, pigment concentration determinations, which use algorithms based upon assumed optical path lengths, may be of limited value. Thus, variability in optical path length may give rise to considerable error in the calculation of cerebral oxygenation in some infants if both absorbance and path length are not contemporaneously measured at each wavelength.

These observations raise questions about the accuracy of quantitative near-infrared spectroscopy methods based upon assumed or estimated optical path lengths. Accurate quantitative measurements in clinical use may require concurrent measurement of both absorbance and optical path length at each wavelength. The current difficulty of performing quantitative NIRS measurements may be related, at least in part, to uncorrected path errors in the method currently used to determine concentration.

Measurement of Cerebral Oxygenation Incorporating the Static Variability of Path Length

We had earlier shown that, through the use of a single, measured optical path length, we could estimate the oxygenation of the cerebral blood in infants undergoing cardiac surgery.[31,45] However, these measurements are at single points in time. Combining continuous path length and absorbance measures have allowed estimates of changes in cerebral oxygenation. Several years of experience with these types of values have been published recently.[45]

Measurement of Cerebral Oxygenation Using Dynamic Variability of Path Length

Given that optical path length varies over time, we set out to test whether taking into account the dynamic variability of optical path length would result in additional information being calculable. We measured transcranial cerebral optical path and absorbance using a dynamically-sensitive TOFA-scope that records absorbance and path length in 30 ms time slices. Path and absorbance were recorded from normal test subjects and from an infant receiving ECMO support (heart/lung bypass) who was monitored for central venous oxygenation using indwelling jugular catheters as part of routine care. We then estimated central venous and arterial saturation using the TOFA data by changing blood volume through positional interventions. The estimates, in many but not all instances, fell near the estimated normal or the measured jugular central venous values. A typical table of calculated values is shown (Table 11–1). The spontaneous path length variability in the cranium was also measured using the TOFA path-determining experiment described above. Again, we were able to estimate central venous saturation using TOFA. Spontaneous variation in path has been noted under several circumstances. This is important as a variable path length source can be localized and imaged, as we have done, and has been reported by Kang.[43]

While quantitative NIRS has been an elusive goal when optical path length is assumed but not measured, the combination of path length and absorbance measurements has allowed quantification. This provides further evidence that there is value in measuring, and not estimating, optical path length at each NIRS wavelength used. Application of such technology to patient care may facilitate the quantitative measurement of oxygenation in organs not currently accessible to study, potentially allowing early warning of

TABLE 11–1.

Oxygen saturation in the brain measured noninvasively in twelve test subjects using time-resolved path correction. Values are near expected ranges, based upon estimates of contributions of arterial, capillary, and venous phases. The equations can, at times, yield inaccurate measures (above 100%, for example) due to patient movement or inaccurate estimates of path length, but such values can be minimized using signal averaging. The lowest value measured (29%) was for an infant with perinatal depression who was actively seizing at the time of measurement and who required ECMO bypass therapy.

Patient Number	Venous Saturation (S_vO_2)
1	78%
2	67%
3	103%
4	70%
5	72%
6	76%
7	60%
8	65%
9	66%
10	83%
11	80%
12	29%

impending or existing ischemic-hypoxic injury, and thus holds exciting clinical potential.[50] Once problems related to quantification have been solved, possible clinical forms for such a device include an ultrasound-like probe that would yield noninvasive saturation images for such tests as noninvasive brain oximetry and noninvasive heart catheterizations that produce images of ventricular and muscle wall oxygenation and maternal transabdominal fetal saturation monitors. Currently, several groups are introducing simultaneous real-time continuous path measurements with their absorbance measurements.

Path-Independent Calculation of Oxygenation

More recently, absorbance has been directly estimated, independent of mean path length and scattering, using time-resolved and frequency-resolved techniques. Devices based upon these direct estimations are expected to be more accurate than conventional oximetry devices. The equations upon which these devices are based are derived from solutions to equations that model the travel of photons through tissue as a diffusion process. The result is absolute absorbance, m_a, in units of absorbance events per centimeter and can be substituted directly into multiparameter analyses for the determination of hemoglobin oxygenation or the oxygenation of other substances in the blood. This use of the diffusion equation means that Beer's Law is no longer being used for absorbance determinations; instead, these values are being derived from a more accurate physical law. The ability to avoid Beer's Law eliminates many inaccuracies in these calculations.

Absolute absorbance measurements have now been used in several laboratories to determine the oxygenation of muscle during exercise in various states of health, such as in normal subjects during exercise, in normal subjects during cuff ischemia (a model for hypoxic injury), in subjects with vascular disease, and in subjects with mitochondrial disorders (Figure 11–1).[51–54] A device with this capability could also be applied to the head for cerebral monitoring, and such a project is in progress at several sites, including at our laboratory. This approach should allow local or regional monitoring of cortical oxygenation.

Once absorbance and scattering have been separated, determination of a scattering-free absorbance measure at 'n' wavelengths then allows the determination of the concentration of up to 'n' substances. Gratton has recently used such measures to monitor absolute oxygenation in the arm and has suggested that even local glucose concentration may be followed using this technique. We have used similar determinations in our time-resolved optical imaging device, described below, to produce images of oxygenation. Using such techniques, monitors are now being designed and tested for clinical use. Such devices would be likely to achieve clinical application within 3 to 5 years.

Oxygenation Measures Alone May Not
Be Sufficient for Brain Monitoring

There are several reasons, however, that even a good oxygenation monitor will need to do more than simply monitor oxygenation.

Brain injury multifactorial

There are many causes of brain injury, and the appearance of the various measured parameters (oxygenation, scattering) may be very different at different stages of disease. For example, even if an episode of hypoxia has resolved, the tissue may be committed to a cell death pathway. Thus, while an operating room monitor to warn of impending injury may be able to rely upon oxygenation as an early sign of brain injury, the same device may fail in a newborn, asphyxiated infant in whom the oxygenation has recovered but cell death is imminent. On the other hand, the signal of scattering may be expected to change with the failure of cellular water and ion transport or changes in the stored calcium status of the cells. Therefore, a scattering monitor may be more relevant in later stages of brain injury. Further, injury may be the result of small cumulative insults, such that no one particular injury is large enough to be detectable using changes in oxygenation, yet the sum total injury over time is great. Such a cumulative loss of neurons, as a

A

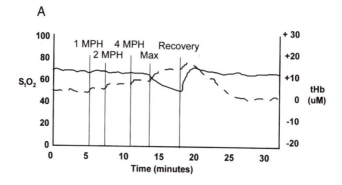

B

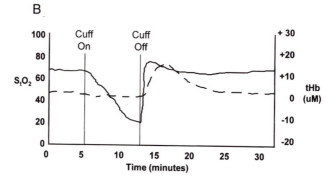

FIGURE 11–1. Optical measurement of muscle hemoglobin oxygenation (solid line) and blood volume (dashed line) in four subjects. (A) In a normal subject, tissue blood volume and flow increase with exercise, and muscle deoxygenation occurs late and only with maximal exercise. Normal, resting hemoglobin oxygenation, measured optically at the capillaries, is about 70%. (B) In cuff ischemia, a model for tissue hypoxia, the blood volume remains constant during vascular occlusion, while the oxygenation drops. After release of the occlusion, there is an overshoot of blood flow during the recovery phase. (C) In a subject with peripheral vascular disease, the oxygenation at baseline is lower than normal. Further, with exercise, there is a failure to increase blood flow, and there is an early decline in tissue oxygenation. (D) In a subject with a mitochondrial disorder, there is a normal increase in blood volume and blood flow with exercise. However, as the oxygen cannot be effectively extracted by the mitochondria, the tissue oxygenation rises instead of falling. Graphs are modified from several sources and are schematic representations of the original data.

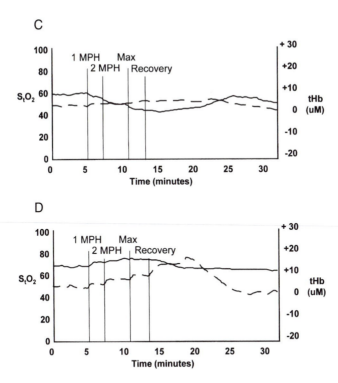

FIGURE 11–1. *(continued)*

result of many small insults over a long period of time, may be detectable using a change in the scattering of the tissue. Alternatively, long-term injury may not require a portable monitor and may also be detectable using chemically-weighted MRS (magnetic resonance spectroscopy), which can image the concentration of, for example, components of intact neurons or markers of neuronal injury, such as choline and N-acetyl-aspartate.

Imaging may be important in determining response to hypoxia

A second limitation is that a nonimaged signal may not be very useful. For example, the average brain oxygenation would be the same if (a) a small region of the brain were to be severely hypoxic, such as during an acute arterial obstruction, or (b) the brain oxygenation of the entire brain dropped in general by a small amount, such as during a drop in cardiac output (Figure 11–2). Although the first situation is an emergency, requiring immediate intervention in order to prevent irreversible brain injury, the second is not. Further, treatment in the two cases would be very different. Thus, imaging may be essential in determining the proper course of medical treatment of an observed oxygenation change.

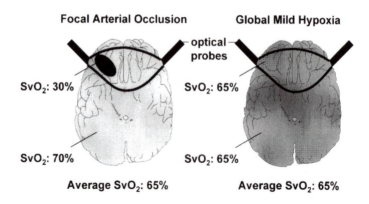

Focal Arterial Occlusion   **Global Mild Hypoxia**

optical probes

SvO$_2$: 30%   SvO$_2$: 65%

SvO$_2$: 70%   SvO$_2$: 65%

Average SvO$_2$: 65%   **Average SvO$_2$: 65%**

FIGURE 11-2. Global v. regional oxygenation measures. A measurement of cerebral oxygenation may need to be in the form of an image in order to provide useful information. A focal, acute arterial occlusion (left), as occurs during an embolic event, and a slight but generalized drop in oxygenation (right), as occurs during a drop in cardiac output, both yield a similar drop in overall brain oxygenation figures. However, each requires a different clinical response; the former constitutes a medical emergency while the latter does not.

Medical Optical Imaging (MOI)

Early Attempts at Optical Imaging

As noted above, imaging may be essential in allowing the physician to determine the proper response to impending or existing brain injury.

Although the power to make good optical tomographic images is only now becoming a reality, light has long been used as a diagnostic imaging tool *in vivo.* Just as dairy farmers used light to candle eggs, light has also been used to transilluminate the body. Curling, an English physician, reported the use of a flare lantern to transilluminate the scrotum of his patients to screen for tumors in 1843.[55] This technique culminated over a century later with the development of a visible light system for detecting breast tumors, known as diaphanography. Unfortunately, this device fell short of its promise, merely generating shadowgrams of superficial structures such as veins while deep structures such as tumors remained lost in a diffuse background glow. These devices failed because they did not take into account the path of photon travel.

Time-resolved optical methods, in which photon transit time affects the image, were first suggested in 1971.[56] Optical imaging of tissue has been difficult to achieve because light is strongly scattered by tissue, producing a wide range in the paths taken by, and the time required for, photons to traverse the tissue. As opposed to conventional radiological methods in which photon travel is linear, scattering produces highly irregular photon paths that degrade image quality, much as detail is lost with distance in a fog. Scattering is also the major attenuator of transmitted photon intensity in tissue.[57] The average photon travels less than 10 mm into tissue before scattering,[58] and multiple scattering events occur for virtually all photons propagating through tissue[59–62] Simple models for this diffusive behavior resemble molecular diffusion equations, while more accurate treatments consider that light scattering has a forward-weighted anisotropy.[58]

Object and Structure Detection

The first step before imaging was to demonstrate that objects are indeed detectable. In order to do this, an optical signal must be identified that indicates when objects are buried in scattering tissue. In some cases, the presence or absence of an object can be optically determined by a characteristic spectral signature or by changes in the path of travel of light through the tissue. For example, a brain hemorrhage may cause the path of light through the hemorrhage to be long, due to the long route around the hemorrhage taken by nonabsorbed photons, or the hemorrhage may be detectable on the basis of the high absorption alone. This detection of hematoma can be sensitive when measurements on one side of the head are compared to measurements taken on the other.

In critically ill infants, illnesses producing maldistributions of heme in the brain have been studied for detectability. After Human Studies Commission approval and parental informed consent were obtained, we studied infants with intraventricular hemorrhage, measuring at multiple skull locations, to see if the presence of bleeding can be detected. Using a comparison of path length on one side of the head versus that on the contralateral side, we found that superficial bleeding (subdural hematomas, cephalohematomas) could be easily identified, and some instances of intraventricular bleeding are detectable as well.[19] Chance, using a path-dependent method in the frequency-domain, found that as little as 50 mL of blood in brain can be detected using his phase system[33] and that by using absorbance alone, with no additional path measurement, hemorrhage in adults can be reliably detected postoperatively.[63]

A clinical device based upon a path length dependent algorithm could take the form of a continuous bedside monitor for a premature infant that displays changes in the structural appearance of the brain, sounding an alarm when a difference over time, such as the appearance of a hemorrhage, is detected. With regard to changes in travel time due to the presence of an object, we defined a detection algorithm to determine the minimal detectable object (MDO). MDO is the smallest object that can be identified as being present with 95% confidence.[64] Based upon model data, TOFA appears to allow detection of solid, 100% absorbing objects as small as an MDO of 3 to 5 mm in diameter in the neonatal brain. This now appears to be confirmed in clinical studies.[65-67]

Imaging of Structure

Once it was clear that path could be used to detect objects, we set out to attempt imaging of structure in scattering media. We developed a laboratory time-of-flight and absorbance (TOFA) laser imaging system. Using power well within safe FDA-established guidelines, we produced MOI images of objects buried within scattering media,[24] generated a whole-body image of an animal, locating major organs and intestinal gas in a rat,[18] imaged hemorrhage in neonatal brain pathology samples,[62] and now have created images of brain structure and oxygenation in newborn infants.[65,66]

The initial laboratory device required measurement by hand at each point of interest. Ultimate use as a clinical tool would require conversion to an automated scanning device, similar in basic arrangement to CT scanning. Therefore, our laboratory device was first converted into a rotational tomographic imaging device.[67] Objects to be imaged were placed upon a 10-cm diameter imaging stage and rotated until imaged. In this method, an object to be scanned is rotated upon a movable rotational stage, while the detector is moved around the object using a second stage that revolves around the first. Pairs of emitter-detector measurements are then made according to a computer-determined pattern. We then made TOFA measurements from up to 10,000 measurement pairs or emitter/detector locations. Data was collected and stored on disk, and images were reconstructed using a variety of methods, including simple back-projection, Radon transforms, and, in the manner of Arridge et al., a recursive transform/inverse transform algorithm.[68,69]

As an example, an image of a 10-cm cylinder containing a single 2-cm diameter rod showed that the center of the rod image was located within 1 mm of the rod's true central location in the cylinder, while the size of the rod in the image was 22 mm. Thus, large, singular fluid collections and clots should be able to be unambiguously detected. An image, taken from a 2-D model containing 4 1-cm nonscattering nonabsorbing cubes placed into a highly scattering nonabsorbing background, showed central cube location within a few mm of their actual location but with some distortion in the shape of the cubes.[67] This data suggested that the imaging of multiple objects was possible, though with some object distortion.

To utilize the device in a clinical setting, a fiber optic headband was constructed. This headband, consisting of a soft rubber backing and a web of fiber optic leads, allowed light to enter the infant's head from all sides, as needed, without the need for mechanical translation (Figure 11–3).[65,66] The complete device is about the size of a standard ultrasound cart. Tomographic reconstruction algorithms performed in the on-board computer

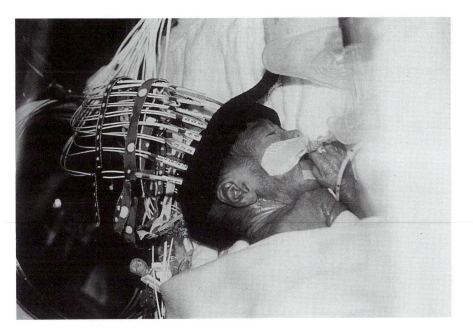

FIGURE 11–3. A time-resolved optical imaging headband in place on an infant. Low-level light enters through the optical fibers and is measured at various points around the head. The data is collected and assembled into an image, much as is done in CT.

were also further developed and refined to allow calculation of an image in a few seconds or minutes. After obtaining Human Studies Commission approval and parental informed consent, infants at high risk for structural disease (such as bleeding) were studied using optical methods. To be included, subjects must have had an additional standard imaging study within 24 hours of the optical scan. The staff performing the optical scans and reading the optical scan results were blinded to the results of the ultrasound examinations. We found that the optical image prediction of the presence and location of bleeding agreed with the formal reading of the ultrasound examinations in 8 out of 9 cases. As there is no gold standard for distribution of oxygenation, the oxygenation images had no such confirming comparison performed.

Several sample images are shown. Infant G.C. had a grade II right-sided intraventricular hemorrhage (IVH), and the corresponding optical image is shown (Figure 11–4A). The localization of the clot to the right side of the brain can be seen from the optical scan. Compare this image to the optical image obtained from infant B.S., who had a left-sided grade III hemorrhage filling much of the left ventricle (Figure 11–4B). Last, compare the image of

A

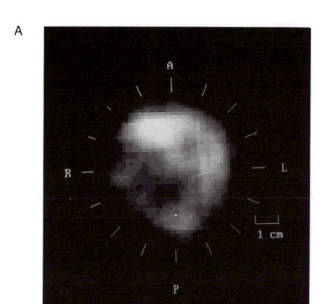

B

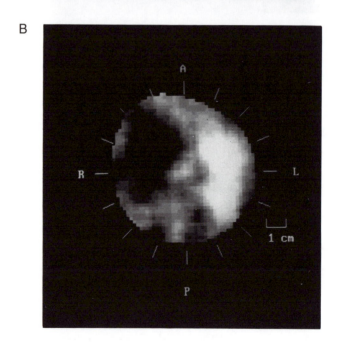

FIGURE 11–4. Optical images of neonates. (A) An
image of a right-sided grade II unilateral intraventricular hemorrhage (white region, upper left of image).
(B) Optical image of a left-sided grade III intraventricular hemorrhage (white region, right side of image).
The intensity of this lesion decreased over two weeks
in the optical scan, while it remained clearly present
in the ultrasound image over the same time period,
raising the possibility that bleeding can also be dated

C

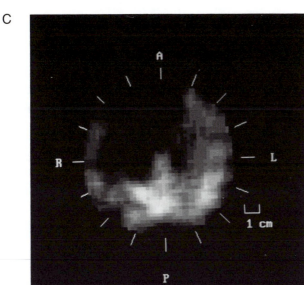

D

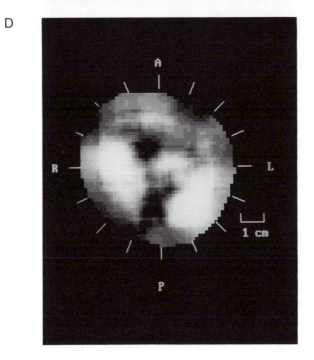

FIGURE 11–4 continued. using optical imaging as an adjunct to ultrasound. (C) Optical image of an infant without intracranial bleeding. No dense white regions are noted, as compared to the images shown in A and B. (D) An optical image of the distribution of oxygenation in a living infant. There is a bilateral symmetry, with darker areas having a relatively lower oxygenation. The clinical significance of such images is not known.

infant B.B., who had no IVH and shows no such highlighted areas on the optical scan (Figure 11–4C).

Using updated imaging algorithms, our images can now be processed by a desktop computer in under two minutes once the data is collected. In theory, a fast version of the program is able to process the images in under 10 seconds. Such images show both substantial distortion of structure and significant error in estimation of absorbance and scattering characteristics, likely a result of imaging algorithms assuming additivity of the measured phenomena. However, images are recognizable and agree with ultrasound examinations as to the presence or absence of bleeding. A fiber optic headband could have immediate application in the monitoring of infants on heart-lung bypass such as ECMO, in which serial ultrasound examinations are performed to detect bleeding. However, such scans are intermittent and may miss the onset of life-threatening intracranial bleeding. Chance,[70] Gratton,[71,72] and others have suggested that similar imaging results can be obtained with phased arrays of light-emitting diodes operating in the frequency domain.

Imaging of Function

The strength of optical techniques comes from the ability to separate absorbance and scattering and thus look at images of brain and tissue function. Such separation allows estimation of chemical content, using absorbance, and estimation of histology, using scattering. To demonstrate that such separation was possible, we constructed 10-cm diameter homogenous tissue phantoms with known but differing levels of scattering and absorbance. Scattering and absorbance were determined using a formula fitting the observed TOFA data to a diffusion-equation approximation of photon travel through tissue. This use of the diffusion equation means that Beer's Law is no longer being used for absorbance determinations, but rather these values are being derived from a more accurate physical law. The ability to avoid Beer's Law eliminates many inaccuracies in these calculations.

The images we obtained from the homogenous phantoms, separated into absorbance and scattering, have different value ranges. Each appears homogeneous, demonstrating that scattering and absorbance can be separated as an image using time-resolved optical tomography and that the imaging algorithms are robust to boundary conditions near the edges of the image. Fine structure of noise in the scattering image can be seen when the scattering scale is expanded. Some of this structure is repeatable from scan to scan, while other features appear randomly. Thus, some of the variations seen may represent fine structure of true inhomogeneities in the model system. The total noise in the image was determined by calculating a value histogram for all pixels of the image. In this histogram ($n = 7,845$), the measured scattering was 2.34 ± 0.030 cm^{-1} (actual scattering coefficient, m_s, was 2.50 cm^{-1}) while the measured absorbance was 0.048 ± .0006 cm^{-1} (actual absorbance coefficient, m_a, was 0.046 cm^{-1}). While there is some error in the estimated mean compared to the actual values (6% for scattering and 2% for absorbance), the standard deviations are much smaller (1.2% for both). Thus, the technique is precise, though not yet accurate.[67]

Other groups have also demonstrated such separation in scattering and absorbance. Delpy and Hebden in London have now demonstrated a time-resolved system allowing the localization and imaging of glass beads in a scattering solution of liquid. The investigators rely upon a solution of the time-resolved data that predicts what would have happened had they been able to measure the very first arriving photons. These first-arriving photons are so rare as to be virtually unmeasurable, but they are of significant interest because they are among the least scattered photons and thus are ideal for imaging. By using a diffusion-based equation, it is possible to predict what the intensity of these photons would have been if the detectors had the sensitivity to detect these photons. These predicted intensities can then be used in the calculations. Arridge and Schweiger, also in the London group, have developed time-resolved imaging algorithms. Recently, a demonstration showing images with resolution comparable to CT and MRI have been shown by this group.

Once it has been demonstrated that scattering and absorbance can be imaged independently, these values can then be used for functional imaging calculations. Although such separations are just now beginning to be possible, many different types of brain function can be imaged. There are several areas that may have importance.

Images of oxygenation

Optical images can be processed for oxygenation. For example, an image of oxygenation for one of the infants with IVH is shown (Figure 11–4D). This image could also be created for a topical map of cortical oxygenation using an array of path-corrected oxygenation probes. However, such an image merely reports average tissue oxygenation, which may not be useful. More important would be the resolution of arterial and venous components of oxygenation. We propose that a head tilt mechanism should be able to resolve venous oxygenation, which should be able to work even when there is no blood flow, such as during cardiac arrest (Figure 11–5). In this type of an approach, a head tilt allows the venous blood volume to change slightly, and subtraction of the "before intervention" image at several wavelengths from the "after intervention" image at several wavelengths should allow an image of oxygenation to be calculated. Early images of this type have been made on critically ill infants at Stanford. A bedside device to rapidly image cerebral venous oxygenation has now been constructed and should be able to generate an image within a few minutes or less.

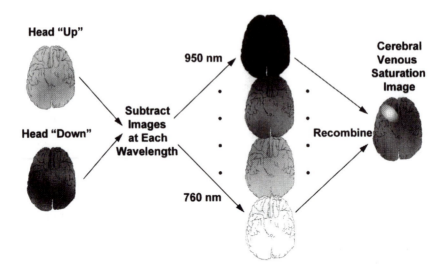

FIGURE 11–5.   Protocol for bedside imaging of stroke. Imaging a stroke can be done at bedside via mapping of venous changes during head tilt, obtained by subtracting before and after images during transition from level and supine to Trendelenberg orientation. Other interventional maneuvers that alter cerebral blood volume may also allow venous oxygenation to be rapidly and inexpensively imaged at the bedside. A venous tilt image can be processed at the bedside in a few minutes.

Images of cerebral blood volume

Provided that blood flow through the brain is present, cerebral blood volume can be determined. This requires use of a marker for blood volume, but fortunately a naturally occurring marker exists. As the oxygenation of the blood changes, as occurs when the inspired oxygen concentration is altered, the blood will change color. The total change in color can be used to determine cerebral blood volume if the starting and ending arterial saturation of the blood with oxygen is known. This is analogous to dissolving a known concentration of a dye in a fluid and predicting the volume of the diluent by measuring the diluted concentration of the dye. Similarly, the change in absorbance of hemoglobin with changes in oxygenation is known, such that the change in absorbance across the entire head during changes in oxygenation allows determination of total blood volume in the head.

Image of cerebral blood flow

Once the blood volume in the head is known, the same information can be used to determine cerebral blood flow. The approach is analogous to the use of injected dyes to determine cardiac output using a Fick-based determination. In this case, the endogenous dye is hemoglobin. By changing the inspired oxygen concentration, and thus altering the hemoglobin saturation in the arterial blood, the rate of rise can be determined and translated into cerebral blood flow. Images of blood flow can be combined with images of oxygenation to produce an image of tissue health (Figure 11–6).

Imaging of non-oxygenation related injury

The brain injury cascade is complex. In some cases, such as if cell death is due to activation of a preprogrammed pathway, the initial causes of the activation may have long since disappeared. For example, oxygenation may have returned to normal, but the cells have already been committed to die at some point in the near future. Thus, it is markers of the impending cell death that need to be detected. Of course, detection of a loss of cytochrome oxidation may be used, but this may be a late sign. We believe that cellular swelling that occurs during edema or cellular injury will result in a dilution of the intracellular components, as well as a change in intracellular storage components such as calcium, or changes in the cell packaging apparatus, all of which are responsible for light scattering. These changes should be detectable using a device that images and quantifies scattering.

It has also been recently shown that there are scattering changes that occur during the process of electrical activity. Such changes occur on a millisecond basis and occur much too rapidly to be explained by changes in

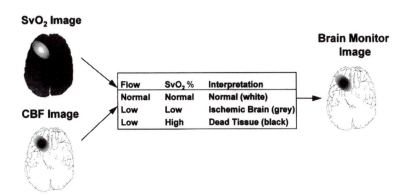

FIGURE 11–6.   Generation of images of brain tissue viability. Combination of venous oxygenation and cerebral blood flow images may allow for a simple-to-interpret image to be generated at the bedside. The combined image in this example differentiates between well-perfused normal tissue, poorly perfused tissue at risk, and metabolically inactive tissue presumed dead. Additional information could be added by mapping static or dynamic scattering, correlated with edema and tissue dysfunction, or chemically mapping metabolites present in injured tissue, via spatially-resolved absorbance spectroscopy.

blood flow or blood volume. We speculate that such changes may be due to a liquid crystal effect of depolarization or other changes within the neuron itself that allow the scattering to rapidly vary. Thus, there is a natural fluctuation in the scattering of active neural tissue. Study of the patterns of these fluctuations may reveal patterns that are indicative of healthy or diseased neural tissues. This approach has already been used by Gratton et al. to demonstrate that different visual quadrants are physically mapped to different regions of the human occipital cortex.[71,72] In these studies, subjects presented with a flashing light in different visual quadrants had externally measurable changes in tissue scattering over area 17 at the occiput of the head. These changes localized to a small area of the scalp overlying area 17, and this area was different for each of the quadrants of photon stimulation. Thus, the receptive areas of the visual cortex have been now functionally mapped using external NIRS in the frequency domain.

Lastly, such images can be made using contrast agents. We have recently shown that measures of pH can be made using contrast agents,[73] and others have used fluorescence as mapping agents.[74] Contrast agents may be important in the detection of tumors because the leaky capillaries and increased blood volume in the tumors may allow for an enhancement of signal localized to the tumors in optical images.

Images of tumors

Images of tumors may be possible using optical methods. For example, although breast tumors are detectable by x ray when there is a 1-mm calcification, at the time that such images can be made there is a much larger functional disturbance in the breast tissue function (e.g., changes in blood flow, oxygenation, scattering, etc.). This allows breast tumor imaging using optics to rival x ray in detection because the 1-cm functional disturbance may be easier to detect than the 1-mm x ray-visible calcification. Two leading manufacturers of imaging equipment are now testing frequency-domain breast scanners, and early results are encouraging. Brain tumors may also be detectable using similar method.

Comparison of Structural and Functional Imaging

The separation of structural and functional imaging has clinical importance. The equations that allow imaging using light can be tuned to give the best structural resolution, or the most accurate determination of quantitative values, but not both at the same time. Therefore, different clinical situations may call for a different optimization.

Structural imaging focuses upon the generation of image with the best physical resolution. The imaged values may not be directly related to known quantitative values, much as in the case of ultrasound, in which the shadows are visible, but these images are not quantitative. This approach would work best if the maximum image resolution were required, such as in the case of identifying and locating hemorrhage, tumors, or other physical lesions. This approach may also prove useful in the identification of margins of disease.

Functional imaging, on the other hand, involves the quantitative determination of body chemistry. The imaged values should thus correlate well with known physical values, but the resolution of such determinations will not be as fine as that using structural imaging approaches. While the resolution on a physical scale will be inferior to structural imaging, the technique has great power in that many of the problems this approach addresses have no discernible physical manifestation. Thus, early stroke, which does not show up on structural scans, will show up clearly on a functional scan. The resolution of a functional image should be sufficient to allow detection of a stroke in the cortex or to identify regional differences in brain oxygenation. Therefore, this approach is potentially useful in the identification and mapping of stroke, ischemic disease, and localized and regional maldistributions of blood volume and blood flow. Based upon variations in chemistry of the tissues, this approach may also be useful in identifying margins of disease. For brain monitoring, it may be that a combination of structural imaging, functional oxygenation, blood volume and blood flow imaging, and scattering monitoring will all be important in determining tissue health and risk of injury.

Directions for Improvement

To improve upon our device, specific features lacking in the TOFA system need to be corrected. First, by adding a more powerful light source (still well within the limits of safety) and by adding detector arrays, image acquisition time can be substantially reduced. A target speed is one image every five minutes. Second, clinical correlation will be essential to verify that such imaging yields improved results over conventional techniques. Such an endeavor will require testing and cross-correlation with outcome measures and existing imaging methodologies. An NIH-NINDS-supported trial is now underway, with a broader multicenter trial planned for late 1995. Last, it is not clear as to whether the time domain or frequency domain is superior, and it is likely that each will have areas in which it works best. These issues will require further study and testing.

Imaging Conclusions

Our results demonstrate that TOFA allows imaging in scattering media such as in animal and human brain. Resolution of subcentimeter objects within brain and brain models appears feasible, and similar or better resolution should be expected for images of tissue function, such as oxygenation, blood flow, blood volume, or for markers of neuronal injury. Others have reported similar progress.[67–73] Given that many functional problems such as stroke and structural problems such as hemorrhage occur on such a scale, it appears that optical imaging and spectroscopy may be a useful clinical tool. The only questions remaining are when this will happen and in what capacity. Such an event could have significant medical consequences by improving our ability to measure problems in tissue function and thus intervene early before the problem leads to permanent injury.

Conclusions

Measurement of cerebral oxygenation, blood flow, and blood volume are possible using near-infrared optical spectroscopy. Imaging of cerebral structure, such as hematoma, has also been demonstrated. Combination of functional and structural imaging now seems likely and is undergoing active study.

As with all new discoveries, the implications for the understanding and practice of medicine are likely to exceed our wildest imagination. X rays, while first used to make funhouse family portraits and to determine shoe sizes, soon offered valuable medical diagnostic potential. MRS, while initially developed as a molecular probe for chemists, has opened new ways of imaging blood flow in formerly unreachable areas. MOS and MOI offer new probes for the measurement of tissue functioning while avoiding harmful exposures. As such, these optical techniques represent a fundamentally new tool in the medical armamentarium. Given the current rate of progress within the optics field, it is hoped that the production of clinically relevant optical imaging devices will be well underway within the next two to five years.

Notes

Portions of this report have been published or presented earlier. Some data presented are new and have not been peer reviewed at this time, and thus are merely speculation or opinions. We thank the NIH (RR-00081, M01-RR-00070-30/1, N43-NS-4-2313, N43-NS-4-2315), the Berry Fellowship Grant, The Zaricor Family Fund, and the Office of Naval Research (N-00014-91-C-0170) for their partial support of the above projects.

References

1. A review of the field, *Optical Tomography,* is available from SPIE (Bellingham, WA). Other excellent collections of topical related articles can be found in SPIE publications 1431 (1991), 1641 (1992), 1888 (1993), 2135 (1994), and 2389 (1995).
2. Ross BD, Kreis R, Ernst T. Cinical tools for the 90s: Magnetic reasonance spectroscopy and metabolite imaging. *Eur J Rad* 1992;14:128–140.
3. Jöbsis FF. Noninvasive infrared monitoring of cerebral and myocardial oxygen sufficiency and circulatory parameters. *Science* 1977;198:1264–1266.
4. McCormick PW, Stewart M, Lewis G, Dujovny M, and Ausman JI. Intracerebral penetration of infrared light. *J Neurosurg* 1992;76:315–318.

5. Kurth CD. Kinetics of hemoglobin oxygenation during hypothermic cardiac arrest in neonates. Presented at NIH workshop on near-infrared spectroscopy, D. Hirtz, Chairperson, April 1992, Chevy Chase, MD.

6. Chance B. Comparison of time-resolved and -unresolved measurements of deoxyhemoglobin in brain. *Proc Natl Acad Sci* 1988; 85:4971–4975.

7. Delpy DT, Cope M, van der Zee P, Arridge SR, Wray S, Wyatt JS. Estimation of optical pathlength through tissue from direct time of flight measurement. *Phys Med Biol* 1988;33:1433–1442.

8. Svaasand LO, Ellingsen R. Optical properties of human brain. *J Cereb Blood Flow Metabol* 1983;3:293–299.

9. Hebden JC, Kruger RA. Transillumination imaging performance: A time-of-flight imaging system. *Med Phys* 1990;17:351–356.

10. Wyatt JS, Cope M, Delpy DT, van der Zee P, Arridge S, Edwards AD, Reynolds EO. Measurement of optical pathlength for cerebral near infrared spectroscopy in newborn infants. *Dev Neurosci* 1990;12:140–144.

11. Benaron DA, Kurth CD, Steven J, Wagerle LC, Chance B, Delivoria-Papadopoulos M. Non-invasive estimation of cerebral oxygenation and oxygen consumption using phase-shift spectrophotometry. *Proc IEEE Eng Med Biol* 1990;12:2004–2007.

12. Benaron DA, Gwiazdowski S, Steven J, Delivoria-Papadopoulos M. Optical path length of 754nm and 816nm light emitted into the heads of infants. *Proc IEEE Eng Med Biol* 1990;12:1117–1119.

13. Drexler B, Davis JL, Schofield G. Diaphanography in the diagnosis of breast cancer. *Radiology* 1985;157:41–44.

14. Marshall V, Williams DC, Smith KD. Diaphanography as a means of detecting breast cancer. *Radiology* 1984;150:339–343.

15. Navarro GA, Profio AE. Contrast in diaphanography of the breasts. *Med Phys* 1988;15:181–187.

16. Edwards AD. Cotside measurement of cerebral blood flow in ill preterm infants by near-infrared spectroscopy. *Lancet* 1988;II:770–771.

17. Smith DS, Levy WJ, Carter S, Wang N, Haida M, Chance B. Time resolved spectroscopy and the determination of photon scattering, pathlength, and brain vascular hemoglobin saturation in a population of normal volunteers. *SPIE* 1993; 1888:511–516.

18. Benaron DA, Stevenson DK. Optical time-of-flight and absorbance imaging of biologic media. *Science* 1993;259:1463–1466.

19. Benaron DA. Imaging neonatal brain pathology using light. *Ped Abstracts* 1993; 33:369A.

20. Material presented at the Society for Pediatric Research, Washington, DC, May 1993.

21. Edwards AD, Wyatt JS, Richardson C, Potter A, Cope M, Delpy DT, Reynolds EO. Effects of indomethacin on cerebral haemodynamics in very preterm infants. *Lancet* 1990;335:1491–1495.

22. McDonnell M, Ives NK, Hope PL. Intravenous aminophylline and cerebral blood flow in preterm infants. *Arch Dis Child* 1992;67:416–418.

23. Delpy DT. Quantitation of pathlength in optical spectroscopy. *Adv Exp Med Biol* 1989;248:41–46.

24. Benaron DA, Lenox MA, Stevenson DK. Two-D and three-D images of thick tissue using time-constrained time-of-flight and absorbance (tc-TOFA) spectrophotometry. *SPIE* 1992;164:35–45.

25. Arridge SR, Cope M, Delpy DT. The theoretical basis for the determination of optical pathlengths in tissue: Temporal and frequency analysis. *Phys Med Biol* 1992;37:1531–1560.
26. Sevick EM, Burch CL, Chance B. Near-infrared optical imaging of tissue phantoms with measurement in the change of optical path lengths. *Adv Exp Med Biol* 1994;345:815–823.
27. Sevick EM, Frisoli J, Burch C, Szmacinski H, Nowacyk K, Johnson M, Lakowicz J. Time-dependent photon migration and imaging in two dimensions: A method of detection and localization of absorbers in tissue-like media. *SPIE* 1993;1888: 428–439.
28. Benaron DA, Stevenson DK. Resolution of near infrared time-of-flight brain oxygenation imaging. *Adv Exp Med Biol* 1994;345:609–617.
29. Lakowicz JR, Laczko GR, Cherek H, Gratton E, Limkeman M. Analysis of fluorescence decay kinetics from variable-frequency phase shift and modulation data. *Biophys J* 1984;46:463–477.
30. Sevick EM, Chance B, Leigh J, Nioka S, Maris M. Quantitation of time- and frequency-resolved optical spectra for the determination of tissue oxygenation. *Analyt Biochem* 1991;195:330–351.
31. Kurth CD, Steven JM, Benaron DA, Chance B. Near-infrared monitoring of the cerebral circulation. *J Clin Mon* 1993;9:163–170.
32. van der Zee P. Experimentally measured optical pathlengths for the adult head, calf, and forearm and the head of the newborn infant as a function of inter optode spacing. *Adv Exp Med Biol* 1992; 316:145–153.
33. Chance B. Early detection of brain ischemia and hemorrhage by optical methods. *SPIE* 1992;1641:162–169.
34. Wang L, Ho PP, Liu C, Zhang G, Alfano RR. Ballistic 2-D imaging through scattering walls using an ultrafast optical Kerr gate. *Science* 1991; 253:769–771.
35. Benaron DA, Kurth CD, Steven JM, Chance B. Cranial optical path length in infants by near-infrared phase-shift spectroscopy. *J Clin Mon* 1995, in press.
36. Benaron DA, Benitz WE, Ariagno RA, Stevenson DK. Noninvasive methods for estimating in vivo oxygenation. *Clin Pediatr* 1992;31:258–273.
37. McCormick PW. Noninvasive cerebral optical spectroscopy for monitoring cerebral oxygen delivery and hemodynamics. *Crit Care Med* 1991;19:89–97.
38. Milikan GA. The oximeter, an instument for measuring continuously the oxygen saturation of arterial blood in man. *Rev Sci Instrum* 1942;13:434–444.
39. Ferrari M, Wei Q, Carraresi L, DeBlasi RA, Zaccanti G. Time-resolved spectroscopy of human forearm. *J Photochem Photobiol* 1992;16:141–153.
40. Kakihana Y, Tamura M. Near-infrared optical monitoring of cardiac oxygen sufficiency through thoracic wall without open-chest surgery. *SPIE* 1991;1431: 314–320.
41. Brazy JE, Lewis DV, Mitnick MG, Jöbsis FF. Monitoring of cerebral oxygenation in the intensive care nursery. *Adv Exp Med Biol* 1986;191:843–847.
42. Wyatt JS, Edwards AD, Azzopardi D, Reynolds EOR. Magnetic reasonance and near infrared spectroscopy for investigation of perinatal hypoxic-ischaemic brain injury. *Arch Dis Child* 1989;64:953–963.
43. Wyatt JS, Cope M, Delpy DT, Richardson CE, Edwards AD, Wray S, Reynolds EO. Quantitation of cerebral blood volume in human infants by near-infrared spectroscopy. *J Appl Physiol* 1990;68:1086–1091.

44. Wickramasinge YA, Livera LN, Spencer SA, Rolfe P, Thorniley MS. Plethysmo-graphic validation of near-infrared spectroscopic monitoring of cerebral blood volume. *Arch Dis Child* 1992;67:407–411.

45. Kurth CD, Steven JM, Nicolson SC, Chance B, Delivoria-Papadopoulos M. Ki-netics of cerebral deoxygenation during deep hypothermic circulatory arrest in neonates. *Anesthesiology* 1992;77:656–661.

46. McCormick PW, Stewart M, Goetting MG, Balakrishnan G. Regional cere-brovascular oxygen saturation measured by optical spectroscopy in humans. *Stroke* 1991;22:596–602.

47. Brazy JE, Lewis DV, Mitnick MH, Jöbsis FF. Noninvasive monitoring of cerebral oxygenation in newborn infants by near-infrared transillumination. *Pediatrics* 1985;75:217–225.

48. Edwards AD. Cotside measurement of cerebral blood flow in ill preterm infants by near-infrared spectroscopy. *Lancet* 1988;II:770–771.

49. Edwards AD. Effects of indomethacin on cerebral haemodynamics in very preterm infants. *Lancet* 1990;335:1491–1495.

50. Cope M, van der Zee P, Essenpreis M, Arridge SR, Delpy DT. Data analysis methods for near infrared spectroscopy of tissue: Problems in determining the relative cytochrome aa3 concentration. *SPIE* 1991;251–262.

51. Maier JS, Fantini S, Franceschini-Fatini MA, Mantulin WW, Walker SA, Grat-ton E. Application of a portable near-infrared spectrometer in the study of sev-eral human tissues. *SPIE* 1995;2387, in press.

52. Quaresima V, Pizzi A, De Blasi RA, Ferrari M. Quadriceps oxygenation changes during walking and running on a treadmill. *SPIE* 1995;2387, in press.

53. De Blasi RA, Fantini S, Franceschini-Fantini MA, Barbieri BF, Ferrari M, Grat-ton M. Cerebral and muscle oxygen saturation measurement by a frequency-domain near-infrared spectroscopic technique. *SPIE* 1995;2387, in press.

54. Bank W, Chance B. Diagnosis of mitochondrial disease by NIRS. *SPIE* 1995; 2389, in press.

55. Muller G, Lazer-Medizin-Zentrum, Berlin, Germany. Personal communication.

56. Duguay MA, Mattick AT. Ultrahigh speed photography of picosecond light pulses and echoes. *Appl Opt* 1971;10:2162–2170.

57. Wilson BC, Patterson MS, Flock ST, Wyman DR. Tissue optical properties in relation to light-propagation models and in vivo dysymmetry. In Chance B (ed.), *Photon migration in tissue.* Plenum, New York: 1989, pp. 25–42.

58. Flock ST, Wilson BC, Patterson MS. Total attenuation coefficients and scatter-ing phase functions of tissues and phantom materials at 633nm. *Med Phys* 1987; 14: 835–841.

59. Patterson MS, Chance B, Wilson BC. Time-resolved reflectance and transmit-tance for the noninvasive measurement of tissue optical properties. *Appl Opt* 1989;28:2331–2336.

60. Bonne RF. Model for photon migration in turbid biological media. *J Opt Soc Am* 1987;4:423–432.

61. van der Zee P, Delpy DT. Computed point spread functions for light in tissue us-ing a measured volume scattering function. *Adv Exp Med Biol* 1988;222:191–197.

62. Yoo KN, Alfano RR. Time-resolved coherent and incoherent components of for-ward light scattering in random media. *Opt Lett* 1990;15:320–322.

63. Gopinath SP, Robertson CS, Grossman RG, Chance B. Near-infrared spectro-scopic localization of intracranial hematomas. *J Neurosurg* 1993;79:43–47.

64. Benaron DA. Noninvasive measurement and imaging of tissue structure and oxygenation using time-of-flight absorbance (TOFA) spectroscopy. *Proc IEEE Eng Med Biol* 1992;14:2402–2404.
65. Benaron DA, Van Houten JP. Results of clinical tomographic imaging using light. *Adv Exp Med Biol* 1995, in press.
66. Van Houten JP, Cheong WF, Spilman SD, Kermit EL, Stevenson DK, Benaron DA. Early results of clinical optical tomography in a neonatal intensive care unit. *SPIE* 1995;2389, in press.
67. Benaron DA, Ho DC, Spilman SD, Van Houten JP, Stevenson DK. Tomographic time-of-flight optical imaging scanner for highly scattering media using non-parallel ray geometry. *App Opt* 1995, in press.
68. Schwieger M, Arridge SR. Near infrared imaging: Photon measurement density functions and reconstruction from phantom data. *SPIE* 1995;2389, in press.
69. Arridge SR. Inverse methods for optical tomography. *Proc Intl Conf Inform Proc Med Imag* 1993;259–277.
70. Chance B, Kang K, He L, Weng J, Sevick E. Highly-sensitive object location in tissue models with linear in-phase and anti-phase multi-element optical arrays in one and two dimensions. *Proc Natl Acad Sci USA* 1993;90:3423–3427.
71. Gratton G, Maier JS, Fabiani M, Mantulin WW, Gratton E. Feasibility of in-tracranial near-infrared optical scanning. *Psychophysiology* 1994;31:211–215.
72. Gratton E, Walker SA. Back projection image reconstruction using photon density waves in tissues. *SPIE* 1995;2389, in press.
73. Cheong W-F, Van Houten JP, Spilman SD, Stevenson DK, Benaron DA. Noninvasive serum pH assay using i.v. phenol red: Studies in vitro. *Pediatr Res* 1995, in press.
74. O'Leary MA. Reradiation and imaging of diffuse photon density waves using fluorescent inhomogeneities. *J Luminescence* 1994;60/61:281–286.

CHAPTER 12

Assessment of CNS Function: Cerebral Blood Flow and Metabolism

William J. Greeley

Current monitors of CNS function include measures of cerebral blood flow, cerebral metabolism, and cerebral electrical activity. This discussion will be confined to the clinical monitoring of cerebral blood flow (CBF) and cerebral metabolism in the operating room. The brain is the most complex organ system to understand and monitor. Our tools to assess brain blood flow and metabolism are crude, simplistic, and usually render global measurements.

So why attempt to monitor the CNS during cardiac surgery in neonates, infants, and children? Outside of the obvious concerns regarding the neuropsychologic sequelae of surgery, there are several other reasons to attempt to monitor the CNS. First, many of the perfusion techniques used during cardiopulmonary bypass (CPB) were empirically derived and based on clinical practice. During CPB, pump flow rate (cardiac output on pump), perfusion temperature, degree of hemodilution, $PaCO_2$, and mean arterial pressure are arbitrarily set. Until recently, the effects of moderately hypothermic CPB, a most fundamental manipulation, have been poorly understood. Moreover, the physiologic extremes of temperature (16° to 18°C) and perfusion (total circulatory arrest) used during neonatal and infant cardiac surgery warrant investigation to determine their effects on the brain.

A second reason to assess the CNS during cardiac surgery is the fact that during CPB many variables of perfusion are controlled. Therefore, the opportunity exists to systematically study the effects of temperature, $PaCO_2$, pump flow rate, etc. in a controlled manner. Viewing cardiac surgery and CPB as a "clinical laboratory" has permitted fundamental clinical observations to be made about hypothermia and circulatory arrest. These observations have not

185

only advanced our knowledge of CPB effects but have also addressed more basic biologic constructs, i.e., temperature effects and the arrested brain. Nowhere else in clinical medicine are the physiologic extremes so pronounced as during infant cardiac surgery. So the opportunity is there to understand the effects of CPB on humans if we systematically evaluate them. A final advantage of systematically monitoring the brain on a regular basis is to understand the potential mechanisms for brain injury in one's own institutional practice. Moreover, protective strategies can be assessed. Because the end points of CBF and metabolism monitoring are immediate, important conclusions can be readily drawn, rather than waiting 3 to 5 years to determine eventual outcome. Since neuropsychologic outcome is the most important measure of successful brain protection, these measures must be linked with the immediate results of CNS monitoring. A number of important observations have been made by our group that have fundamentally altered our practice and improved cerebral outcome. Cerebral blood flow monitors use either a direct tracer methodology based on the Fick principle or infer cerebral blood flow from Doppler measurements of cerebral blood velocity. Cerebral metabolism, which is probably the single most important aspect of monitored cerebral physiology, can be assessed through direct measurements of $CMRO_2$ or through noninvasive near-infrared technology.

Methods of CBF Measurement

Most methods of determining CBF are based on the Fick principle. The classic reference method of measuring CBF[1] requires the administration of a freely diffusible, insoluble, inert tracer substance (133xenon, N20, krypton, and Evans blue dye) and sampling of the cerebral venous system (catheter in the jugular venous bulb) and arterial blood during its wash in or washout of the cerebral circulation. If the time until equilibration of arterial and cerebral venous tracer substance is calculated, the blood-brain partition coefficient of the tracer known, and steady state conditions over the study period obtained, a quantitative determination of CBF can be made.[2-4] The greater the CBF, the less time it takes for the arterial and cerebral venous concentrations to equilibrate. The 133xenon clearance technique is a simple, noninvasive method of determining CBF which has been validated[5] and is widely used for CBF measurements during CPB. Clinically, we have used 133xenon because it has a short half-life, has proven reliability, can be used to obtain serial measurements in a single patient, and involves minimal radiation exposure.[6-7] CBF is measured by injecting 1.5 μCi of xenon dissolved in 2 mL of sterile saline into the aorta or the arterial limb of the pump-oxygenator. Two extracranial cadmium telluride gamma emission detectors are placed over the right and left temporal lobes to detect the radioactive decay from the brain after injection. The cadmium telluride gamma emission detectors are wide-angle construction and are placed on either side of the patient's head. Wide-angle detectors are selected to minimize detection of scalp blood flow and maximize detection of flow to the cortical gray and white matter structures.

Cerebral blood flow is measured using the initial slope index (ISI) of the tracer washout curve or by measuring the area underneath the washout curve. Both methods provide a reproducible measure of global hemispheric flow.[5,6] We use the ISI method because it is more accurate at the low temperatures used during infant heart surgery, does not require a full 10 to 15 minutes of time to accumulate data, and therefore has less impact on the surgeon's need to alter pump flow during measurement periods. The equation describing the ISI is

$$\text{CBF ISI (mL/100 g/min)} = -\log \text{ slope} \times (\lg) \times (100)$$

where log slope is the natural logarithm of ^{133}Xe clearance after the peak of the curve; lg is the gray-matter blood partition coefficient for xenon, corrected for temperature and hematocrit;[3] and 100 converts mL/g/min to mL/100 g/min. In addition to the initial slope index, area under the curve can also be used to determine flow.[4] Clinically we have observed, on occasion, abnormally low flow in the right hemisphere immediately after commencement of CPB. This has correlated clinically with the tip of the aortic cannula extending too distally into the aortic arch.

Although ^{133}Xe clearance is an effective technique for measuring CBF, there are several limitations of this methodology. These include:

1. A need to correct the clearance curve for background ^{133}Xe or perform CBF determinations when counts return to baseline values.
2. [133]Xe does not provide a continuous measurement of cerebral blood flow.
3. The methodology assumes steady state conditions for the duration of the sampling period, a minimum of 5 minutes using ISI methodology.
4. [133]Xe is a radioactive tracer.
5. Electrocautery interference can occur.
6. There is a potential for extracranial scalp blood flow contamination of clearance results. We have quantified this latter limitation in our earliest studies and found the contribution to flow by the scalp vessels to be minimal.

Transcranial Doppler (TCD) is another method currently being used to monitor cerebral blood flow during pediatric cardiac surgery.[8,9] This technology for assessing CBF is discussed more in depth in Part II, Burrows, chapter 9 and will only be highlighted here. Transcranial Doppler (TCD) sonography was introduced by Aaslid in 1982.[10] TCD technology uses the Doppler principle to detect shifts in the frequency of reflected signals from blood in the middle cerebral artery to calculate blood flow velocity.[11] Since the diameter of this large cerebral artery is relatively constant, flow velocity should approximate cerebral blood flow. However, quantitative CBF values cannot be obtained because blood flow through a vessel is equal to the mean blood flow velocity multiplied by the cross-sectional area of that vessel, which is unknown.[12] Typically, the temporal ultrasonic window (1.5 cm anterior to the ear and just above the zygomatic arch) is used to interrogate the middle cerebral artery, although any large cerebral vessel may be evaluated. Probe position, however, is crucial to obtaining reproducible information, and this limits its reliability in the clinical setting where even minute movements of the patient's head can dramatically alter the signal intensity.

The principle advantages of TCD include (1) its noninvasive nature, (2) the absence of radiation exposure, and (3) its application as a continuous monitor. An additional advantage of this technique is the capability of assessing rapid alterations in blood flow velocity due to temperature or perfusion changes, as commonly occur during cardiac surgery. The limitations of transcranial Doppler monitoring include (1) reproducibility, especially at low flows, where minute movement of the patient's head can dramatically alter signal intensity and alter baseline measurements, and (2) the lack of validating studies of TCD during hypothermic CPB, where temperature, reduced flow rates, and the laminar flow characteristics of nonpulsatile perfusion may limit the accuracy of cerebral blood flow velocity measurements. While CBF velocity measurements by TCD have a reasonable correlation with more standard measures of CBF during normothermia, there have been few studies examining its validity during hypothermic cardiopulmonary bypass.

TCD has been used to investigate the effect of CPB and deep hypothermic circulatory arrest on cerebral hemodynamics in children, as well as to assess the incidence of cerebral emboli. Recent studies examining the brain using TCD have enabled several investigative groups to provide important information regarding questions of normal and abnormal brain perfusion during cardiac surgery in children. Questions regarding cerebral perfusion pressure, autoregulation, effect of $PaCO_2$, and temperature have been addressed using TCD in children and are discussed below.[9] TCD has also provided qualitative information regarding the presence of gaseous emboli in the middle cerebral artery during cardiac surgery.[13,14] Quantification of this important mechanism of cerebral injury during cardiac surgery would be instructive. Future investigations using TCD should address this mechanism of injury as well.

Cerebral Metabolic Rate Measurements

The most important measurement of brain function is metabolism. The capability now exists of measuring cerebral metabolic activity during cardiac surgery. Methods for monitoring cerebral metabolic activity include the determination of the cerebral metabolic rate for oxygen (CMRO$_2$), jugular venous bulb saturation, and the use of near-infrared spectroscopy (NIRS). CMRO$_2$ is determined by multiplying the oxygen content difference between the arterial (radial artery) and cerebral venous effluent and the radioisotopically determined CBF. Retrograde cannulation of the jugular venous bulb is a safe and technically simple method of obtaining the cerebral equivalent of mixed venous blood.[15] The equation describing CMRO$_2$ is

$$CMRO_2(mL/100g/min) = CBF \times 1.39 \times Hgb\ ([SaO_2-SvO_2]$$
$$+ .003\ [PaO_2-PvO_2]\ )/100$$

SaO$_2$ and SvO$_2$ are the arterial and venous oxygen saturation of the radial arterial and jugular venous bulb blood, respectively. Hgb is hemoglobin and PvO$_2$ is venous oxygen tension.[16]

The primary effect of cooling during cardiac surgery is to reduce energy metabolism so that low flow states and DHCA can be used. Monitoring the efficacy of brain cooling can be performed by measuring the venous oxygen saturation of the brain. The higher the saturation level during cooling, the greater the oxygen metabolic suppression and the protective cooling effects. A jugular venous bulb catheter is easily placed in the right internal jugular vein, threaded retrograde to the venous bulb, and positioned to assess the cerebral venous effluent.[15,16] The blood obtained from the jugular bulb is the effluent from many regions of the brain. Consequently, the oxygen content and saturation difference between the arterial and jugular venous bulb blood is a global average and may not reflect areas of regional cerebral perfusion. Therefore, a normal or elevated jugular venous saturation does not necessarily ensure adequate cerebral blood flow, but a low saturation suggests ongoing cerebral metabolism.[17]

The recovery of cerebral metabolism may reflect the quality of cerebral protection during CPB and TCA. Using this technique, potential mechanisms for brain injury have been identified and effective protection strategies developed. Some of our current work suggests that measures of cerebral venous lactate and cerebral venous saturation provide data which is similar to metabolic recovery data and are helpful in measuring the patient's response to an event such as cooling or rewarming. Measurements of jugular venous lactate or jugular venous saturation are easily obtained in the clinical setting through the use of a jugular venous bulb catheter. On-line monitoring of jugular venous oxyhemoglobin saturation is possible using commercially available oximeter catheters. However, current catheters frequently contact the wall of the jugular bulb and must be frequently recalibrated and repositioned.[18,19]

NIRS has the capability of measuring regional brain tissue oxyhemoglobin, deoxyhemoglobin, and cytochrome aa3, the terminal mitochondrial enzyme in the respiratory chain. Near-infrared spectroscopy is a noninvasive method of monitoring brain oxygen saturation (cerebral oximetry).[20-22] The principle is based upon the ready transmission of near-infrared wavelengths of light through biological tissue; attenuation is attributed to oxyhemoglobin, deoxyhemoglobin, and cytochrome aa3. Changes in the wavelength of near-infrared light that penetrates the skull and is transmitted through or reflected from brain tissue are proportional to the relative concentrations of oxy- and deoxyhemoglobin or cytochrome. Near-infrared spectroscopy has been used to monitor cerebral oxygenation during cardiac surgery with cardiopulmonary bypass and during periods of hypothermic arrest.[22,23] It is not inconceivable that cerebral oxygenation during CPB will be monitored using near-infrared technology as routinely as arterial oxygen saturation is currently monitored with pulse oximetry. Additionally, refinements in this technique will make CBF determinations clinically feasible.

References

1. Kety S, Schmidt C. The nitrous oxide method for the quantitative determination of cerebral blood flow in man: Theory, procedure and normal values. *J Clin Invest* 1948;27:476–483.
2. Bering EAJ. Effect of body temperature change on cerebral oxygen consumption during hypothermia. *Am J Physiol* 1961;200:417–422.
3. Chen RYZ, Foun-Chung F, Syngeuk K, Kung-Ming J, Shunichi V, Shu C. Tissue-blood partition coefficient for xenon: Temperature and hematocrit dependence. *J Appl Physiol* 1980;49:178–183.
4. Olesen J, Paulson OB, Lassen NA. Regional cerebral blood flow in man determined by the initial slope of the clearance of intraarterially injected 133Xe. *Stroke* 1971;2:519–524.
5. Spahn DR, Quill TJ, Hu W, Lu J, Smith LR, Reves JG, McRae RL, Leone BJ. Validation of 133Xe clearance as a cerebral blood flow measurement during cardiopulmonary bypass. *J Cereb Blood Flow Metab* 1992;12:155–161.
6. Greeley WJ, Ungerleider RM, Smith LR, Reves JG. The effects of deep hypothermic cardiopulmonary bypass and total circulatory arrest on cerebral blood flow in infants and children. *J Thorac Cardiovasc Surg* 1989;97:737–745.
7. Greeley WJ, Ungerleider RM, Kern FH, Brusino FG, Smith LR, Reves JG. Effects of cardiopulmonary bypass on cerebral blood flow in neonates, infants, and children. *Circulation* 1989;80(1):1209–1215.
8. Lundar T, Lindberg H, Lindegaard KF, Tjonneland S, Rian R, Bo G, Nornes H. Cerebral perfusion during major cardiac surgery in children. *Pediatr Cardiol* 1987;161–165.
9. Hillier SC, Burrows FA, Bissonnette B, Taylor RH. Cerebral hemodynamics in neonates and infants undergoing cardiopulmonary bypass and profound hypothermic circulatory arrest: Assessment by transcranial Doppler sonography. *Anesth Analg* 1991;72:723–728.
10. Aaslid R. The Doppler principle. *Transcranial Doppler sonography.* New York: Springer-Verlag, 1986.
11. Bishop CCR, Powell S, Rutt D, Browse NL. Transcranial Doppler measurement of middle cerebral artery blood flow velocity: A validation study. *Stroke* 1986; 17:913–915.

12. van der Linden J, Wesslen O, Ekroth R, Tyden H, von Ahn H. Transcranial Doppler-estimated versus thermodilution-estimated cerebral blood flow during cardiac operations. *J Thorac Cardiovasc Surg* 1991;102:95–102

13. Padayachee TS, Parsons S, Theobold R, Linley J, Gosling RG, Deverall PB. The detection of microemboli in the middle cerebral artery during cardiopulmonary bypass: A transcranial Doppler ultrasound investigation using membrane and bubble oxygenators. *Ann Thorac Surg* 1987;44:298–302.

14. van der Linden J, Casimir AH. When do cerebral emboli appear during open heart operations? A transcranial Doppler study. *Ann Thorac Surg* 1991;51: 237–241.

15. Goetting MG, Preston G. Jugular bulb catheterization: Experience with 123 patients. *Crit Care Med* 1990;18:1220–1223.

16. Greeley WJ, Kern FH, Ungerleider RM, Boyd JL, Quill T, Smith LR, Baldwin B, Reves JG. The effect of hypothermic cardiopulmonary bypass and total circulatory arrest on cerebral metabolism in neonates, infants, and children. *J Thorac Cardiovasc Surg* 1991;101:783–794.

17. Kern FH, Jonas RA, Mayer JE, Hanley FL, Castaneda AR, Hickey PR. Temperature monitoring during infant CPB: Does it predict efficient brain cooling? *Ann Thor Surg* 1992;54:749–754.

18. Schell RM, Kern FH, Reves JG. The role of continuous jugular venous saturation monitoring during cardiac surgery with cardiopulmonary bypass. *Anesth Analg* 1992;74:627–629.

19. Nakajima T, Kuro M, Hayashi Y, Kitaguchi K, Uchida O, Takaki O. Clinical evaluation of cerebral oxygen balance during cardiopulmonary bypass—On-line continuous monitoring of jugular venous oxyhemoglobin saturation. *Anesth Analg* 1992;74:630–635.

20. Jobsis A, vander Vliet FF. Niroscopy: Non-invasive near infrared monitoring of cellular oxygen sufficiency in vivo. *Adv Exp Med Biol* 1986;191:833–836.

21. Brazy JE, Lewis DV, Mitnick MH, Jobsis A, vander Vliet FF. Noninvasive monitoring of cerebral oxygenation in preterm infants: Preliminary observations. *Pediatrics* 1985;75:217–225.

22. Greeley WJ, Bracey VA, Ungerleider RM, Greibel JA, Kern FH, Boyd JL, Reves JG, Piantadosi CA. Recovery of cerebral metabolism and mitochondrial oxidation state is delayed after hypothermic circulatory arrest. *Circulation* 1991;84: 400–415.

23. Kurth CD, Steven JM, Nicolson SC. Changes in brain oxygenation during cardiopulmonary bypass and hypothermic arrest in neonates. *Anesthesiology* 1989; 71:A1035.

CHAPTER 13

Cerebral Evaluation with Nuclear Magnetic Resonance Spectroscopy

Julie A. Swain

This chapter will review the acquisition and analysis of phosphorus-31 nuclear magnetic resonance (P-31 NMR) spectra in biological systems. P-31 NMR spectroscopy has the advantages of being relatively nondestructive and giving a nearly continuous measurement of relative concentrations of phosphocreatine, ATP, and intracellular pH. NMR of biological systems is a relatively recent development. In the late 1970s, Gadian and Radda, at Oxford, made important advances in the ability to use radiofrequency coils on intact rats and to obtain NMR spectra of the heart, brain, and other organs.[1] There are several excellent reviews of the principles of NMR in biological systems.[2,3]

Principles of NMR

Elements with odd atomic mass and/or odd atomic numbers act like spinning electrical charges and have a magnetic moment. The elements that we are most interested in, as biologists, are phosphorus-31, which is a naturally abundant isotope, and carbon-13, which has a low natural abundance and requires doping of the isotope. Phosphorus-31 is extremely important for tracking the high-energy phosphate compounds and energy production in cells. Proton NMR has been used for many years for imaging and spectroscopy and gives data on lactate metabolism, fatty acid concentrations (especially in the brain), and the water content of organs.

When a phosphorus-containing compound, such as ATP, is not in a magnetic field, the magnetic moment (which is the sum of the individual magnetic moments) is oriented randomly. When phosphorus-containing compounds are placed in a magnet, the magnetic spins line up parallel and antiparallel in the magnet. In an NMR experiment, the compound is excited to a higher energy level with a radiofrequency pulse from a coil placed on the tissue. The difference in energy between basal and excited states is proportional to the frequency of the energy that is emitted when the nucleus undergoes transition from the higher energy state to baseline. Energy and frequency are related by a proportionality constant. The frequency of this radiation depends on two factors: the gyromagnetic ratio, which is a constant but is unique to each compound, and the effective magnetic field. The effective magnetic field is a function of both the intensity of the external magnetic field and a shielding constant, which reflects the environment of the atoms. The shielding constant allows a spectrum of many peaks because of the differences in the effective magnetic field of the same element (such as phosphorus) in different locations in a biological compound (such as ATP).

Biological NMR

ATP is one of the most important compounds in biological systems. It contains three phosphates that are shielded differently. Because these three phosphates are in different effective magnetic fields, we can differentiate them in a spectrum. Figure 13–1 demonstrates a biological phosphorus-31 NMR spectrum. The three phosphates in ATP are well defined, as is phos-

SHEEP BRAIN (15ºC)

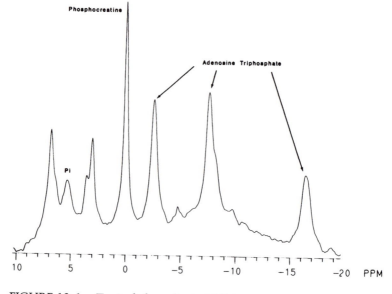

FIGURE 13–1.   Typical sheep brain 31-P NMR spectrum at 15°C.

phocreatine (PCr), the high energy phosphate most sensitive to ischemia. The information from the NMR spectrum gives the unique fingerprint of the compound, which includes the frequency and number of peaks. The amplitude of a peak is proportional to the concentration of the compound. Using energy absorption as a marker, the rates of chemical reactions, such as the creatine kinase reaction, can be determined. The relaxation time, or time it takes the compound to return to a basal energy state, reflects the environment of the compound and is important in NMR imaging.

The measurement of intracellular pH from the NMR spectrum is possible. The resonance position of the inorganic phosphate peak is exquisitely sensitive to intracellular pH, down to the 0.01 level. By measuring this resonance position, which is an amalgam of the relative concentrations of HPO_4 and H_2PO_4, we can measure intracellular pH in a very sensitive manner.

The effect of ischemia on the NMR spectrum is illustrated in Figure 13–2. Phosphocreatine is the most sensitive compound to ischemia and decreases first, followed by a decrease in ATP. At the same time, inorganic phosphate (Pi) increases, and the resonance frequency shifts, thus reflecting intracellular acidosis during ischemia.

The NMR Equipment

The equipment needed to perform an NMR experiment includes a strong magnet, which is usually a superconducting magnet cooled by liquid helium and liquid nitrogen. The normal clinical magnets have a strength of 2.0 Tesla. Research magnets are up to 4.7 Tesla for large animal studies. The biological system, e.g., a cell culture or a sheep on cardiopulmonary bypass, is placed in the bore of the magnet, and a radiofrequency coil is put on the organ to be studied. A radio transmitter is used to create a radiofrequency pulse to excite the tissues up to the next energy level. The coil then becomes a radiofrequency receiver and is used to detect the very low-intensity energy pulses emitted when the compounds relax back to the basal state. The energy decay is mathematically analyzed to produce a computer-generated spectrum, virtually on-line. The signal-to-noise ratio is such that many spectra must be added together to get a well resolved spectrum.

In Vivo NMR Experiments

The animal preparation that we use is adolescent sheep, peripherally cannulated for cardiopulmonary bypass without opening the chest. The radiofrequency coil is placed on the skull for brain experiments.

The problem, technically, is that all electronic or metal equipment has to be at least 15 to 20 feet away from the bore of the magnet. This makes manipulation of the animal difficult. There are three special dangers involved in working with these strong magnets. The first is that ferromagnetic objects

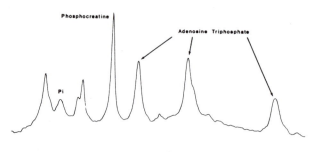

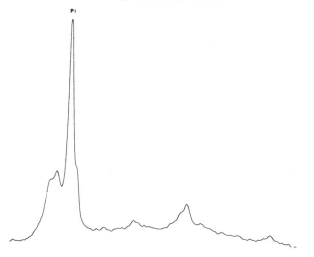

FIGURE 13–2. Phosphorus-31 nuclear magnetic resonance spectra of sheep brain (4.7 Telsa at 15°C on full-
flow cardiopulmonary bypass (*top*) and after 2 hours of
circulatory arrest (*bottom*). Notice near-complete depletion of ATP and PCr and accumulation of Pi. Spectral
peaks are labeled. Unlabeled peaks to the left and right of
the Pi peak are attributed to phosphomonoesters and
phosphocholine diesters, respectively. (All spectra represent 320 acquisitions for 20 minutes, are processed with
10 Hz of line broadening, and are scaled to each other).

fly! There have been numerous injuries in NMR laboratories from airborne
metal-containing objects. The magnets cannot be safely turned off quickly.
The second danger is that the high energy used to power the radiofrequency
coil results in electrical injuries if one is not extremely careful. The final

problem is that we do not know the effects of high magnetic fields on humans who work for long periods around these fields. Because all biological systems rely on small electrical fields, which interact with magnetic fields, we do not know the long-term effects on cell division and function.

In summary, nuclear magnetic resonance spectroscopy has been extremely valuable in allowing us to study biological systems. The advances in technology on the horizon will enable us to get even more detailed biochemical and structural information about organ systems.

References

1. Gadian DG, Radda GK. NMR studies of tissue metabolism. *Ann Rev Biochem* 1981;50:69–83.
2. Balaban RS. The application of nuclear magnetic resonance to the study of cellular physiology. *Am J Physiol* 1984;246 (cell Physiol 15):C10–19.
3. Osbakken M, Haselgrove J, Liegeti L. Introduction to NMR techniques. In Osbakken M, Haselgrove J (eds.), *NMR techniques in the study of cardiovascular structure and function.* New York: Futura, 1988, pp. 3–33.

PART III

Mechanisms of Neurological Injury

CHAPTER 14

Mechanisms of Perinatal Ischemic Brain Damage

Robert C. Vannucci

Introduction

The brain damage that results from cerebral ischemia is a major cause of perinatal mortality and of chronic neurologic morbidity in the survivors of such insults. Research over the past decade has expanded our knowledge of those critical cellular metabolic events that eventually lead to tissue injury arising from cerebral ischemia. Investigations have shown that ischemia sets in motion a cascade of biochemical alterations that are initiated during the course of the insult and that proceed well into the recovery period after resuscitation. This review will highlight those cellular processes that are perturbed by the tissue oxygen and substrate (glucose) debt arising from cerebral ischemia and will explain how these alterations evolve into perinatal brain damage.

Oxidative Metabolism and Excitatory Amino Acids

Ischemic insults to brain have been investigated largely in experimental animals, using a variety of models under diverse circumstances in an attempt to uncover pathophysiologic mechanisms responsible for the production of tissue injury. In all animal models studied, whether the event studied is ischemia alone or a combination of hypoxia and ischemia, the fundamental observation has been an uncoupling of cerebral blood flow from oxidative metabolism.[1-4] Thus, in situations where blood flow to all or part of the brain is reduced below a critical level, oxygen and substrate delivery to the tissue is curtailed, leading to a shift from aerobic to anaerobic metabolism. However, anaerobic glycolysis is unable to keep pace with cellular energy needs, and high-energy phosphate stores are rapidly depleted. Either prior to, concurrent with, or following the onset of the energy failure, other metabolic alterations occur, which include the activation of excitatory amino acid cell surface receptors, the intracellular accumulation of calcium (Ca^{2+}) ions, and, in selected neurons, the production of the free radical gas, nitric oxide. Catabolic processes also proceed with ribosomal disaggregation, protein degradation, and the liberation of free fatty acids from membrane phospholipids. All of these metabolic events culminate in cellular disintegration if the circulation and blood supply to the brain are not promptly and adequately restored. Even with recirculation and reoxygenation of the tissue, either spontaneous or by resuscitation, the metabolic perturbations occurring during the course of the insult might worsen during the recovery period. Whatever the final common denominator of tissue injury, alterations in cerebral perfusion and metabolism are the early—and probably late—critical events that ultimately determine the presence and severity of ischemic brain damage.

Recent years have witnessed a shift from investigations of those cerebrovascular and metabolic disturbances which occur during the course of cerebral ischemia to those lingering alterations which characterize the brain during recovery from the insult. One rationale for this shift in approach relates to the possibility of uncovering therapeutic modalities, applied during the early recovery period, which might prevent or minimize brain damage. Numerous investigators in separate laboratories have focused on distinct aspects of the neurotoxic capacity of specific metabolic events which occur post ischemia. These lingering alterations in cellular homeostasis include (1) a persistent energy debt due to an uncoupling of oxidative phosphorylation, (2) a lingering cellular acidosis, (3) the continued accumulation of cytosolic Ca^{2+} ions, (4) the formation of oxygen free radicals, (5) the accumulation of free fatty acids, and (6) the continued accumulation of excitatory neurotransmitters and of nitric oxide, which are cytotoxic in nature. Many, if not all, of these disturbances in metabolism are interrelated through specific biochemical reactions, with Ca^{2+} possibly playing a pivotal role.

Currently, there are two theories concerning those critical metabolic events that initiate the process of neuronal necrosis arising from cerebral ischemia, which have been labeled the "energy debt" and "excitotoxic" theories. In the first, more traditional proposal, ischemia produces an immediate cellular oxygen debt to the extent that the electron transport chain of mitochondria can no longer oxidize reducing equivalents to generate ATP required for endergonic reactions and the maintenance of transmembrane ion potentials.[1-4] The altered energy state (decreased phosphocreatine and ATP, increased ADP) activates anaerobic glycolysis with the production of cytosolic lactic acid and an associated intracellular acidosis. However, anaerobic glycolysis cannot keep pace with cellular energy demands, and endogenous energy reserves continue to decline, leading to a cellular energy debt (Figure 14–1). The rate of energy utilization might actually decrease as neuronal activity is curtailed in the cell's attempt to conserve energy.[5-8] The loss of cellular ATP severely compromises those metabolic processes that require energy for their completion. Thus, ATP-dependent Na^+ extrusion through the plasma membrane and concomitant exchange for K^+ is disrupted, resulting in the intracellular accumulation of Na^+ and

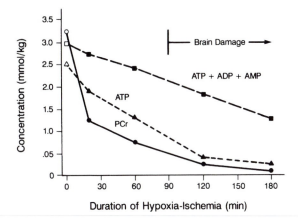

FIGURE 14–1. Changes in cerebral high-energy phosphate reserves during hypoxia-ischemia in the immature rat. Seven-day postnatal rats were subjected to unilateral common carotid artery ligation followed by exposure to systemic hypoxia with 8% oxygen at 37°C. Symbols represent means for ATP, phosphocreatine (PCr), and total adenine nucleotides (ATP + ADP + AMP). All values are significantly different from control (zero time point). Histologic brain damage commences at approximately 90 minutes of hypoxia-ischemia, with increasing severity thereafter. (Reprinted by permission of the publisher from Vannucci RC. Experimental biology of cerebral hypoxia-ischemia: Relation to perinatal brain damage. *Pediatr Res* 1990;27:317–326.)

Cl⁻ ions, as well as water (cytotoxic edema). Equally vital to cellular function is the prompt restoration of the energy reserves during and after resuscitation. Without regeneration of ATP, endergonic reactions cannot resume, especially those involving ion pumping at plasma and intracellular membranes. Intracellular Na^+ and Cl^- ions and water will continue to accumulate, and electrochemical gradients cannot be reestablished. Just how long the cell can survive in this situation is not entirely known, and it is likely that other factors are called into play that adversely influence ultimate cellular integrity (Figure 14–1).

The excitotoxic theory of neuronal death stems from the original investigations of Lucus and Newhouse[9] and Olney[10] who showed that the amino acid, glutamate, is toxic to the developing retina and brain. With this and other experiments, Olney[10] championed the excitotoxic nature of glutamate and its analogs. The mechanism by which glutamate exerts its toxic effect has not been entirely clarified, but altered ion fluxes across the plasma membrane of neurons, and possibly glia, undoubtedly play a role.[11,12] Based primarily on their investigations in neuronal cell cultures, Rothman and Olney[13] have proposed two mechanisms of ion-mediated neuronal injury (Figure 14–2). The first or early toxicity relates to glutamate-induced Na^+ influx into neurons during depolarization and is initiated by cerebral ischemia. Depolarization disturbs the intra-/extracellular balance of Cl^-, and the anion flows down its electrochemical gradient into the cell. The entry of Na^+ and Cl^- increases cell osmolality, necessitating the influx of water. Subcellular edema ensues, which if severe enough leads to lysis of the neuron. A delayed neurotoxicity also occurs, as has been observed *in vivo* in selected neurons of the hippocampus in adult animals[14,15] and possibly in immature animals as well.[16] This delayed neuronal necrosis presumably relates to excessive

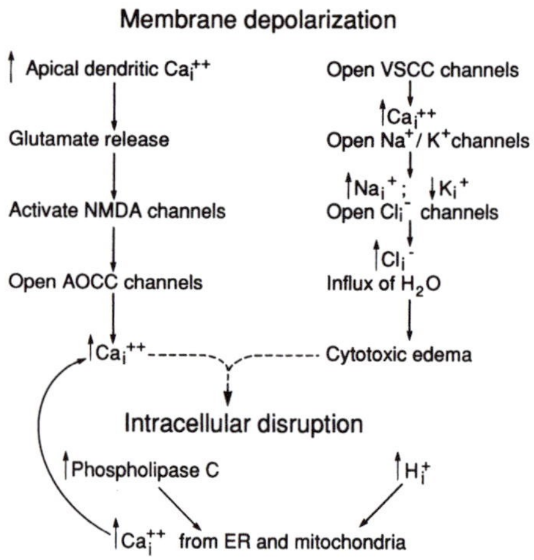

Membrane depolarization

$\uparrow$ Apical dendritic Ca_i^{++} Open VSCC channels

Glutamate release $\uparrow Ca_i^{++}$
Open Na^+/K^+ channels

Activate NMDA channels $\uparrow Na_i^+ : \downarrow K_i^+$
Open Cl_i^- channels

Open AOCC channels $\uparrow Cl_i^-$
Influx of H_2O

$\uparrow Ca_i^{++}$ -------- ------- Cytotoxic edema

Intracellular disruption

$\uparrow$ Phospholipase C $\uparrow H_i^+$

$\uparrow Ca_i^{++}$ from ER and mitochondria

FIGURE 14–2. Transmembrane ionic fluxes during cerebral ischemia. During cerebral ischemia, glutamate-induced Na^+ influx into neurons occurs during depolarization. The intra-/extracellular balance of Cl^- is disturbed, and the ion flows down its electrochemical gradient into the neuron. Water follows the influx of Na^+ and Cl^-, leading to cytotoxic edema. Both an early and late intracellular Ca^{2+} accumulation also occurs due to activation of NMDA channels. The excessive Ca^{2+} entry into the neuron sets in motion a cascade of biochemical events that culminate in death of the cell (see Figure 14.3).

Ca^{2+} entry into the cell via NMDA receptor-mediated channels. Ca^{2+}, in turn, sets in motion a cascade of biochemical events that culminate in death of the neuron (Figure 14–3).

Recent experiments suggest that the free radical gas, nitric oxide (NO), is involved in the cascade of metabolic events that cause or contribute to the

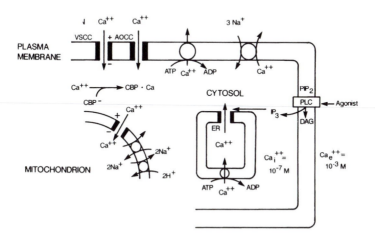

FIGURE 14–3. Transcellular and intracellular calcium fluxes. Ca^{2+} influx from the extracellular space into the cytosol of the neuron occurs via both voltage-sensitive calcium channels (VSCC) and agonist-operated calcium channels (AOCC). Ca^{2+} efflux from the cytosol into the extracellular fluid occurs via an energy-dependent uniport system and an antiport system involving Na$^+$. Intracellular Ca^{2+} sequestration occurs primarily within mitochondria and the endoplasmic reticulum (ER). Ca^{2+} is also bound by a specific calcium-binding protein (CBP-). Ca^{2+} release from the ER occurs upon stimulation by inositol trisphosphate (IP$_3$), whereas Ca^{2+} release from mitochondria involves an antiport system with Na$^+$, which is influenced by the hydrogen ion concentration.

Cerebral ischemia increases the free cytosolic concentration of Ca^{2+}. The elevation of Ca^{2+} arises from two sources, specifically, release of intracellular stores and increased influx (or decreased efflux) across the plasma membrane. An intracellular Ca^{2+} overload activates numerous intracellular reactions—including the activation of several lipases, proteases, and endonucleases—all of which attack the structural integrity of the cell. Excessive Ca^{2+} also activates phospholipase C, contributes to the formation of oxygen free radicals, and leads to an uncoupling of oxidative phosphorylation within mitochondria. Taken together, the toxic effects of excessive Ca^{2+} accumulation are adequate to cause membrane disintegration and the death of the neuron.

occurrence of ischemic brain damage.[17,18] NO is produced in selected neurons of the brain. The pathway for its synthesis involves the direct conversion of L-arginine to citrulline by the catalytic, cytosolic enzyme, NO synthase. NO production is linked to activation of glutamate and related excitatory amino acid surface receptors, especially NMDA receptors. The activation of these receptors leads to Ca^{2+} influx into cells and its binding to calmodulin. Once formed, NO influences numerous metabolic events, primarily through an activation of the second messenger enzyme, guanylate cyclase, with the formation of cGMP. In excessive concentrations, NO can act as a neurotoxic agent and may constitute a final common pathway for amino acid excitotoxicity in the brain, as has also been proposed for Ca^{2+}.[1] Experiments in adult animals suggest that NO mediates neuronal death following focal cerebral ischemia[19] and that the severity of neuronal loss can be reduced by the prior administration of inhibitors of NO synthase activity.[20] A similar protective effect also has been observed in the immature rat subjected to cerebral hypoxia-ischemia.[21,22] The mechanisms by which NO functions as a neurotoxin are numerous. Being a free radical, NO can react with other free radicals to form even more active species, including the hydroxyl free radical[23] (see below). NO also inactivates the glycolytic enzyme, glyceraldehyde-3-phosphate dehydrogenase.[24] Paralysis of the glycolytic pathway would curtail the cytosolic production of ATP and prevent the production of reducing equivalents available to mitochondria for further energy production. NO also inhibits components of the mitochondrial electron transport chain as well as the Krebs cycle enzyme, aconitase.[25] Thus, the neurotoxic effect of NO in part relates to its capacity to disrupt oxidative metabolism.

Superficially, the two theories of ischemic death of neurons appear to have opposing mechanisms of action. In the energy debt theory, the rate of cerebral energy utilization is inhibited to conserve energy, while in the excitotoxic theory, the rate of energy utilization might actually be stimulated[26,27] as a result of massive transmembrane ion fluxes produced by glutamate receptor activation. Furthermore, the excitotoxic theory implies that neuronal destruction occurs without a major disruption of cellular energy reserves. In reality, tissue culture experiments have shown that excitotoxic death does not occur unless cellular energy levels (ATP) are at least partially depleted.[28] Furthermore, it is now apparent that an intimate relationship exists between glutamate-mediated transmembrane ion regulation and oxidative metabolism[27-30] (Figure 14–4). However, several questions remain. First, what is the initiating biochemical event that sets in motion further processes which culminate in neuronal death? Second, what is the sequence of the biochemical events and how are they interrelated? Third, what is the relative role of oxygen versus substrate debt in initiating or perpetuating the process of cellular metabolic demise? Last, can neuronal death occur during the course of ischemia as a result of these metabolic perturbations, or is a period of reperfusion and reoxygenation necessary for cellular injury to occur? Answers to these questions are critical to our understanding the basic mechanisms of perinatal ischemic brain damage.

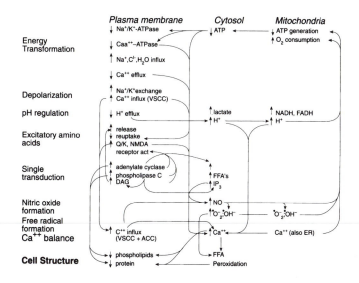

FIGURE 14–4. Interrelationships between cellular and molecular events leading to ischemic brain damage. Cerebral ischemia sets in motion a cascade of biochemical events commencing with a shift from oxidative to anaerobic metabolism, which leads to an accumulation of NADH, FADH, and lactic acid plus H+ ions. Anaerobic glycolysis cannot keep pace with cellular energy demands, resulting in a depletion of high-energy phosphate reserves, including ATP. Transmembrane ion pumping fails, leading to an accumulation of intracellular cations, anions, and water (cytotoxic edema). Ischemia also stimulates release of excitatory amino acids (glutamate) from axon terminals. The glutamate release, in turn, activates kainate/quisqualate (K/Q) and NMDA cell surface receptors, resulting in an influx of Na+ and Ca2+ ions. Within the cytosol, free fatty acids (FFA) accumulate from increased membrane phospholipid turnover and thereafter undergo peroxidation by oxygen free radicals, which arise from reductive processes within mitochondria and as by-products in the synthesis of prostaglandins, xanthine, and uric acid. Nitric oxide (NO) contributes to the formation of oxygen free radicals (especially the hydroxyl radical) as well as to the disruption of oxidative metabolism. Ca2+ ions accumulate within the cytosol as a consequence of increased plasma membrane influx via VSCC and AOCC and decreased efflux across the plasma membrane combined with release from mitochondria and the ER; the latter process is stimulated by IP3 (see Figure 14.3). The combined effects of cellular energy failure, acidosis, free radical formation, Ca2+ accumulation, and lipid peroxidation serve to disrupt structural components of the cell resulting in its ultimate death. (Modified with permission of the publisher from Vannucci RC. Experimental biology of cerebral hypoxia-ischemia: Relation to perinatal brain damage. *Pediatr Res* 1990;27:317–326.)

Free Radical Formation

As mentioned previously, experiments in animal models of ischemic brain damage have shown that tissue injury is initiated during the course of the ischemia and might worsen during recovery. The term *secondary injury* often is applied to describe the brain damage that evolves after the primary insult. Recent studies in immature animals have shown that ischemic brain damage can be reduced by interventions initiated during the recovery period following resuscitation.[31-33] Indeed, the hallmark of secondary brain injury is that it can be ameliorated by interventions initiated during the recovery interval.

Of the mechanisms that potentially cause or accentuate ischemic brain damage during the recovery period, the formation of oxygen free radicals plays a major role. Oxygen free radicals are generated during and following cerebral ischemia in several ways.[1,34,35] During partial cerebral ischemia, when at least a small amount of oxygen is available to the tissue, the low oxygen concentration at the site of cytochrome oxidase impedes the acceptance of electrons, thereby liberating free radicals at the more proximal steps in the electron transport chain. These oxygen free radicals cannot be consumed further within mitochondria and leak out into the cytoplasm. Two other potential sources of oxygen free radicals are as by-products in the synthesis of prostaglandins and of xanthine and uric acid during cerebral ischemia and upon reoxygenation of the tissue.[4] Finally, NO also acts as a free radical and is capable of interacting with other free radicals to form even more active species, including especially the hydroxyl free radical (see above).

The manner in which free radicals cause or contribute to tissue injury presumably relates to their ability to attack the fatty acid moiety of cellular membranes.[1,3,34,35] Polyunsaturated fatty acids seem especially prone to peroxidative attack by free radicals that initiate and perpetuate chain reactions within the hydrophobic core of the lipid bilayer, leading ultimately to membrane fragmentation. The chain reaction is promoted by excessive concentrations of intracellular free fatty acids and Ca^{2+} ions.

Protective Effect of Hypothermia on Ischemic Brain Damage

Studies conducted several years ago suggested a protective influence of hypothermia on hypoxic survival and on hypoxic-ischemic brain damage in immature animals.[36-38] More recently, Young et al.[39] subjected immature rats to cerebral hypoxia-ischemia and showed that brain damage was far less extensive in those rat pups exposed to hypoxia-ischemia at 29°C rather than 37°C. Neuronal injury was prevented entirely in those animals exposed to hypoxia-ischemia at 21°C. Therefore, moderate hypothermia (29°C) affords partial, and deep hypothermia (21°C) complete, protection from perinatal hypoxic-ischemic brain damage. Recent experiments in adult animals have suggested that even mild hypothermia (33° to 35°C) affords protection from ischemic brain damage.[40-42] Indeed, some investigators have suggested that the beneficial effects of calcium channel blockers and glutamate receptor antagonists might act, at least in part, through a curtailment of systemic and cerebral metabolic rates, thereby producing mild tissue hypothermia.[42]

To investigate the effect of mild hypothermia on perinatal hypoxic-ischemic brain damage, Yager et al.[43] subjected immature rats to cerebral hypoxia-ischemia at either 37°, 34°, or 31°C. Temperatures were recorded every 15 minutes from thermistor probes placed rectally and in the cerebral hemisphere undergoing hypoxia-ischemia. Neuropathologic alterations were assessed in surviving animals. A strong direct correlation existed between rectal and brain temperatures. Under normoxic conditions, the rat pups maintained their core temperature at 35°C irrespective of the ambient temperature. During systemic hypoxia, both rectal and brain temperatures rapidly equilibrated with that of the environment (Figure 14–5). There were no deaths during hypoxia-ischemia in either the 34° or 31°C groups compared to a 10% mortality in the 37°C group. Brain damage occurred in 90% of those rat pups exposed to hypoxia-ischemia at 37°C, with a 50% incidence of cystic infarction. Cerebral injury decreased linearly with decreasing temperature (Figure 14–6). Only 40% of rats exhibited brain damage at 34°C, none of which showed evidence of infarction. Rat pups exposed to hypoxia-ischemia at 31°C had no brain damage, even though the insult was extended to an interval twice as long as that used for animals exposed to hypoxia-ischemia at 34° or 37°C. The results indicate that in the immature rat (1) rectal temperature closely reflects brain temperature, (2) hypoxia-ischemia induces a state of poikilothermia, and (3) minor reductions in rectal/brain temperature (3° to 6°C) substantially reduce brain damage arising from hypoxia-ischemia.

Selective cooling of the brain also appears to be protective to the perinatal animal subjected to hypoxia-ischemia. Towfighi et al.[44] devised a technique in which the subcutaneous space of the scalp was irrigated with cool water to produce focal cerebral hypothermia in the immature rat. During the irrigation, the immature rats were exposed to cerebral hypoxia-ischemia and were maintained at an environmental temperature of 37°C. Neuropathologic examination of the animals showed that focal cooling of the scalp to temperatures lower than 28°C completely protected the animal from brain damage, with lesser damage occurring at higher temperatures than that expected at normothermia (37°C). The findings suggest that focal selective surface cooling protects the perinatal brain from ischemic damage to an extent roughly equivalent to that of total body cooling to comparable temperatures.

The mechanism for the protective effect of either systemic or focal hypothermia on brain tissue subjected to ischemic stress undoubtedly relates to a reduction in cerebral energy demands that are relatively proportionate

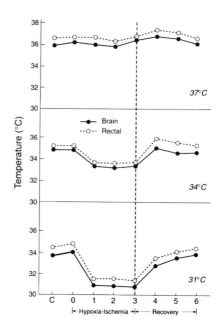

FIGURE 14–5. Brain and core temperature during normoxia, hypoxia-ischemia, and recovery at environmental temperature of either 37°, 34°, or 31°C in immature rats. Seven-day postnatal rats underwent unilateral common carotid artery ligation, followed thereafter by exposure to systemic hypoxia with 8% oxygen for 3 hours. (Modified with permission of the publisher from Yager J, Towfighi J, Vannucci RC. Influence of mild hypothermia on hypoxic-ischemic brain damage in the immature rat. *Pediatr Res* 1993;34:525–529.)

to a reduction in cerebral blood flow.[45–47] Of necessity, a mismatch occurs between cerebral blood flow and metabolism during hypothermic cerebral ischemia, because with a reduction in cerebral perfusion, metabolism must continue at least at a basal rate to maintain ion gradients. Basal metabolism would be expected to continue for extended intervals in immature animals, owing to physiologically low rates of cerebral energy utilization combined with high endogenous stores of carbohydrates—specifically glucose and glycogen—which serve as organic fuels for anaerobic glycolysis and energy production.[48,49] Indeed, ATP concentrations in the brains of poikilothermic animals (turtles, frogs, fish) are not exhausted for many hours of total cere-

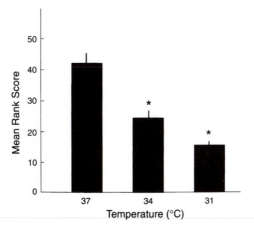

FIGURE 14–6. Rank score analysis of brains of rats previously subjected to hypoxia-ischemia at environmental temperature of either 37°, 34°, or 31°C. The animals were subjected to hypoxia-ischemia at 7 days of postnatal age. Columns represent means; vertical lines denote 1 S.E. (Modified with permission of the publisher from Yager J, Towfighi J, Vannucci RC. Influence of mild hypothermia on hypoxic-ischemic brain damage in the immature rat. *Pediatr Res* 1993;34:525-529.)

bral ischemia, and brine shrimp exposed to total anoxia maintain ATP levels for up to one month.[50] It follows that the lower the cerebral metabolic rate of an animal at normothermia, the greater the ischemic resistance promoted by hypothermia. Other factors undoubtedly also play a role in the hypothermic protection of the brain from ischemic damage, including blunting of excitatory amino acid neurotoxicity, free radical formation, cerebral edema, no-reflow phenomenon, or hyperviscosity.

References

1. Siesjo BK. Cell damage in the brain: A speculative synthesis. *J Cereb Blood Flow Metab* 1981;1:155–185.
2. Hossmann K-A. Treatment of experimental cerebral ischemia. *J Cereb Blood Flow Metab* 1982;2:275–297.
3. Raichle ME. The pathophysiology of brain ischemia. *Ann Neurol* 1983;13:2–10.
4. Vannucci RC. Experimental biology of cerebral hypoxia-ischemia: Relation to perinatal brain damage. *Pediatr Res* 1990;27:317–326.

5. Fowler JC. Escape from inhibition of synaptic transmission during in vitro hypoxia and hypoglycemia in the hippocampus. *Brain Res* 1992;573:169–173.

6. Bickler PE. Cerebral anoxic tolerance in turtles: Regulation of intracellular calcium and pH. *Am J Physiol* 1992;263:R1298–R1302.

7. Perez-Pinzon MA, Rosenthal M, Sick TJ, Lutz PL, Pablo J, Mash D. Down regulation of sodium channels during anoxia: A putative survival strategy of turtle brain. *Am J Physiol* 1992;262:R712–R715.

8. Corbett RJT, Laptook AR, Garcia D, Ruley JI. Energy reserves and utilization rates in developing brain measured in vivo by 31p and 1H nuclear magnetic resonance spectroscopy. *J Cereb Blood Flow Metabol* 1993;13:235–246.

9. Lucas DR, Newhouse JP. The toxic effect of sodium-L-glutamate on the inner layers of retina. *AMA Arch Ophthalmol* 1957;58:193–201.

10. Olney JW. Brain lesions, obesity and other disturbances in mice treated with monosodium glutamate. *Science* 1969;164:719–721.

11. Siesjo BK, Bengtsson F. Calcium fluxes, calcium antagonists, and calcium-related pathology in brain ischemia, hypoglycemia, and spreading depression: A unifying hypothesis. *J Cereb Blood Flow Metabol* 1989;9:127–140.

12. Meldrum B. Excitatory amino acids and anoxic-ischemic brain damage. *Trends Neurosci* 1985;8:47–48.

13. Rothman SM, Olney JW. Glutamate and the pathophysiology of hypoxic-ischemic brain damage. *Ann Neurol* 1986;19:105–111.

14. Kirino T. Delayed neuronal death in the gerbil hippocampus following ischemia. *Brain Res* 1982;239:57–69.

15. Pulsinelli WA, Brierley JB, Plum F. Temporal profile of neuronal damage in a model of transient forebrain ischemia. *Ann Neurol* 1982;11:491–498.

16. Hattori H, Wasterlain CG. Posthypoxic glucose supplementation reduces hypoxic-ischemic brain damage in the neonatal rat. *Ann Neurol* 1990;28:122–128.

17. Johns RA. EDRF/nitric oxide. The endogenous nitrovasodilator and a new cellular messenger. *Anesthesiology* 1991;75:927–931.

18. Dawson TM, Dawson VL, Snyder SH. A novel neuronal molecular messenger in brain: The free radical, nitric oxide. *Ann Neurol* 1992;32:297–311.

19. Nowicki JP, Duval D, Poignet H, Scatton B. Nitric oxide mediates neuronal death after focal cerebral ischemia in the mouse. *Eur J Pharmacol* 1991;204:339–340.

20. Nagafuji T, Matsui T, Koide T, Asano T. Blockade of nitric oxide formation by N-omega-nitro-L-arginine mitigates ischemic brain edema and subsequent cerebral infarction in rats. *Neurosci Lett* 1992;147:159–162.

21. Trifiletti RR. Neuroprotective effects of NG-nitro-L-arginine in focal stroke in the 7-day old rat. *Eur J Pharmacol* 1992;218:197–198.

22. Hamada Y, Hayakawa H, Hattori H, Mikawa H. Inhibitor of nitric oxide synthesis reduces hypoxic-ischemic brain damage in the neonatal rat. *Pediatr Res* 1994;35:10–14.

23. Beckman JS, Beckman TW, Chen J, Marshall PA, Freeman BA. Apparent hydroxyl radical production by peroxynitrite: Implications for endothelial injury from nitric oxide and super oxide. *Proc Natl Acad Sci* 1990;87:1620–1624.

24. Molina y Vedia L, McDonald B, Reep B, Brune B, DiSilvio M, Billiar TR, Lapetina EG. Nitric oxide-induced S-nitrosylation of glyceraldehyde-3 phosphate dehydrogenase inhibits enzymatic activity and increases endogenous ADP-ribosylation. *J Biol Chem* 1992;267:24929–24932.

25. Granger DL, Lehninger AL. Sites of inhibition of mitochondrial electron transport in macrophage-induced neoplastic cells. *J Cell Biol* 1982;95:527–535.

26. Uematsu D, Greenberg JH, Reivich M, Karp A. Cytosolic free calcium and NAD/NADH redox state in the cat cortex during in vivo activation of NMDA receptors. *Brain Res* 1989;482:129–135.

27. Katayama Y, Kawamata T, Kano T, Tsubokawa T. Excitatory amino acid antagonist administered via microdialysis attenuates lactate accumulation during cerebral ischemia and subsequent hippocampal damage. *Brain Res* 1992;584: 329–333.

28. Novelli A, Reilly JA, Lysko PG, Henneberry RC. Glutamate becomes neurotoxic via the N-methyl-D-aspartate receptor when intracellular energy levels are reduced. *Brain Res* 1988;451:205–212.

29. Simon R, Shiraishi K. D-methyl-D-aspartate antagonist reduces stroke size and regional glucose metabolism. *Ann Neurol* 1990;27:606–611.

30. Shimizu H, Graham SH, Chang LH, Mintorovitch J, James TL, Faden AI, Weinstein PR. Relationship between extracellular neurotransmitter amino acids and energy metabolism during cerebral ischemia in rats monitored by microdialysis and in vivo magnetic resonance spectroscopy. *Brain Res* 1993;605:33–42.

31. Hattori H, Morin AM, Schwartz PH, Fujikawa DG, Wasterlain CG. Post-hypoxic treatment with MK-801 reduces hypoxic-ischemic damage in the neonatal rat. *Neurology* 1989;39:713–718.

32. Palmer C, Towfighi J, Roberts RL, Heitjan DF. Allopurinol administered after inducing hypoxia-ischemia reduces brain injury in 7-day-old rats. *Pediatr Res* 1993;33:405–411.

33. Thordstein M, Bagenholm R, Thiringer K, Kjellmer I. Scavengers of free oxygen radicals in combination with magnesium ameliorate perinatal hypoxic-ischemic brain damage in the rat. *Pediatr Res* 1993;34:23–26.

34. McCord JM. Oxygen-derived free radicals in postischemic tissue injury. *N Engl J Med* 1985;312:159–163.

35. Palmer C, Vannucci RC. Potential new therapies for perinatal cerebral hypoxia-ischemia. *Clin Perinatol* 1993;20:411–432.

36. Mott JC. The ability of young mammals to withstand total oxygen lack. *Br Med Bull* 1961;17:144–148.

37. Daniel SS, Dawes GS, James LS, Ross RB, Windle WF. Hypothermia and the resuscitation of the asphyxiated fetal rhesus monkeys. *J Pediatr* 1966;68:45–53.

38. Heideger PM, Miller FS, Miller JA. Cerebral and cardiac enzymatic activity and tolerance to asphyxia during maturation in the rabbit. *J Physiol* 1970;206:25–40.

39. Young RS, Olenginski TP, Yagel SK, Towfighi J. The effect of graded hypothermia on hypoxic-ischemic brain damage: A neuropathologic study in the neonatal rat. *Stroke* 1983;14:929–934.

40. Busto R, Dietrich WD, Globus MY-T, Valdes I, Scheinberg P, Ginsberg MD. Small differences in intra-ischemic brain temperature critically determine the extent of ischemic neuronal injury. *J Cereb Blood Flow Metabol* 1987;7:729–738.

41. Busto R, Globus MY, Dietrich WD, Martinez E, Valdes I, Ginsberg MD. Effect of mild hypothermia on ischemia induced release of neurotransmitters and free fatty acids in rat brain. *Stroke* 1989;20:904–910.

42. Buchan A, Pulsinelli WA. Hypothermia but not the N-methyl-D-aspartate antagonist MK-801, attenuates neuronal damage in gerbils subjected to transient global ischemia. *J Neurosci* 1990;10:311–316.

43. Yager J, Towfighi J, Vannucci RC. Influence of mild hypothermia on hypoxic-ischemic brain damage in the immature rat. *Pediatr Res* 1993;34:525–529.
44. Towfighi J, Housman C, Heitjan DF, Vannucci RC, Yager JY. The effect of focal cerebral cooling on perinatal hypoxic-ischemic brain damage. *Acta Neuropathol* 1994;65:108–118.
45. Astrup J, Sorensen PM, Sorensen HR. Inhibition of cerebral oxygen and glucose consumption in the dog by hypothermia, pentobarbital and lidocaine. *Anesthesiology* 1981;55:263–268.
46. Steen PA, Newberg L, Milde JH, Michenfelder JD. Hypothermia and barbiturates: Individual and combined effects on canine cerebral oxygen consumption. *Anesthesiology* 1983;58:527–532.
47. Palmer C, Vannucci RC, Christensen MA, Brucklacher RM. Regional cerebral blood flow and glucose utilization during hypothermia in newborn dogs. *Anesthesiology* 1989;71:730–737.
48. Vannucci RC, Plum F. Pathophysiology of perinatal cerebral hypoxia-ischemia. In Gaull E (ed.), *Biology of brain dysfunction.* New York: Plenum Press, 1975, pp. 1–45.
49. Vannucci RC. Vulnerability of the immature brain to hypoxia-ischemia. In *Cold Spring Harbor Symposium, Banbury Report 11: Environmental effects of maturation.* Cold Spring Harbor, NY: Cold Spring Harbor Laboratory, 1982, pp. 2691–2698.
50. McDougal DB, Holowach J, Howe MC, Jones EM, Thomas CA. The effect of anoxia upon energy sources and selected metabolic intermediates in the brains of fish, frog and turtle. *J Neurochem* 1968;15:577–588.

CHAPTER 15

Endothelial and White Cell Activation in Bypass and Reperfusion Injury: Brain Injury

Paul R. Hickey

The role of endothelial and leukocyte adhesion molecules in the vascular damage and subsequent organ dysfunction related to cardiopulmonary bypass is an emerging area of interest that is based on the intense and continuing basic discoveries in the area of cellular adhesion research. The bulk of these discoveries has been made in the past decade as molecular biology has come of age. It is clear that adhesion between cells controls many aspects of cellular function and response. In the area of the inflammatory response, adhesive interactions between formed elements of the blood and the endothelium play a large, if not a dominant, role in modulating the subsequent inflammatory processes. Our increasingly sophisticated biotechnology industry is producing monoclonal antibodies that have significant potential for influencing these processes. The potential for the use of such monoclonal antibodies to prevent bypass-related vascular injury stemming from the inflammatory response to bypass and ischemia/reperfusion is now becoming clear. It is up to those of us interested in brain injury related to cardiac surgery in children to apply these discoveries to this field. Leukocyte and endothelial adhesion and subsequent activation underlie both the vascular injury resulting from extracorporeal circulation *per se* as well as that resulting from the ischemia and reperfusion that occur during bypass and circulatory arrest.

Bypass Vascular Injury

The pathophysiology of cardiopulmonary bypass has been characterized as a generalized vascular injury and subsequent inflammatory response; this

215

results in endothelial dysfunction, increased microvascular permeability, and other, poorly characterized microcirculatory disturbances.[1-3] This vascular injury results ultimately in varying degrees of dysfunction in vital organs. Clinical studies have demonstrated disturbances in the cerebral circulation following cardiopulmonary bypass and circulatory arrest in children. It is likely that such disturbances in the cerebral circulation resulting from bypass and circulatory arrest are related to vascular injury, inflammatory responses, and endothelial dysfunction in the cerebral microcirculation. Such injury may well underlie a substantial proportion of the brain injury resulting from pediatric cardiac surgery.

Accumulated evidence shows that exposure of blood to abnormal surfaces and conditions during bypass results in systemic activation of the complement, coagulation, and kallikrein-kinen cascades; activation of leukocytes and platelets; and accumulation of activated leukocytes in the microcirculation. Leukocytes accumulated in target organs at least partially mediate the endothelial injury and inflammation seen, particularly in the microcirculation. Complement is initially activated during cardiopulmonary bypass by the alternate pathway, resulting in the release of anaphylatoxins C3a and C5a.[4] High levels of C3a during bypass are associated with increased morbidity in a variety of vital organs, including heart, lung, brain, and kidney.[5] Specific binding sites have been demonstrated on neutrophils for C5a;[6] another product of the cleavage of C5, C5b-9 complex, binds to neutrophils during cardiopulmonary bypass and also promotes activation.[7] These events stimulate leukocyte shape changes and decreased cellular deformability. These changes, together with leukocyte aggregation and adherence, all contribute to sequestration of leukocytes during and after bypass in the microcirculation of organ beds. Activation, adherence, and accumulation of leukocytes in the microcirculation all have been demonstrated to accompany cardiopulmonary bypass.[4,8-10] Circulation of blood through extracorporeal circuits *in vitro*, where organ beds and potential ischemic-reperfusion stimuli are not factors, still results in neutrophil activation.[9,11]

Events immediately following cardiopulmonary bypass may also contribute to mechanisms of injury involving leukocyte/endothelial adhesion molecules. After bypass, protamine administration for reversal of heparin anticoagulation further activates the complement system by the classical pathway.[12] Such heparin-protamine interactions in humans have been shown to immediately increase plasma levels of C3a and C4a, confirming the occurrence of nonimmunological complement activation *following* clinical cardiopulmonary bypass.[13,14] In sheep, such heparin-protamine interaction has resulted in profound leukopenia and transpulmonary leukosequestration, along with increases in C3a plasma levels,[15] and in man, transient leukopenia, predominantly in granulocytes. Thus even after bypass is completed, further activation of complement and leukocytes may occur, with protamine administration resulting in yet additional accumulation of leukocytes in the microcirculation.

Release of C5a and kallikrein, and contact with plastic, nonendothelial surfaces during bypass stimulate and activate leukocytes by promoting expression of a variety of leukocyte surface adhesion molecules including Mac-1 (CD11b/CD18).[16] Subsequent adherence to specific endothelial ligands plays a role in localization of leukocytes in specific vascular beds in poorly understood ways and also appears to result in secretory functions by the leukocyte. Leukocyte proteases are released, oxygen free radicals are generated, and other cytotoxic mediators are produced when neutrophil-endothelial adherence occurs, as well as when stimulated neutrophils adhere to protein-coated plastic surfaces such as those found in extracorporeal circuits.[17,18] Close adherence between neutrophil and endothelium may create microenvironments wherein high concentrations of proteases and oxygen free radicals are protected from circulating free radical scavengers and antiproteases. During and after cardiopulmonary bypass, circulating levels of elastase, myeloperoxidase, superoxide, and lactoferrin are increased, presumably due to ongoing leukocyte activation, adherence, and secretory activity.[10,19,20] Levels of interleukin-1 are also increased with cardiopulmonary bypass.[21] Interleukin-1 is a cytokine known to upregulate an important endothelial ligand (ICAM-1) for leukocyte adhesion molecules in inflammatory processes other than bypass.[22] Taken together, this entire body of work suggests strongly that leukocytes and leukocyte-mediated processes at the endothelium play key roles in bypass-related vascular injury.

Leukocyte/Endothelial Adhesion in Inflammation and Bypass

Another substantial body of work has demonstrated that leukocyte adhesion molecules, in combination with their endothelial ligand receptors, play a key role in a wide variety of inflammatory processes. Briefly, this work shows that after stimulation by cytokines and complement, leukocytes are activated, marginate, and adhere progressively more intimately to endothelium in the microcirculation. Eventually the leukocytes adhere firmly, damaging endothelium and migrating through the endothelium into the tissues where leukocyte-mediated damage progresses. On the endothelial surface a variety of selectin proteins, such as CD62 and ELAM-1, and other carbohydrate ligands are expressed and are thought to play major roles in the attachment of activated leukocytes, particularly neutrophils, during shear flow. Initial interaction of endothelial surface ligands with leukocyte adhesion molecules such as LAM-1, even in unactivated leukocytes, results in rolling of marginated leukocytes along the endothelial surface, upregulation of other leukocyte adhesion molecules such as Mac-1, and subsequent shedding of the LAM-1 molecule.[23] Further interaction of upregulated adhesion molecules Mac-1 and LFA-1 on activated leukocytes with Ig-family-related endothelial surface ligands ICAM-1 and ICAM-2 are thought to strengthen leukocyte adhesion, triggering subsequent endothelial injury and eventually leading to transendothelial migration of leukocytes into the tissues and direct tissue injury. In the case of the brain, these processes should cause substantial disruption of the blood-brain barrier, and indeed there is substantial experimental and clinical evidence that the blood-brain barrier function is disrupted as a result of cardiopulmonary bypass.

The role of specific leukocyte surface adhesion molecules, Mac-1, LFA-1, and LAM-1 or lymphocyte-specific adhesion molecules, such as VLA-4, in these processes as they occur during and after cardiopulmonary bypass has not been investigated. Correspondingly, on the endothelial side, the role of a variety of leukocyte adhesion molecule ligands, such as the selectins CD62 and ELAM-1, and the Ig-family-related molecules ICAM-1 and ICAM-2 in bypass-related vascular and organ damage has not been investigated. Likewise unknown is the possible role of another Ig-family-related endothelial adhesion molecule, VCAM-1, which appears to be specific for lymphocyte endothelial adhesion.

The role of CD62, an endothelial selectin protein, in bypass-related vascular damage may be particularly important because it is an adhesion molecule found in platelets as well as on the endothelium. Blood contact with nonendothelial surfaces, as occurs during cardiopulmonary bypass, leads to CD62 expression on the platelet surface, as well as CD18 expression on leukocytes, leading to aggregation and other neutrophil/platelet amplifying interactions such as leukotriene transcellular synthesis. Synthesis and release of known chemoattractants such as leukotrienes promote further neutrophil activation and attraction. Platelets are known to be activated during clinical cardiopulmonary bypass; the percentage of platelets expressing CD62 (GMP-140) has been recently shown to increase progressively during bypass in humans.[24] As platelet activation increases on bypass, the absolute platelet numbers and percentage of aggregated platelets both decrease, reaching a nadir at 2 to 4 hours after bypass when neutrophil accumulation in postischemic, reperfused tissue reaches a maximum. These events suggest progressive deposition of aggregated platelets and leukocytes in the microcirculation during and after bypass. At the same time, CD62 stored within endothelial cells is rapidly mobilized to the endothelial surface by a variety of stimuli including thrombin.[25] Thrombin is formed during bypass by activation of the coagulation cascade; microcoagulation occurs during bypass even in the presence of adequate heparin levels[26] and may lead to continued endothelial CD62 expression. Thus the adhesion molecule CD62 may contribute to both endothelial adhesion and platelet adhesion during cardiopulmonary bypass, leading to the plugging of vessels by platelet/leukocyte aggregates and subsequent "no reflow" phenomenon following reperfusion. This mechanism of damage might augment the probable role of CD62 in initial "rolling" adherence of neutrophils and its subsequent consequences: neutrophil attachment, endothelial damage, and transendothelial migration. During cardiopulmonary bypass there is abundant evidence of systemic activation of both complement and platelets, and it is likely that such activation plays a substantial role in subsequent vascular damage in the brain and other organs that occurs with cardiopulmonary bypass.

Ischemia/Reperfusion Injury During Cardiopulmonary Bypass

In addition to damage and leukocyte/endothelial interactions triggered by extracorporeal circulation *per se*, both the pulmonary circulation and the coronary circulation are made deliberately ischemic and are subsequently reperfused during clinical cardiopulmonary bypass. Deliberate, hypothermic ischemia with subsequent reperfusion is used routinely during clinical cardiopulmonary bypass in specific organ beds and, as total circulatory arrest, in the entire body including the brain. Some damaging effects of bypass are certainly related to ischemia and reperfusion. The most frequent sites of bypass-related damage are those organs frequently made ischemic during bypass, the lung and the heart.[5] Leukocyte and endothelial interactions, mediated by adhesion molecules, are now known to play a large role in ischemic/reperfusion injury.[27] Abundant evidence documents the role of leukocytes in myocardial ischemia/reperfusion injury.[28–31] Experimental myocardial reperfusion injury has been reduced by the use of two monoclonal antibodies that inhibit leukocyte adhesion, anti-CD11b[32] and anti-CD18 (components of Mac-1),[33] and also by leukocyte depletion.[21]

Ischemia and reperfusion also routinely occur in the pulmonary circulation during clinical bypass; damaging effects of CPB are frequently seen in the lung.[1] Leukocyte depletion has been shown to ameliorate such bypass-related lung injury seen with cardiopulmonary bypass.[34] Lung injury follows ischemia and reperfusion in the lung despite the ready availability of alveolar oxygen to the pulmonary microcirculation. Such reperfusion lung injury in animals subjected to pulmonary ischemia without bypass can be reduced by decreasing leukocyte adhesion with anti-CD18.[35,36] Extensive leukosequestration in the lung commonly occurs during bypass with subsequent reperfusion of the ischemic pulmonary circulation,[4] and leukocyte-mediated endothelial damage in the pulmonary microcirculation is a major component of lung injury.[37–40] After sequestration of activated leukocytes in pulmonary vessels, electron microscopy shows large numbers of neutrophils in close contact with pulmonary endothelium, together with focal destruction of endothelial cells and basement membrane of pulmonary capillaries.[41]

Total Circulatory Arrest

When total circulatory arrest techniques are used during bypass, all organs, including the brain, are subjected to ischemia/reperfusion and potential subsequent damage. Leukocytes, and increased leukocyte adhesiveness, have been shown to be important in the development of microvascular injury and tissue injury following warm ischemia and reperfusion in tissues as diffuse as those in the ear,[42] lungs,[43,44] liver, kidney,[45] gastrointestinal mucosa,[46] skeletal muscle,[47,48] heart,[28,30–33] and the central nervous system.[49] In these tissues, neutrophil adherence to the vascular endothelium appears to be essential in the postischemic microvascular dysfunction that occurs, possibly contributing to the simple mechanical plugging of capillaries that occurs in the no-reflow phenomenon found in virtually all reperfused organs, particularly in the brain, after ischemic injury including hypothermic circulatory arrest. Adherence of activated, nondeformable leukocytes to capillary endothelium and adherence of aggregations of activated leukocytes and platelets in larger arterioles and venules are likely to account for the no-reflow. It is unclear to what extent simple mechanical plugging of the microcirculation by leukocytes,[50] direct endothelial injury,[51] or more complex leukocyte-mediated damage in tissues after transendothelial migration is responsible for tissue damage. Either depletion of neutrophils[28,34] or inhibition of leukocyte adherence (by using a monoclonal blocking antibody directed against leukocyte adhesion molecule CD18[33,52] or CD11b[32]) effectively reduced ischemia/reperfusion injuries in virtually all tissues studied, including the central nervous system.[49]

Despite the potential for bypass-related amplification or alteration of these adhesive injury mechanisms with ischemia and reperfusion, the role of adhesion molecules in bypass-related ischemia/reperfusion injury has not been studied. It is now unclear how much of bypass-related vascular injury is due to extracorporeal circulation and how much is due to ischemia/reperfusion. Studies of adhesion molecules in ischemia and reperfusion injury during cardiopulmonary bypass are clearly needed because of the potential amplifying or modifying influence of the systemic activation of complement and platelets during bypass.

The Effects of Hypothermia on Adhesion
Molecules and Interactions

Because hypothermia is protective against ischemic/reperfusion injury and bypass-related organ injury, clinical cardiopulmonary bypass is frequently used in conjunction with hypothermia. When total circulatory arrest techniques are used, profound degrees of hypothermia are employed approaching 10°C in some cases. The effect of hypothermia on leukocyte and endothelial adhesion molecules and their interactions is unknown, particularly with regard to those interactions occurring during cardiopulmonary bypass and those related to ischemia and reperfusion. Preliminary work, outlined below, has demonstrated that blocking leukocyte adhesion molecules in the setting of hypothermic cardiopulmonary bypass with circulatory arrest will reduce injury in a variety of organs.

Current Studies

Preliminary studies suggest that monoclonal antibodies against one leukocyte adhesion molecule, CD18, can prevent organ dysfunction in a whole-body bypass model of hypothermic total circulatory arrest.[53] These pilot studies are the initial demonstration that monoclonal antibodies against leukocyte adhesion molecules are effective against *hypothermic* ischemia and reperfusion injury in the setting of systemic activation of complement and platelets with cardiopulmonary bypass. The role of leukocyte and endothelial adhesion molecules in vascular injury associated with cardiopulmonary bypass and circulatory arrest have not been widely investigated despite the abundant evidence outlined above that interactions between activated complement, platelets, leukocytes, and endothelium are likely to be key components in the vascular injury and organ damage seen with cardiopulmonary bypass.

Model and Methods

These recent studies utilized a cardiopulmonary bypass and circulatory arrest model in the neonatal pig and have demonstrated the feasibility of attenuating the deleterious effects of cardiopulmonary bypass with a monoclonal antibody directed against the leukocyte cell adhesion glycoprotein CD18. In this model, an anesthetized neonatal piglet undergoes sternotomy and is placed on cardiopulmonary bypass. Intracardiac monitoring catheters and sampling catheters are placed together with flow probes around the aorta and carotid trunk to measure blood flow, and radioactive microsphere injections at timed intervals are used to measure regional blood flows. Control measurements are taken and repeated after warm cardiopulmonary bypass is instituted. The animal is core-cooled to 20°C and the entire circulation arrested for 1 hour. Repeat flow and metabolic measurements during reperfusion on bypass are taken periodically as the animal is warmed to 37°C. The animal is then maintained on warm cardiopulmonary bypass for 3 hours with hourly measurements. After 3½ hours of bypass following reperfusion, the animal is sacrificed.

The control group of 8 piglets received no treatment (Group C); the treatment group of 9 piglets (Group MAb) received anti-CD18 monoclonal antibody (Robert Rothlein, Bohringer Ingelheim) in a concentration of 20ug/mL of estimated total circulating blood volume on bypass. Simple measures of the integrity of the microcirculation and of organ function were used to compare bypass and hypothermic circulatory arrest-related damage between anti-CD18 treated and untreated groups. Preliminary res
ults in this small group of animals indicate considerable potential for this therapeutic approach to the prevention of damage from clinical bypass and circulatory arrest.

Results

As would be expected with activation and leukosequestration of white cells as a result of cardiopulmonary bypass and circulatory arrest, total white blood cell count and neutrophil count decreased significantly after initiation of CPB in group C, whereas the decrease was substantially less in group MAb (p<.05). The platelet count also decreased after CPB, but there was no difference between the two groups, as would be expected with this particular monoclonal antibody which blocks an adhesion receptor not present on platelets.

Body weight gain during bypass is a substantial clinical problem during cardiopulmonary bypass, particularly in infants. Weight gain during bypass is thought to be related to microvascular damage and subsequent increases in endothelial permeability resulting from leukocyte activation, adhesion, and secretory activity. In our studies, the relative mean changes in body weight (expressed as %) at the conclusion of bypass was less in group MAb (24.6±2.1%) than in group C (36.8±4.6%)(p=.03). Likewise, water content of the heart and the lungs at the end of the experiment was significantly less in group MAb than in group C (p<.05). However, there were no significant differences between the groups in the water content in the brain or in other organs tested.

Endothelial function was assessed by using an endothelium-dependent vasodilator, acetylcholine (ACh) and an endothelium-independent vasodilator, nitroglycerine (TNG). There was no difference between groups in either ACh or TNG vasodilation response at 10 minutes of initial normothermic CPB in either the systemic or the carotid circulation. However, carotid vasodilation response to ACh was more pronounced in group MAb than group C at 60 minutes after reperfusion, and systemic response to ACh was better in group MAb than group C at 230 minutes of reperfusion (p<.05). Vasodilator responses to TNG in the two groups were no different at any time. These results suggest that in the carotid circulation, as well as in the whole body circulation, pretreatment with a monoclonal antibody better preserves endothelial function and prevents at least some endothelial damage.

Regional vascular resistance was calculated from regional blood flow (mL/min/100g tissue) and mean systemic blood pressure(mmHg) assuming a venous pressure of zero, expressed in mmHg/mL/min/100g tissue. The vascular resistance was lower in group MAb in the brain at 5 minutes of reperfusion (group C: 2.34±0.30 vs group MAb: 1.48±0.12), and in the renal cortex at 225 minutes of reperfusion (group C: 0.70±0.07 vs group MAb: 0.50±0.04) (p<.05). By considering the values at 20 minutes after initiation of CPB as the bypass baseline, subsequent changes in regional vascular resistance were calculated as percent change in vascular resistance during the time course of the experiment. There was less elevation of vascular resistance at 5 minutes of reperfusion in the brain (group C: 197±20% vs group MAb: 122±8%) and the liver (group C: 138±13% vs group MAb: 96±10%); at 5 minutes and 45 minutes of reperfusion in the heart (group C: 44±5% vs group MAb: 30±3%, group C: 72±11% vs group MAb: 44±5%, respectively); at 225 minutes of reperfusion in the renal cortex (group C: 224±21% vs group MAb: 148±16%); and at 5 minutes and 225 minutes of reperfusion in the intestine (group C: 60±7% vs group MAb: 41±6%) (p<.05).

Regional Blood Flow in the Brain

The regional blood flow in the brain showed differences between the two groups, but this varied among the different brain regions examined.[53] The basal ganglia, midbrain, and brainstem (pons and medulla oblongata) had a transient hyperemia at 5 minutes of reperfusion (greater flow compared with the flow prior to circulatory arrest during hypothermia and compared with the flow at 45 minutes of reperfusion). The MAb group showed greater blood flow to the basal ganglia and midbrain during hypothermia (58.3±8.1 vs 35.4±5.2 mL/min/100g tissue, p=.01 and 34.1± 4.8 vs 20.4±2.7 mL/min/100g tissue, p=.04, respectively) and at normothermic reperfusion (40.3±2.6 vs 32.7±1.4 mL/min/100g tissue, p=.03). At 5 minutes of reperfusion the MAb group showed better regional blood flow in the brainstem, basal ganglia, and the midbrain (108.9±12.1 vs 67.7± 12.0 mL/min/100g tissue, p=.03; 56.6±6.3 vs 35.6±7.6 mL/min/100g tissue, p=.05; 80.8±10.7 vs 50.4±8.4 mL/min/100g tissue, p=.05, respectively). No differences were apparent between groups in the cortex of the cerebral hemispheres.

In view of problems with choreoathetosis that are reported sporadically in children undergoing cardiac surgery, where lesions in the basal ganglia are thought to be responsible for the clinical picture seen, these regional alterations in cerebral blood flow are of particular interest. In particular, the apparent effect of monoclonal antibody treatment in improving cerebral blood flow early in the reperfusion period in the subcortical brain structures is intriguing in this regard.

Significance

The data obtained in these preliminary studies are consistent with progressive endothelial injury and dysfunction, which are prevented by blocking leukocyte adhesion with anti-CD18. The time course of this developing endothelial dysfunction, as reflected in the systemic response to acetylcholine, is more prolonged than the response reported by Lefer and colleagues that occurs within minutes in normothermic animals.[54,55] However, it is probable that hypothermia in the piglets we studied prevented the early endothelial injury seen in the normothermic ischemia/reperfusion studies of Lefer and colleagues. The time course of the endothelial dysfunction with reperfusion in the piglets was more consistent with the accumulation of neutrophils at 3 hours reported in the Lefer, and other, studies.[30,31] These data suggest that endothelial injury after hypothermic circulatory arrest on bypass may be delayed and may result from a different mechanism than that seen in normothermic ischemia/reperfusion. During and after cardiopulmonary bypass there is continued production of activated neutrophils, complement, and platelets, providing a continuing source of potential mediators of endothelial damage. Even though the immediate endothelial injury seen in normothermic studies was apparently largely prevented in both the control and treated groups by hypothermia, anti-CD18 treatment probably prevented progressive late endothelial damage during continued reperfusion by the extracorporeal circuit.

Data from these initial studies, although only suggestive and preliminary, when taken together with the persuasive body of clinical and experimental evidence of mechanisms of function, provide a strong argument that a variety of leukocyte and endothelial adhesion molecules play critical, but poorly understood, roles in the cerebrovascular injury associated with cardiopulmonary bypass and circulatory arrest in children. This field is currently exploding in the basic science area as new adhesion receptors on white cells, platelets, endothelium, and tissue cells in organs are discovered and their roles are explored. The role of a variety of cytokines in promoting expression of such adhesion receptors is becoming progressively apparent, further complicating the picture. What ultimate picture will emerge of the role of these mechanisms in vascular and tissue damage in the brain as well as in other organs is certainly unclear. However, work in these areas has much to contribute to our knowledge of brain injury during pediatric cardiac surgery. There is promise of therapeutic avenues coming out of this work, and these may eventually have substantial impact on the clinical problem of brain injury associated with pediatric cardiac surgery.

References

1. Kirklin JK. Prospects for understanding and eliminating the deleterious effect of cardiopulmonary bypass. *Ann Thorac Surg* 1991;51:529–531.
2. Smith EEJ, Naftel DC, Blackstone EH, Kirklin JW. Microvascular permeability after cardiopulmonary bypass. *J Thorac Cardiovasc Surg* 1987;94:225–233.
3. Kirklin JW. The postperfusion syndrome: Inflammation and the damaging effects of cardiopulmonary bypass. In John Tinker (ed.), *Cardiopulmonary bypass: Current concepts and controversies.* Monograph. Philadelphia: Saunders, 1989: pp. 131–146.
4. Chenoweth DE, Cooper SW, Hugli TE, et al. Complement activation during cardiopulmonary bypass. Evidence for generation of C3a and C5a anaphylatoxins. *N Engl J Med* 1981;304:497–403.
5. Kirklin JK, Westaby S, Blackson EH, et al. Complement and damaging effects of cardiopulmonary bypass. *J Thorac Cardiovasc Surg* 1983;86:845–857.
6. Chenoweth DE, Hugli TE. Demonstration of specific C5a receptor on intact human polymorphonuclear leukocytes. *Proc Natl Acad Sci USA* 1978; 753943–753947.
7. Salama A, Hugo F, Heinrich D, et al. Deposition of terminal C5b-9 complement complexes on erythrocytes and leukocytes during cardiopulmonary bypass. *N Engl J Med* 1988;318:408–414.
8. Unarska M, Robinson GB. Adherence of human leukocytes to synthetic polymeric surfaces. *Life Support Syst* 1987;5:283–292.
9. Colman RW. Platelet and neutrophil activation in cardiopulmonary bypass. *Ann Thorac Surg* 1990;49:32–34.

10. Faymonvile ME, Pincemail J, Duchateau J, et al. Myeloperoxidase and elastase as markers of leukocyte activation during cardiopulmonary bypass in humans. *J Thorac Cardiovasc Surg* 1991;102:309–317.

11. Wachtfogel YT, Kuici U, Greenplate J, et al. Human neutrophil degranulation during extracorporeal circulation. *Blood* 1987;69:324–330.

12. Rent R, Ertel N, Eisenstein R, Gewurz H. Complement activation by interaction of polyanions and polycations: I, Heparin-protamine induced consumption of platelet. *J Immunol* 1975;114:120–124.

13. Cavarocchi NC, Schaff HV, Orszulak TA. Evidence for complement activation by protamine-heparin interaction after cardiopulmonary bypass. *Surgery* 1985; 98:525–530.

14. Kirklin JK, Chenoweth DE, Naftel DC, et al. Effects of protamine administration after cardiopulmonary bypass on complement, blood elements, and hemodynamic state. *Ann Thorac Surg* 1986;41:193–199.

15. Morel DR, Lowenstein E, Nguyenduy T, Robinson DR, Repine JE, Chenoweth DE, Zapol WM. Acute pulmonary vasoconstriction and thromboxane release during protamine reversal of heparin anticoagulation in awake sheep. *Circ Res* 1988;62:905–912.

16. Anderson DC, Miller LJ, Schmalstieg FC, Rothlein R, Springer TA. Contributions of the Mac-1 glycoprotein family to adherence-dependent granulocyte structure-function assessment employing subunit-specific monoclonal antibodies. *J Immunol* 1986;137:15–27.

17. Smedly LA, Tonnesen MG, Sandhaus RA, et al. Neutrophil mediated injury to endothelial cells: Enhancement by endotoxin and essential role of neutrophil elastase. *J Clin Invest* 1986;77:1233–1243.

18. Shappell SB, Toman C, Anderson DC, Taylor AA, Entman ML, Smith CW. Mac-1(CD11b/CD18) mediates adherence-dependent hydrogen peroxide production by human and canine neutrophils. *J Immunol* 1990;144:2702–2711.

19. Stahl RF, Fisher CA, Kucich U, et al. Effects of simulated extracorporeal circulation on human leukocyte elastase release, superoxide generation, and procoagulant activity. *J Thorac Cardiovasc Surg* 1991;101:230–239

20. Riegel W, Spillner G, Schlosser V, Horl WH. Plasma levels of main granulocyte components during cardiopulmonary bypass. *J Thorac Cardiovasc Surg* 1988; 95:1014–1019.

21. Haeffner-Cavaillon N, Roussellier N, et al. Induction of interleukin-1 production in patients undergoing cardiopulmonary bypass. *J Thorac Cardiovasc Surg* 1989;98:1100–1106.

22. Smith CW, Marlin SD, Rothlein R, Toman C, Anderson DC. Cooperative interactions of LFA-1 and Mac-1 with intercellular adhesion molecule-1 in facilitating adherence and transendothelial migration of human neutrophils in vitro. *J Clin Invest* 1989;83:2008–2017.

23. Griffin JD, Spertini O, Ernst TJ, et al. Granulocyte-macrophage colony-stimulating factor and other cytokines regulate surface expression of the leukocyte adhesion molecule-1 on human neutrophils, monocytes, and their precursors. *J Immunol* 1990;145:576–584.

24. Rinder CS, Bohnert J, Rinder HM, et al. Platelet activation and aggregation during cardiopulmonary bypass.*Anesthesiology* 1991;75:388–393.

25. Hattori R, Hamilton KK, McEver RP, Sims PJ. Complement proteins C5b-9 induce vesiculation of the endothelial membrane and expose catalytic surfaces. *J Biol Chem* 1989;26:9053–9060.

26. Kirklin JW, Barratt-Boyes BG. *Cardiac surgery.* New York: John Wiley & Sons, 1986, p. 55.
27. Harlan JM, Winn RK, Vedder NB, Doerschuk CM, Rice CL. In vivo models of leukocyte adherence to endothelium. In Harlan JM, Liu D (eds.), *Adhesion: Its role in inflammatory disease.* New York: Freeman, 1992, pp. 117–150.
28. Romson JL, et al. Reduction of the extent of ischemic myocardial injury by neutrophil depletion in dogs. *Circulation* 1983;67:1016.
29. Simpson PJ, et al. Reduction of experimental canine myocardial infarct size with prostaglandin E1 inhibition of neutrophil migration and activation. *J Pharmacol Exp Ther* 1988;244:619–624.
30. Engler RL, Dahlgren MD, Peterson MA, et al. Accumulation of polymorphonuclear leukocytes during 3-h experimental myocardial ischemia. *Am J Physiol* 1986;251:H93–100.
31. Smith EF III, Egan JW, Bugelski PJ, et al. Temporal relation between neutrophil accumulation and myocardial reperfusion injury. *Am J Physiol* 1988;255:H1060–1068.
32. Simpson PJ, et al. Reduction of experimental canine myocardial reperfusion injury by a monoclonal antibody (anti-Mo1, anti-CD11b) that inhibits leukocyte adhesion. *J Clin Invest* 1988;81:624–629.
33. Ma X-L, Johnson G III, Tsao PS, Lefer AM. Antibody to CD-18 β-chain preserves endothelium and myocardium in myocardial ischemia and reperfusion. *Circ* (Suppl) 1990;82:III–701 (abstract).
34. Bando K, Pillai R, Cameron DE, et al. Leukocyte depletion ameliorates free radical-mediated lung injury after cardiopulmonary bypass. *J Thorac Cardiovasc Surg* 1990;99:873–877.
35. Horgan MJ, Wright SD, Malik AB. Antibody against leukocyte integrin (CD18) prevents reperfusion induced lung vascular injury. *Am J Physiology* 1990;259:L315–319.
36. Bishop MJ, Kowalski TF, Guidotti SM, Harlan JM. *J Surg Research* 1991, in press.
37. Martin WJ. Neutrophils kill pulmonary endothelial cells by a hydrogen peroxide-dependent pathway: An in vitro model of neutrophil mediated lung injury. *Am Rev Respir Dis* 1981;130:209–214.
38. Sacks T, et al. Oxygen radical-mediated endothelial cell damage by complement-stimulated granulocytes: An in vivo model of immune vascular damage. *J Clin Invest* 1978;61:1161–1168.
39. Tvedten HW, Till GO, Ward PA. Mediators of lung injury in mice following systemic activation of complement. *Am J Pathol* 1985;H119:92–105.
40. Flick MR, Perel A, Staub NC. Leukocytes are required for increased lung microvascular permeability after microembolization in sheep. *Circ Res* 1981;48:344–349.
41. Weiss SJ, Ward PA. Immune complex-induced generation of oxygen metabolites by human neutrophils. *J Immunol* 1982;129:309–316.
42. Vedder NB, Winn RK, Rice CL, et al. Inhibition of leukocytes adherence by anti-CD18 monoclonal antibody attenuates reperfusion injury in the rabbit ear. *Proc Natl Acad Sci USA* 1990;87:2643–2646.
43. Johnson A, et al. Superoxide dismutase prevents the thrombin-induced increase in lung vascular permeability: Role of superoxide in mediating the alteration in lung fluid balance. *Circ Res* 1986;59:405–415.
44. Vedder NB, Winn RK, Rice CL, Chi EY, Arfors KE, Harlan JM. A monoclonal antibody to the adherence-promoting leukocyte glycoprotein, CD18 reduces organ

injury and improves survival from hemorrhagic shock and resuscitation in rabbits. *J Clin Invest* 1988;81:939–944.

45. Linas SL, Shanley PF, Whittemburg D, et al. Neutrophils accentuate ischemia-reperfusion injury in isolated perfused rat kidneys. *Am J Physiol* 1988;255: F728–735.

46. Goisham MB, Herandez LA, Granger DN. Xanthine oxidase and neutrophil infiltration in intestinal ischemia. *Am J Physiol* 1986;251:G567–575.

47. Korthuis RJ, Goisham MB, Granger DN. Leukocyte depletion attenuates vascular injury in postischemic skeletal muscle. *Am J Physiol* 1988;254:H823–834.

48. Carden DL, Smith JK, Korthuis RJ. Neutrophil-mediated microvascular dysfunction in postischemic canine skeletal muscle. Role of granulocyte adherence. *Circ Res* 1990;66:1436–1444.

49. Clark WM, Madden KP, Rothlein R, Zivin JA. Reduction of central nervous system ischemic injury in rabbits using leukocyte adhesion antibody treatment. *Stoke* 1991;22:877–83.

50. Schmid-Schonbein GW. Capillary plugging by granulocytes and the no-reflow phenomenon in the microcirculation. *Fed Proc* 1987;46:2397–2401.

51. Kloner R, Ganote CE, Jennings RB. The "no-reflow" phenomenon after temporary occlusion in the dog. *J Clin Invest* 1974;54:1496–1508.

52. Mileski WJ, Winn RK, Vedder NB, Pohlman TH, Harlan JH, Rice CL. Inhibition of CD-18 dependent neutrophil adherence reduces organ injury after hemorrhagic shock in primates. *Surgery* 1990;108:206–212.

53. Aoki N, Jonas RA, Namura F, Kawata H, Hickey PR. "Anti-CD18 Attenuates deleterious effects of cardiopulmonary bypass and hypothermic circulation arrest in piglets." *J. Card. Surg.* (1995), 10:407–417.

54. Lefer AM, Tsao PS, Lefer DJ, Ma X-L. Role of endothelial dysfunction in the pathogenesis of reperfusion injury after myocardial ischemia. *FASEB J* 1991;5: 2029–2034.

55. Tsao PS, Aoki N, Lefer DJ, Johnson G III, Lefer AM. Time course of endothelial dysfunction and myocardial injury during myocardial ischemia and reperfusion injury in the cat. *Circulation* 1990;82:1402–1412.

CHAPTER 16

Excitotoxicity and Nitric Oxide

Stuart A. Lipton

NMDA Receptor Antagonists As Neuroprotectants

In an earlier chapter Dr. Michael Johnston explained that a large portion of ischemic damage, and probably several other neurological diseases, is mediated by overexcitation of glutamate receptors. One of the predominant types of glutamate receptors involved is the N-methyl-D-aspartate (NMDA) receptor (Figure 16–1). It is an important receptor because the channel associated with the receptor is permeable not only to sodium, but also to calcium. If the receptor is excessively excited, the cell becomes overloaded with calcium. Then a series of processes can result, ending up initially with what John Olney has termed excitotoxicity, or neuronal injury, and then neuronal death. This chapter will further develop this theme.

Our strategy is to develop clinically tolerated antagonists to the NMDA receptor. There are many antagonists, some of which you read about in earlier chapters, but until very recently, none of them have been able to be tolerated by an adult, let alone by an infant. There are some drugs indicated for other reasons that are already on the market, but which are not available in the United States, that are actually quite potent and effective NMDA antagonists.

When glutamate and glycine bind to the NMDA receptor, the associated ion channel's gate swings open. Sodium and calcium pour in. However, there are various sites on the channel where we know substances can bind and modulate the activity of the channel. Memantine is a German drug used for Parkinson's disease. It is almost a familiar drug to physicians in the United States. It looks like amantadine, but amantadine is not quite potent enough. Memantine can clog the NMDA receptor-associated channel and prevent excessive Ca^{2+} influx at the NMDA receptor.

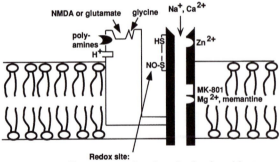

FIGURE 16–1. Schematic diagram of the NMDA receptor/channel complex. This subtype of glutamate receptor is stimulated by NMDA or glutamate. Glycine acts as a co-agonist. There are several modulatory sites that regulate the degree of cation (Na$^+$ and Ca^{2+}) influx. These modulatory sites include (a) the channel, where Mg^{2+} or various drugs, such as MK-801, phencyclidine, and memantine, bind; (b) a pH-sensitive region where H$^+$ exerts an effect; (c) a polyamine binding site; (d) a Zn^{2+} binding site; and (e) a redox site consisting of one or more thiol (–SH) groups, which may react with an oxidized congener of nitric oxide (supplied, for example, by nitroglycerin) and may facilitate disulfide bond formation. (Modified from Lipton SA, Rosenberg RA. Mechanisms of disease: Excitatory amino acids as a final common pathway in neurologic disorders. *N Engl J Med* 1994;330:613–622; and Lipton SA. Prospects for clinically-tolerated NMDA antagonists: Open-channel blockers and alternative redox states of nitric oxide. *Trends Neurosci* 1993;16: 527–532.)

Another drug that acts as an NMDA antagonist, surprisingly, is an old friend, nitroglycerin, which can bind to a sulfhydryl group on the NMDA receptor. It has been termed by our group a redox modulatory site because redox factors, namely, factors that give or take away electrons, can modulate this site. Oxidizing agents facilitate disulfide bond formation on the NMDA receptor/channel complex. This reaction decreases the opening frequency of the channel and limits the influx of calcium. Interestingly, it does not totally block the channel, so some function can continue. However, nitroglycerin prevents excessive excitation of the receptor, as manifested by too many openings of the channel.

Nitric Oxide and the NMDA Receptor

In order to really understand how these drugs work, it is necessary to understand the pathophysiology explaining why we think calcium can be bad, why we need to stop it, and how forms of nitroglycerin, which were previously thought to work through nitric oxide, work at a redox modulatory site.

Much of this work began in tissue culture experiments. How is this relevant to the infant brain? This work has recently been extended to animal models, but the reason to start in a culture dish is because it is simpler. We do not have to worry about blood vessel effects or about hypotension or hypertension. Using tissue culture, we can look directly at the neurons, the contiguous glial elements, and see how they are affected. Also there is very tight control over the various receptors on a neuron in a culture dish. We can electrically record from them with patch electrodes and thereby visualize the calcium influx into the neurons by an electrical measurement. We can apply various drugs by rapid perfusion techniques. That is why many of the experiments start out with this simple system. Then one can build upon this *in vitro* model to develop animal models.

When the NMDA receptor is excited by glutamate, calcium fluxes through the channel. This, in turn, activates a series of processes, one of which is the activation of nitric oxide synthase. However, there are many other enzymes that are turned on, and they are also potentially important in excitotoxicity. Although nitric oxide synthase might be involved in one of the neurotoxic systems, it is certainly not the only enzyme. There are various calcium-dependent enzymes, such as calpains, that can degrade proteins. Calcium can also activate endonucleases that degrade DNA and contribute to apoptosis and activate phospholipase A_2, which can eventually lead to the production of reactive oxygen species.

In Dr. Solomon Snyder's laboratory, Valina and Ted Dawson showed that at least one of the important components in neurotoxicity is the activation of the enzyme nitric oxide synthase because it is calcium-sensitive.[1,2] Calcium comes in and activates the enzyme, which produces nitric oxide (Figure 16–2). I have represented nitric oxide NO˙. The dot symbolizes one free electron, i.e., a free radical. The Snyder group postulated that NO˙ went on to mediate neurotoxicity. Further, they reasoned, if one could limit the production of nitric oxide, perhaps nerve cells could be protected.

In fact, workers in Dr. Snyder's laboratory and many other workers have considerable evidence for this hypothesis. Interestingly, the very same month that Dr. Snyder's paper was published, we found that forms of NO protected neurons. The findings seemed to create a paradox.

How could this be? This was clearly confusing. It turns out that quite a bit is known about the chemistry of NO because it is a component of smog. NO is one of the components besides carbon monoxide that is emitted as automobile exhaust. So our chemistry colleagues actually knew a great deal

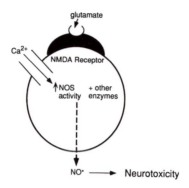

FIGURE 16–2. Model of activation of nitric oxide synthase
by NMDA receptor stimulation
and consequent Ca^{2+} influx.

about NO, dating back at least to the 1920s. In contrast, biologists knew relatively little about it.

Redox Modulation of the NMDA Receptor

To understand the actions of the NO moiety one has to review some chemistry. As you will see, the bottom line is that an old friend, nitroglycerin, can
actually be used to prevent damage mediated by excessive activation of the
NMDA receptor. First, we need to review the properties of the redox site of
the NMDA receptor because that is actually one of the sites where the NO
group can react (see Figure 16.1). This site modulates the activity of the
NMDA receptor and limits calcium influx. If a disulfide bond is formed at
this site, an oxidation reaction is produced. This limits the influx of calcium
by decreasing the opening frequency of the NMDA receptor-associated channel. This can protect neurons from Ca^{2+} mediated damage.

Conversely, a chemical reducing agent used to break a disulfide bond
results in two free –SH groups, or sulfhydryl or thiol groups. This causes the
channel to open more frequently, more calcium fluxes through, and more
neuronal injury results.[3,4] This is actually quite relevant because, as we have
known for over 20 years from the pioneering work of Raivich and Ginsberg
and others, during a stroke a chemically reducing state exists. Although we
worry about redox states for diabetic ketoacidosis, we don't worry about
them in ischemia, and we should. In a reducing state, a disulfide bond on the
NMDA receptor may break, resulting in more calcium influx and, consequently, more damage.

What does this mean in terms of the nerve cell? We began a quest for a mild oxidizing agent that would reform a disulfide bond and downregulate the activity of the NMDA receptor. We used everything on the shelf that ended in oxide, figuring it was an oxidizing agent. Eventually, we got to nitric oxide.

Nitric oxide is thought to be a neurotransmitter. It is involved in several activities that are important to all of us: learning and memory, penile erection, vascular relaxation, and various other important functions. However, we have been interested in NO because of the finding that we can protect neurons with certain redox-related forms of the NO group.

Several of the drugs we give to patients every day have nitric oxide embedded in them. I will only mention three or four of these drugs, although there are another half dozen NO donors that we use.

One is S-nitrosocysteine, which is comprised of NO coupled to the amino acid cysteine. When NO is liberated, two cysteines react together to form cystine. Control experiments are therefore performed with cystine. If cystine has no effect, then the effects observed were most likely due to the NO group. There are also various other controls that one can do with hemoglobin to complex NO. However, none of these are perfect controls. That is why it is very important, with these kinds of experiments, to use a variety of NO donors and to make sure that they yield concordant results.

Another NO donor is nitroglycerin. It has been used for over 150 years. It has a glycerol backbone composed of three carbons. Glutathione can prevent the release of the NO group from nitroglycerin and can therefore be used in control experiments to provide convincing evidence that the NO moiety of nitroglycerin is mediating the observed effects.

Another famous NO donor is sodium nitroprusside, the antihypertensive agent. However, it is a complicated drug because not only does it have NO embedded in it, but it also has iron and cyanide, two very reactive molecules. Sometimes it is very difficult to tell which is the active ingredient in sodium nitroprusside. Therefore, a study that tries to investigate mechanism, that only uses sodium nitroprusside, may have to be interpreted with caution because several NO donors should be used to be sure the NO group is involved.

One might use NO as a gas. We can quantify nitric oxide with a nitric oxide-specific electrode. However, it is still very hard to control NO gas. It tends to lower the pH, which also affects glutamate receptor function. Also, it forms a very toxic product called peroxynitrite, when it combines with superoxide anion. In my view, it is much better to use several different NO donors.

Redox-Related Forms of NO

That is what biologists knew until mid-1993. It turns out, however, what we biologists have been calling nitric oxide is not always nitric oxide at all.

An analogy can be made with oxygen. Everybody knows it's O_2. We would never make the mistake of calling oxygen, superoxide anion, whose chemical formula is $O_2^{\cdot-}$. Superoxide is also a free radical with one free electron.

It turns out that NO, which we generally call nitrogen monoxide, is just like ice cream that comes in several flavors, because the properties of NO depend on how many electrons it has. Physiologically there is indeed nitric oxide, which is $NO^{\cdot}$, but if you take away one electron, the resulting substance is called nitrosonium ion, or NO^+. In fact, all nitroso-compounds have nitrosonium ion or an equivalent in them. They do not have nitric oxide.

I do not want to give the false impression that there are free nitrosonium ions. Under most physiological conditions, there are not. However, consider the structure of the NO group within one of these molecules, sodium nitroprusside, nitroglycerin or S-nitrosocysteine, or the more general cases of any protein that has an NO attached to a cysteine (RSNO). All of these are similar or identical to NO^+, as can be seen by counting the electrons associated with the NO group. Therefore, they tend to donate NO^+.

It is true in some cases that these drugs can gain an electron to become $NO^{\cdot}$, and they can do this in fairly simple ways. Vitamin C can donate an electron. Cysteine, or another thiol group, can donate an electron. Under those conditions, some of these drugs can become legitimate nitric oxide, $NO^{\cdot}$, particularly S-nitrosocysteine and sodium nitroprusside.

However, nitroglycerin is very reluctant to accept an electron. It really prefers what can be called NO^+ character. It is not exactly NO^+, but it acts like NO^+. It turns out that $NO^{\cdot}$ leads to a neurotoxic pathway, and nitrosonium ion or NO^+ can lead to a neuroprotective pathway.

Nitroglycerin appears to oxidize the NMDA receptor and makes NMDA-evoked currents smaller.[4,5] Consequently, less Ca^{2+} enters the neurons.[4,5] In parallel experiments, nitroglycerin protects neurons in culture from NMDA receptor-mediated toxicity.[4,5]

What is the mechanism for this? Nitroglycerin has a 3-carbon backbone with 3 attached $-ONO_2$ groups. It actually does not generate $NO^{\cdot}$. But what it can do is transfer one or possibly more of these NO groups to the –SH groups on what is referred to as a redox site(s) on the NMDA receptor. That reaction facilitates disulfide bond formation.[5] (See left-hand side of Figure 16–3.) Because of that, the channels open less frequently, and therefore less neuronal killing occurs.

We get a very similar result to nitroglycerin using sodium nitroprusside under certain conditions. If our cultures are incubated with sodium nitroprusside, the next day they are essentially not any different from controls with respect to the number of nerve cells. If, however, NMDA alone is added, neuronal killing occurs. If the two are incubated together—sodium nitroprusside and NMDA for just a few minutes—then washed out, the next day there is much less killing than with NMDA alone.

Sodium nitroprusside has a pentocyanoferrate moiety and an NO^+ moiety. The NO^+ can be transferred to a redox site on the NMDA receptor by a

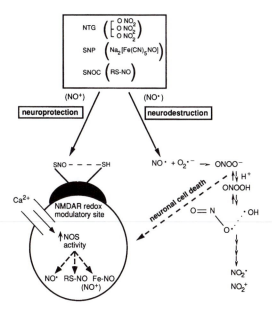

FIGURE 16–3. Proposed model of action of the NO group on neurons. The NMDA receptor's redox modulatory site can be downregulated by NO group transfer (S-nitrosylation with NO+ to form RSNO), which may facilitate disulfide bond formation. This reaction, which leads to less NMDA-evoked Ca²⁺ influx and thus neuroprotection, involves NMDA receptor thiol because it is blocked by specific sulfhydryl alkylating agents. In contrast, if the NO group is chemically reduced to NO˙ it can react with superoxide anion and become neurotoxic via peroxynitrite (ONOO⁻) formation, or its decomposition products. Exogenous nitroso-compounds or endogenous synthesis (via the Ca²⁺-activated enzyme, neuronal nitric oxide synthase) can supply NO—in one of several redox states—for these reactions. NTG, nitroglycerin; SNP, sodium nitroprusside; SNOC, S-nitrosocysteine; NMDAR, NMDA receptor-channel complex; NOS, nitric oxide synthase; Fe–NO, iron-nitrosyl. (Reprinted with permission from Lipton SA, Choi Y-B, Pan Z-H, Lei SZ, Chen H-SV, Sucher NJ, Singel DJ, Loscalzo J, Stamler JS. A redox-based mechanism for the neuroprotective and neurodestructive effects of nitric oxide and related nitroso-compounds. *Nature* (London) 1993;364:626–632.)

complicated chemical reaction with an intermediate.[5] That reaction can facilitate disulfide bond formation.

Another example is the NO donor, S-nitrosocysteine. Its NO group can be transferred in the form of NO^+. NMDA increases calcium in cells. But by interposing an incubation in S-nitrosocysteine, the NO group is transferred to a sulfhydryl on the NMDA receptor and facilitates disulfide bond formation. Then, when the same amount of NMDA is administered, less calcium rushes into the cell.[4,5]

Thus all three of these NO donors can generate NO^+. Each has a slightly different chemical mechanism, but the bottom line is, it appears to reform the putative disulfide bond of the NMDA receptor.

Because many laboratories were finding, under certain conditions, that the NO group could kill, we started doing experiments with the same drugs under slightly different conditions to see if we could get killing or saving. S-nitrosocysteine incubated in a culture causes, in a dose-dependent fashion, neuronal cell killing.[5] But I just mentioned that S-nitrosocysteine can protect neurons. What is going on here?

It turns out to depend on what else is going on in the culture dish. Superoxide dismutase is an enzyme we have heard a lot about recently because it is abnormal in familial forms of amyotrophic lateral sclerosis and perhaps in other diseases. It scavenges superoxide anions. Superoxide dismutase can prevent killing by S-nitrosocysteine (SNOC). The mechanism is as follows: If SNOC does not react with an NMDA receptor thiol and transfer its NO group, it quickly decomposes by homolytic cleavage from an RSNO—that is, a cysteine and an NO group—to produce nitric oxide (NO·). The nitric oxide is only toxic when it combines with superoxide. We know that, because when we put in superoxide dismutase to scavenge the superoxide, SNOC is not toxic. In fact, under those conditions, there is more nitric oxide because it no longer reacts with the endogenous superoxide anions.

What results from putting nitric oxide and superoxide together? The product is called peroxynitrite. Since our paper on this subject was published,[5] a member of the IUPAC nomenclature committee wrote to us. He wrote that the systematic name for peroxynitrite should be oxoperoxonitrate (1−). Our group has suggested another name, "Oh NO" representing that $ONOO^-$ is the bad substance under these conditions. Either $OONO^-$ or a breakdown product of $OONO^-$ kills nerve cells. It appears to kill by lipid peroxidation or, more likely, nitration of tyrosines, thus destroying cellular membranes (right side of Figure 16.3).

Interestingly, as one would predict, if superoxide dismutase (SOD) is added after $OONO^-$ has already formed, SOD no longer protects. So we really know the toxic product is peroxynitrite ($OONO^-$).

Some groups have found that sodium nitroprusside can kill neurons. How can we rationalize that it can save under our conditions but kill under others? The answer is that in the presence of electron donors that can donate an electron to its NO^+ moiety to make NO·, to make real nitric oxide, then sodium nitroprusside kills.[5] Therefore, sodium nitroprusside can become a killer, but only if there is an available donor that can give it an electron, for example, either a thiol or ascorbate (Vitamin C).

In contrast, nitroglycerin will not take an electron from cysteine. In fact, it actually prevents killing under a variety of conditions because nitroglycerin transfers its NO^+-like moiety to the NMDA receptor. Unlike sodium nitroprusside, nitroglycerin is very hesitant to make nitric oxide directly.[5]

To summarize, there are various clinically available NO group donors. Under different conditions, they can enter one of two pathways (see Figure 16.3). One is an NO^+ pathway, where the NO group is added to a redox site of the NMDA receptor. If an NO group is added there, it facilitates disulfide bond formation and limits the influx of calcium. That action actually turns off nitric oxide synthase and the neurons make less $NO^{\cdot}$, representing a form of feedback inhibition. It also turns off the other enzymes that may be deleterious to neuronal survival.

Conversely, some of these NO donors can gain an electron. For example, S-nitrosocysteine or sodium nitroprusside can produce $NO^{\cdot}$ and thus enter the nitric oxide neurodestructive pathway; in this case $NO^{\cdot}$ combines with superoxide to form neurotoxic $OONO^-$ (peroxynitrite).

Obviously, for neuroprotection what one would like is a drug that prefers nitrosonium character and avoids nitric oxide. Nitroglycerin seems to be one such drug. In collaboration with our colleagues, Drs. Frank Wang, Frances Jensen, and Phil Stieg, we have begun a series of experiments on rat pups and adult rats, administering nitroglycerin during acute ischemia. We can do this in a variety of ways. We can give it acutely, with a pressor agent so we do not lower the blood pressure—one obviously does not want to lower blood pressure acutely during ischemia. Another paradigm for nitroglycerin administration invokes making an animal tolerant to the systemic effects of nitroglycerin. If a person forgets to take a nitroglycerin patch off at night, it does not work for the heart by the next morning. The person may awaken with angina because of tolerance to the cardiovascular effects of nitroglycerin. However, one does not become tolerant to the central nervous system effects. In fact, the more nitroglycerin given, the more –SH groups are tied up on the NMDA receptor and the better neuroprotection is provided. In our experiments, we slowly acclimate an animal to nitroglycerin by simply putting on pieces of a nitroglycerin patch over a few days and increasing the dose. There is very little, if any, drop in blood pressure. Then we induce a stroke. Under these conditions, the size of focal cerebral infarcts appears to be smaller than in control animals.

Is this so new? Nitroglycerin was written about in the *Lancet* in 1879. It stated that nitroglycerin was a remedy for angina. So nitroglycerin has been around for quite a while.

However, the *Lancet* went on to state that the actions of nitroglycerin, as reported in the *Medical Times and Gazette* 20 years earlier, were quite controversial. I think this controversy has continued. A hundred years ago, it was controversial, and I suspect that someone looking back on our work will say it remains controversial. But I think we are making some progress, simply by talking to our chemistry colleagues. It is really a case where our mutual ignorances have complemented one another, as we begin to understand the chemistry of how nitroglycerin and other nitroso-compounds might work in the brain.[5]

References

1. Dawson VL, Dawson TM, London ED, Bredt DS, Snyder SH. Nitric oxide mediates glutamate neurotoxicity in primary cortical cultures. *Proc Natl Acad Sci USA* 1991;88:6368–6371.
2. Dawson TM, Dawson VL, Snyder SH. A novel neuronal messenger molecule in brain: The free radical, nitric oxide. *Ann Neurol* 1992;32:297–311.
3. Aizenman E, Lipton SA, Loring RH. Selective modulation of NMDA responses by reduction and oxidation. *Neuron* 1989;2:1257–1263.
4. Lei SZ, Pan ZH, Aggarwal SK, et al. Effect of nitric oxide production on the redox modulatory site of the NMDA receptor-channel complex. *Neuron* 1992;8: 1087–1099.
5. Lipton SA, Choi YB, Pan ZH, et al. A redox-based mechanism for the neuroprotective and neurodestructive effects of nitric oxide and related nitroso-compounds. *Nature* 1993;364:626–632.

PART IV

Clinical and Laboratory Studies of Cardiopulmonary Bypass, Hypothermia, and Circulatory Arrest

CHAPTER 17

A Newborn Canine Model of Hypothermic Circulatory Arrest

Robert C. Vannucci

Introduction

In this chapter, a canine model of hypothermic circulatory arrest with cerebral ischemic damage, which was developed in our laboratory over the past several years, will be described. The rationale for conducting research in the newborn dog relates to the well established observation that acute brain damage secondary to systemic hypoxia, hypotension, or cardiac arrest is prevented, or at least reduced, by prior or concurrent hypothermia.[1–3] The observation is especially true of immature animals, and also human infants, and forms the basis of present day open heart surgery in infants and children. At many institutions throughout the United States and abroad, infants harboring surgically correctable congenital malformations of the heart are subjected to hypothermic circulatory arrest to provide optimal surgical repair of the cardiac defect. It is the duration of cardiac arrest during hypothermia and its attendant total cerebral ischemia that is limiting for the prevention of brain damage. It is not entirely clear how long an infant can tolerate hypothermic circulatory arrest without sustaining ischemic brain injury, although clinical practice suggests a safe interval of 60 to 70 minutes.[4–6] Unfortunately, infants occasionally sustain brain damage even when the duration of cardiac arrest is well within the therapeutic window.[7,8] It has not been established whether such brain damage arises as a complication of the surgical procedure itself (e.g., postoperative hypotension, air emboli, etc.) or as a result of cerebral ischemia beyond the safety margin for any specific individual infant. Given the fact that 0.5% to 1.0% of all infants are born with surgically correctable cardiac lesions, it is not surprising that investigators have developed animal models of hypothermic circulatory arrest to answer many clinically relevant questions.

Over the past several years, we have developed a model of hypothermic circulatory arrest with brain damage in the newborn dog. There are several scientific reasons why dogs are an optimal species to study the protective effect of hypothermia on the perinatal brain during complete circulatory arrest. First, newborn dogs of 3 to 5 days postnatal age exhibit physiologic, anatomic, and functional characteristics similar to those of newborn human infants. In this regard, the brain of the newborn dog is histologically equivalent to that of the human fetus or newborn infant at 34 to 36 weeks gestation. Specifically, the cerebral cortex is a six-layered structure, white matter is undergoing myelination, and the germinal matrix has involuted. The newborn dog brain, like the brain of the human infant, is metabolically immature, with cerebral blood flow and cerebral metabolic rate for oxygen approximating 40% of the values measured in the adult dog.[9] From a functional perspective, the newborn dog less than 1 week of postnatal age exhibits predominantly brainstem and subcortical functions, including sucking and postural reflexes and sensitivity to pain and temperature. Thermoregulation, responses to auditory and visual stimuli, and neocortical activity, as reflected by the electroencephalogram, are primitive.[10,11]

Preparation of the Canine Model

In our initial and subsequent experiments, newborn dogs were anesthetized with halothane, paralyzed, and artificially ventilated with 70% nitrous oxide/30% oxygen. Under local anesthesia, a femoral artery and vein were catheterized, and the arterial catheter was connected to a dynographic recorder for continuous monitoring of systemic blood pressure and heart rate. A side arm of the arterial catheter allowed for intermittent blood sampling for measurements of PaO_2, $PaCO_2$, and PHa as well as of specific metabolites. When the animals were in physiologic oxygen and acid-base balance, they were surface cooled with ice packs to 20°C core temperature. Preliminary studies indicated that a reduction in core temperature from 37° to 20°C in newborn dogs was associated with a decrease in mean arterial blood pressure (MABP) from 75 to 47 mmHg and in heart rate from 240 to 60 beats/min.[12] $PaCO_2$ was reduced from 38 to 31 mmHg (corrected to 37°C), whereas pHa was unchanged from control (7.40). The electroencephalogram slowed progressively and became isoelectric at 22° to 25°C. During normothermia, cerebral blood flow (CBF) to 16 component structures of the brain varied from 17 to 65 mL/100 g/min, whereas during hypothermia, blood flow was lower in all regions at remarkably uniform levels (8.3 to 10.3 mL/100 g/min) (Figure 17–1). The greatest reductions in CBF occurred in those structures with the highest intrinsic flows during normothermia and were proportionately less in low-flow structures. The cerebral metabolic rate for glucose (CGU) also decreased in all brain regions. Normothermic rates of glucose utilization varied from 9 to 24 μmol/100 g/min, whereas during hy-

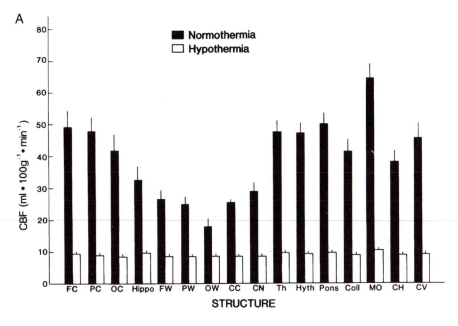

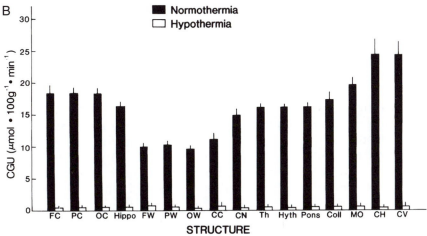

FIGURE 17–1.   Regional cerebral blood flow (rCBF) shown in A and cerebral glucose utilization (rCGU) shown in B during normothermia (37°C) and hypothermia (20°C) in newborn dogs. Bars represent means of 5 to 6 animals; vertical lines denote ± 1 S.E. All hypothermic values were significantly different from normothermia with p <.001. Abbreviations: FC = frontal cortex; PC = parietal cortex; OC = occipital cortex; Hippo = hippocampus; FW = frontal white; PW = parietal white; OW = occipital white; CC = corpus callosum; CN = caudate nucleus; Th = thalamus; Hyth = hypothalamus; Coll = colliculi; MO = medulla oblongota; CH = cerebellar hemisphere; CV = cereballar vermis. (Reprinted with permission from Palmer C, Vannucci RC, Christensen MA, Brucklacher RM. Regional cerebral blood flow and glucose utilization during hypothermia in newborn dogs. *Anesthesiology* 1989;71:730–737.)

pothermia, glucose utilization, like CBF, was within a narrow range (0.47 to 0.57 μmol/100 g/min). The percent reductions in regional CGU were always greater than corresponding reductions in regional CBF. These initial findings indicate that the CGU is globally depressed during deep hypothermia, but that CBF remains more than adequate to support the energy needs of the immature brain, as is also indicated by the maintenance of physiologic concentrations of high-energy phosphate reserves during hypothermia.[13]

Once the newborn dogs were cooled to 20°C, complete circulatory arrest was produced with intravenous KCl. Dogs remained asystolic without ventilation for 1 to 2 hours, following which resuscitation was accomplished with closed chest compressions, resumption of artificial ventilation, the intravenous injection of epinephrine and NaHCO₃, and slow surface rewarming to 37°C. These maneuvers typically resulted in spontaneous heart action within 5 to 15 minutes, with progressively increasing heart rate and systemic blood pressure thereafter. Once rewarming to 37°C was complete, the animals were weaned from the ventilator as the effect of the paralytic agent subsided. Thereafter, the animals were placed in a warmer and received an intravenous infusion of 5% to 10% glucose to maintain optimal glucose and fluid balance. In selected animals, orogastric feedings with simulated bitch's milk was initiated at 8 hours of recovery. Animals were maintained for up to 72 hours of recovery.

Neuropathologic Responses to Hypothermic Circulatory Arrest

To characterize the presence and extent of ischemic brain damage following hypothermic circulatory arrest in newborn dogs, puppies were subjected to cardiac arrest at 20°C for 1.0, 1.5, 1.75, or 2.0 hours following which they were allowed to recover for up to 72 hours.[14,15] Animals arrested for 1.0 hours exhibited no evidence of ischemic brain damage at any interval of recovery, and this was also the case for animals subjected to 1.5 hours of circulatory arrest unless they exhibited early post-ischemic systemic hypotension.[15] Newborn dogs subjected to circulatory arrest for greater than 1.5 hours were universally brain damaged. Those sustaining cardiac arrest for 1.75 hours showed brain damage predominantly of the cerebral cortex but also of the basal ganglia and amygdaloid nucleus. Injury to these structures ranged from mild to severe (5%–majority of neurons involved). In animals arrested for 2.0 hours, brain damage was more extensive (>50% neurons involved) and involved not only cerebral cortex, basal ganglia, and amygdaloid nucleus, but the hippocampus as well. White matter was occasionally involved. In all brain-damaged animals, tissue injury was characterized by selective neuronal necrosis with eosinophilic cytoplasm and pyknotic or karyorrhexic nuclei. Within cerebral cortex, injury was focused on layers 3 and 5 + 6, especially at the arterial boundary zones (Figures 17–2 and 17–3). Within the

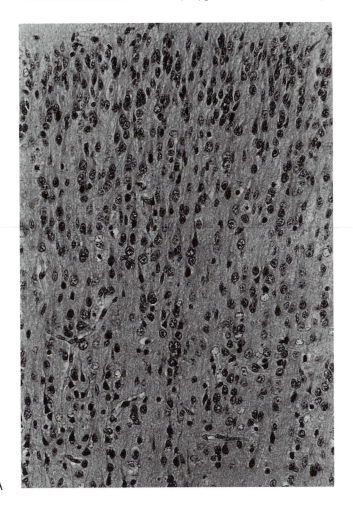

A

FIGURE 17–2. Representative sections of cerebral cortex showing moderate (A) and severe (B) ischemic damage with selective neuronal necrosis in newborn dogs subjected to hypothermic circulatory arrest. In both brains, neuronal alterations are apparent, either localized on layers 3 and 5 + 6, or scattered throughout the cerebral cortex. In the severely damaged brain (B), neuronal necrosis is associated with rarefaction of the neuropile, suggesting laminar necrosis. (Hematoxylin and eosin; 200X magnification).

hippocampus, injury was focused predominantly upon the subiculum with relative sparing of the remainder of the pyramidal cell layer. Within the basal ganglia, the striatum (caudate nucleus and putamen) as well as the claustrum were damaged, especially in their dorsal regions. The amygdaloid nucleus

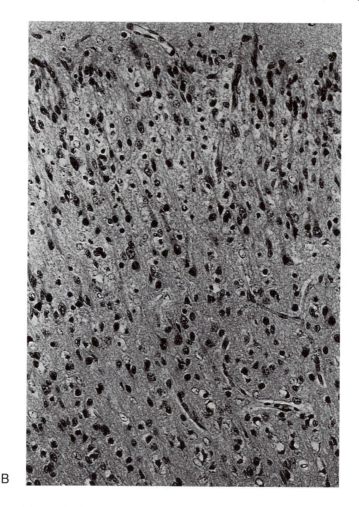

B

FIGURE 17–2.   continued

also was consistently involved, showing many damaged neurons, especially in its lateral aspect. In all involved structures, neuronal injury was apparent even at 4 hours of recovery, with little or no increase in severity thereafter for up to 72 hours; suggesting that delayed neuronal necrosis, especially of the hippocampus, is not a feature in this model of hypothermic circulatory arrest in newborns.

Cerebral Blood Flow and Metabolism During and Following Hypothermic Circulatory Arrest

To ascertain alterations in cerebral metabolism that occur during hypothermic circulatory arrest, additional experiments were conducted in anes-

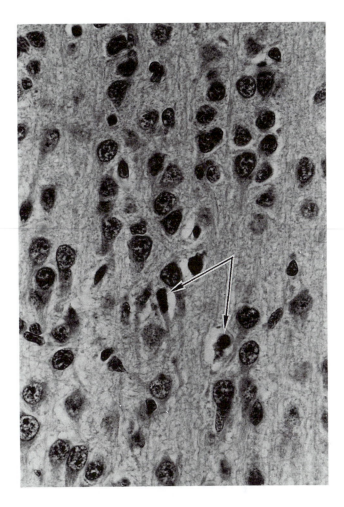

FIGURE 17–3. High power view of damaged cerebral cortex. Shown are shrunken pyramidal neurons with dense pyknotic nuclei (arrows). (Hematoxylin and eosin; 520X magnificiation).

thetized, paralyzed, and artificially ventilated newborn dogs that were surface-cooled to 20°C followed by cardiac arrest with KCl for up to 1.75 hours.[13] Hypothermia alone was associated with optimal preservation of labile metabolites in brain, even in caudal brainstem and cerebellum, as compared to barbiturate-anesthetized littermates (Figure 17–4). After onset of hypothermic circulatory arrest, glucose decreased progressively in cerebral cortex, caudate nucleus, hippocampus, and subcortical white matter to negligible levels by 30 minutes. Pyruvate increased transiently (+50%) at 10 minutes, whereas lactate increased and plateaued at 10 to 11 mmol/kg at 30 minutes (Figure 17–5). The disproportionate increases in pyruvate and

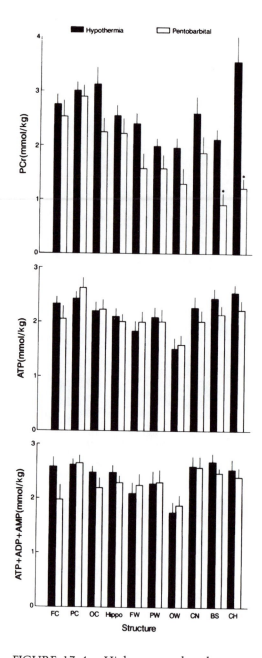

FIGURE 17–4. High-energy phosphate reserves in newborn dog brain during hypothermia or barbiturate anesthesia. Hypothermia was effected by surface cooling to 20°C, and barbiturate anesthesia was produced by the i.v. injection of pentobarbital adequate to produce systemic hypotension comparable to that of the hypothermic animals. Bars represent means for 4 newborn dogs in each

lactate resulted in a progressive rise in the lactate/pyruvate ratio in all analyzed structures. The high-energy phosphate reserve, phosphocreatine, fell precipitously to <0.05 mmol/kg in all structures, with a preservation of ATP for the first 10 minutes of cerebral ischemia (Figure 17.5). Thereafter, ATP decreased to <0.1 mmol/kg in cerebral cortex and to between 0.1 and 0.2 mmol/kg in caudate nucleus, hippocampus, and white matter. Total adenine nucleotides (ATP + ADP + AMP) were partially depleted by 30 minutes in the gray matter structures but were unchanged from control for 60 minutes in white matter. The findings show a direct correlation between preservation of cerebral energy stores during hypothermic circulatory arrest and the selective resistance of subcortical white matter to ischemic damage. However, no such correlation existed for the hippocampus. Other factors must influence the resistance of the hippocampus to ischemic injury during hypothermia, including possibly a paucity of excitatory neurotransmitter cell surface receptors at this early age.

To ascertain alterations in regional CBF during and following hypothermic circulatory arrest, newborn dogs were surgically prepared as described above and surface-cooled to 20°C followed by complete circulatory arrest with KCl for either 1.0 or 1.75 hours. Obviously, the brains of these animals are totally ischemic during the entire arrest interval. Following resuscitation, regional CBF was measured by the indicator fractionation technique, using [^{14}C]-iodoantipyrine as the radioactive tracer.[16] No alterations in CBF at either 2 or 18 hours of recovery were present in any of 16 analyzed structures in animals previously subjected to hypothermic circulatory arrest compared to controls rendered hypothermic alone (Figure 17-6). A direct linear correlation existed between mean arterial blood pressure and blood flow within cerebral cortex, subcortical white matter, hypothalamus, and cerebellum in animals arrested for 1.75 hours and recovered for 2 hours, suggesting a loss of CBF autoregulation at this interval. No such correlation between systemic blood pressure and CBF was apparent at 18 hours of recovery. The findings suggest that maintenance of adequate systemic blood pressure and hence cerebral perfusion in the early postoperative period are

---

FIGURE 17–4 continued. group; vertical lines denote ± 1 S.E. p < .05 compared to hypothermia. Abbreviations:FC = frontal cortex; PC = parietal cortex; OC = occipital cortex; Hippo = hippocampus; FW = frontal white; PW = parietal white; OW = occipital white; CN = caudate nucleus; BS = brainstem; CH = cerebellar hemisphere. (Reprinted with permission from Yager JY, Brucklacher RM, Mujsce DJ, Vannucci RC. Cerebral oxidative metabolism during hypothermia and circulatory arrest in newborn dogs. *Pediatr Res* 1992;32:547–552.)

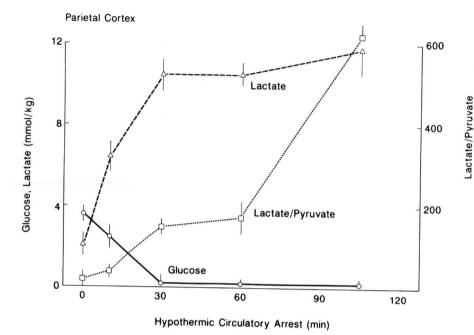

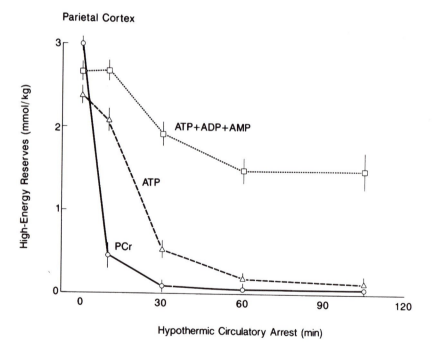

FIGURE 17–5. Glycolytic intermediates and high-energy reserves of newborn dog cerebral cortex during hypothermic circulatory arrest. Symbols represent means of 3 to 5 brains at each interval; vertical lines denote ± 1 S.E. (Reprinted with permission from Yager JY, Brucklacher RM, Mujsce DJ, Vannucci RC. Cerebral oxidative metabolism during hypothermia and circulatory arrest in newborn dogs. *Pediatr Res* 1992;32:547–552.)

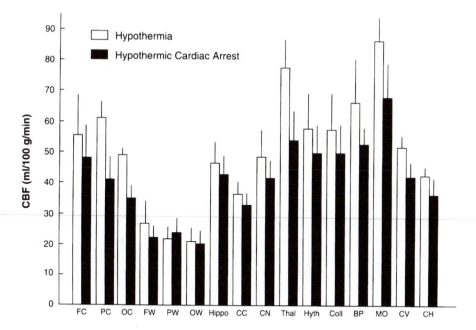

FIGURE 17–6. Cerebral blood flow (CBF) to 16 component structures of newborn dog brain at 18 hours of recovery from either hypothermia alone or hypothermic circulatory arrest of 1.75 hours duration. Bars represent means ± 1 S.E. for 3 dogs in the hypothermia alone group and 4 dogs in the 1.75 hour arrested group. Abbreviations: FC = frontal cortex; PC = parietal cortex; OC = occipital cortex; FW = frontal white; PW = parietal white; OW = occipital white; Hippo = hippocampus; CC = corpus callosum; CN = caudate nucleus; Thal = thalamus; Hyth = hypothalamus; Coll = colliculi; BP = basis pontis; MO = medulla oblongata; CV = cerebellar vermis; CH = cerebellar hemisphere.

important to prevent or minimize ischemic brain damage in newborn infants subjected to hypothermic circulatory arrest.

Influence of Differences in Intra-ischemic Temperature on Neurologic Outcome

As mentioned previously, hypothermia to a core temperature varying from 16° to 24°C, combined with either complete circulatory arrest or low circulation (low-flow state), accomplished with cardiopulmonary bypass, is the established procedure for the surgical correction of congenital heart defects. What presently is not established is the optimal core temperature during ischemia that allows complete recovery of all organs, including the brain, without untoward postoperative complications. Too warm a core temperature shortens the safe interval for surgical repair during circulatory arrest, while too cold a temperature increases the risk of cellular injury arising from hypothermia *per se* as well as the risk of greater difficulty in reestablishing cardiac activity. Accordingly, experiments were accomplished that were designed to ascertain whether or not small differences in core temperature during hypothermic circulatory arrest influence the presence and extent of ischemic brain damage in newborn dogs.[17] Puppies were anesthetized and surgically prepared as described above, following which they were surface-cooled to either 16°, 20°, or 24°C. The animals then were subjected to circulatory arrest for 1.75 hours, following which all animals were successfully resuscitated, rewarmed to 37°C, and ultimately weaned from anesthesia and ventilatory support. Of 20 dogs, 4 sustained secondary cardiopulmonary collapse and death between 4 and 7 hours of recovery. Of the 16 surviving animals, all but one (surface-cooled to 16°C) showed histologic evidence of brain damage at 8 hours of recovery. Morphometric analysis of the number of damaged neurons in the vulnerable gray matter structures showed the greatest injury to cerebral cortex at 24°C and the least injury to this structure at 16°C (p = .008). The extent of damage to the caudate nucleus was similar in the three temperature groups, while damage to the amygdaloid nucleus was greater at 24°C compared to 20°C, but with no difference in the severity of injury between 20° and 16°C. A close correlation existed between neurobehavioral deficits in the surviving dogs and the severity of damage to especially the cerebral cortex (r = .72; p = .001). The findings indicate that differences in intra-ischemic core temperature during deep hypothermic circulatory arrest influence the severity of damage especially to the cerebral cortex of newborn dogs. Specifically, the lower the temperature below 24°C, the more protected the structure from ischemic injury. Furthermore, the greater the cortical damage, the more severe the neurobehavioral deficits. Accordingly, differences in core temperature, even at very low levels, appear critical for optimal protection of the newborn brain during hypothermic circulatory arrest.

Conclusion

The experiments accomplished to date clearly demonstrate an ability to produce and completely reverse hypothermic circulatory arrest in the newborn dog, allowing for a comprehensive evaluation of those physiologic variables and therapeutic endeavors which potentially reduce or accentuate ischemic brain damage. Further experiments will allow for a determination of whether or not specific modalities of therapy will reverse secondary systemic complications, thereby potentially allowing for more complete recoverability and ultimately reduced brain damage. The systemic physiologic and regional cerebral blood flow and metabolic responses to hypothermia alone, as well as during and following hypothermic circulatory arrest, have now been well characterized. Further experiments will focus on the immature brain's response to hypothermic circulatory arrest and those critical events that occur during recovery from the ischemic stress.

References

1. Treasure T, Naftel DC, Conger KA, Garcia JH, Kirklin JW, Blackstone EH. The effect of hypothermic circulatory arrest time on cerebral function, morphology and biochemistry. *J Thorac Cardiovasc Surg* 1983;86:761–770.
2. O'Connor JV, Wilding T, Farmer P, Sher J, Ergin MA, Griepp RB. The protective effect of profound hypothermia on the canine central nervous system during one hour of circulatory arrest. *Ann Thorac Surg* 1986; 41:225–259.
3. Hickey PR, Anderson NP. Deep hypothermic circulatory arrest: A review of pathophysiology and clinical experience as a basis for anesthetic management. *J Cardiothorac Anesth* 1987;1:137–155.
4. Stevenson JG, Stone EF, Dillard DH. Intellectual development of children subjected to prolonged circulatory arrest during hypothermic open heart surgery in infancy. *Circulation* 1974;49:54–59.
5. Dickinson DF, Sambrooks JE. Intellectual performance in children after circulatory arrest with profound hypothermia in infancy. *Arch Dis Child* 1979; 54:1–6.
6. Wells FC, Coghill S, Caplan HL. Duration of circulatory arrest does influence the psychological development of children after cardiac operations in early life. *J Thorac Cardiovasc Surg* 1983;86:823–831.
7. Brunberg JA, Reilly EL, Doty DB. Central nervous system consequences in infants of cardiac surgery using deep hypothermia and circulatory arrest. *Cardiovasc Surg* 1974;49:60–68.
8. Ferry PC. Neurologic sequelae of cardiac surgery in children. *Am J Dis Child* 1987;141:309–312.
9. Hernandez MJ, Brennan RW, Vannucci RC, Bowman GS. Cerebral blood flow and oxygen consumption in the newborn dog. *Am J Physiol* 1978;234: R209–R215.
10. Fox MW. The postnatal growth of the canine brain and correlated anatomical and behavioral changes during neuro-ontogenesis. *Growth* 1964;28:135–141.
11. Scott JP, Fuller JL. *Genetics and the social behavior of the dog.* Chicago: University of Chicago Press, 1965.
12. Palmer C, Vannucci RC, Christensen MA, Brucklacher RM. Regional cerebral blood flow and glucose utilization during hypothermia in newborn dogs. *Anesthesiology* 1989;71:730–737.
13. Yager JY, Brucklacher RM, Mujsce DJ, Vannucci RC. Cerebral oxidative metabolism during hypothermia and circulatory arrest in newborn dogs. *Pediatr Res* 1992;32:547–552.
14. Mujsce DJ, Towfighi J, Vannucci RC. Physiologic and neuropathologic aspects of hypothermic circulatory arrest in newborn dogs. *Pediatr Res* 1990;28: 354–360.
15. Mujsce DJ, Towfighi J, Yager JY, Vannucci RC. Neuropathologic aspects of hypothermic circulatory arrest in newborn dogs. *Acta Neuropathol* 1993;85: 190–198.

16. Yager JY, Christensen MA, Vannucci RC. Regional cerebral blood flow following hypothermic circulatory arrest in newborn dogs. *Brain Res* 1993;620: 122–126.
17. Mujsce DJ, Towfighi J, Heitjan DF, Vannucci RC. Differences in intra-ischemic temperature influence neurologic outcome following deep hypothermic circulatory arrest in newborn dogs. *Stroke* 1994;25:1433–1442.

CHAPTER 18

Effects of CPB, Hypothermia, and Circulatory Arrest on Cerebral Blood Flow and Metabolism

William J. Greeley

The use of deep hypothermic cardiopulmonary bypass (DHCPB) with or without deep hypothermic circulatory arrest (DHCA) has substantially improved operating conditions for children undergoing congenital heart surgery, resulting in improved survival and reduced cardiac morbidity. As overall surgical outcome has improved, neuropsychiatric dysfunction has become a more prominent and visible complication of the congenital heart patient. Recent reports suggest that transient and permanent neuropsychiatric injuries occur in as many as 25% of all infants undergoing hypothermic cardiopulmonary bypass with or without circulatory arrest.[1,2] This uncomfortably high incidence of neuropsychiatric impairment is becoming a major focal point for current research into the mechanism of cerebral injury during CPB. Currently the most effective means of protecting the brain from CPB- or DHCA-induced injury is hypothermia.[3-6] Hypothermia reduces cerebral blood flow and metabolism and preserves cellular stores of high-energy phosphates. The hypothermic methods that can be employed—either moderate hypothermia, deep hypothermia, or deep hypothermia with circulatory arrest—have differing effects on cerebral physiology and should be considered separately.

Moderate Hypothermia

The cerebral impact of moderate hypothermic CPB on children is similar to that observed in adults.[7] The systemic vasculature constricts with temperature reduction and thereby directs a larger proportion of flow toward the brain. Although a larger portion of total flow is directed toward the brain, CBF and metabolism decrease with cooling.[8] The normal principles of cerebral autoregulation that are present during normothermia are maintained during moderate hypothermic CPB. Cerebral blood flow remains dependent on brain metabolism. If metabolism is high, the cerebral vascular resistance falls and cerebral blood flow increases. This is known as flow/metabolism coupling, and it remains intact during moderate hypothermic CPB.[3,7]

Pressure/flow autoregulation or the ability to maintain a constant CBF despite wide ranges in mean arterial pressure also remains intact during moderate hypothermic CPB. The cerebral vasculature remains capable of dilating during low perfusion pressure and constricts when perfusion pressure is high.[9]

Deep Hypothermia

During deep hypothermic CPB (using alpha-stat blood gas strategy) the normal vascular responses that are present during moderate hypothermic CPB are lost.[9] In the brain, the cerebral vasculature cannot dilate in response to low mean arterial pressure. Therefore reductions in systemic pressure result in a fall in CBF, i.e., a loss of pressure/flow autoregulation. This loss of pressure/flow autoregulation is most likely due to the influence of deep hypothermic temperatures on vascular reactivity. Severe temperature reductions impair vascular relaxation.[9,10] This has been described as a cold induced *cerebrovasoparesis*.

Cerebral blood flow decreases linearly with reductions in temperature. In contrast, cerebral metabolism decreases exponentially with reductions in temperature. Therefore flow/metabolic ratios must increase with decreasing temperature during CPB in children. In the awake healthy child, cerebral blood flow (CBF) and metabolism ($CMRO_2$) are regulated by the metabolic needs of regional areas of the brain. This has been termed *cerebral flow/ metabolism coupling* and is an important regulatory feature of cerebral homeostasis.[4,11-13] In humans, a mean $CMRO_2$ of 3.0 to 4.0 mL/100g/min is coupled to a CBF of 45 to 80 mL/100g/min, for a $CBF/CMRO_2$ ratio of 13 to 20/1. In neonates $CMRO_2$, CBF, and the $CBF/CMRO_2$ ratio are generally higher than older children and adults. This is believed to be due to increased metabolic demand for neuronal growth, myelinization, etc.[14]

Deep hypothermic temperatures affect CBF and cerebral metabolism differently. CBF decreases in a linear fashion with cooling, and cerebral metabolism decreases in an exponential fashion. The net result is that CBF becomes more luxuriant at deep hypothermic temperatures and flow metabolism coupling is lost. At normothermia the mean ratio of CBF to $CMRO_2$ is 20/1, and at deep hypothermia the ratio increases to 75/1.[3] This becomes important when low-flow CPB is used.

In theory, low-flow CPB could provide an indefinite period of effective cerebral perfusion during hypothermia, if adequate cerebral oxygen delivery is supplied. Since cerebral blood flow becomes increasingly luxuriant with temperature reduction, pump flow requirements should decrease with lower temperatures.[8] An exponential equation describing the relationship between $CMRO_2$ and temperature was described by our group.[3] With the assumption that 100 mL/kg/min is a minimal acceptable flow rate for infants at normothermia, an equation estimating minimal acceptable pump flow rates at any temperature can be formulated. Solving this equation for various temperatures, we can provide an estimate of acceptable minimal perfusion flow rates. At the typical hypothermic temperatures used during deep hypothermic CPB, one would predict that flow rates as low as 20 to 30 mL/kg/min should meet cerebral demands. This is slightly higher than the experimental findings obtained from Swain, et al., who demonstrated that flow rates of 5 mL/kg/min were inadequate to maintain cerebral ATP stores at 15°C, whereas flow rates of 10 mL/kg/min were adequate.[5]

Elevated CO_2 tension is a potent cerebrovasodilator in both the awake and anesthetized state, with or without CPB. During CPB, multiple groups have independently shown that CBF increases with increasing arterial carbon dioxide tension.[7,15-17] In children, however, the response to increases in CO_2 tension is diminished by two factors, deep hypothermia and age less than one year. The attenuated response of deep hypothermia is not surprising in view of the previous discussion of cold-induced cerebrovasoparesis.[17] The blunted CBF response to elevations in $PaCO_2$ in children under one year of age is consistent with experimental data which show an age-dependent increase in CBF response to CO_2 from fetus to newborn to adults in unanesthetized animals.[14]

Despite the blunting of the CBF response to CO_2, global CBF significantly increases with the addition of CO_2 to the gas mixture in children during CPB. Although somewhat attenuated by age, the major differences between CO_2 management in adults and children relates to the lower temperatures used, periods of circulatory arrest, and the increased risk for air embolism in pediatric CPB.

Deep Hypothermic CPB with Circulatory Arrest

Arresting the circulation at deep hypothermic temperatures introduces the question of how well deep hypothermia preserves organ function, with the brain being at greatest risk. Several authors have demonstrated ongoing basal cerebral metabolism during deep hypothermic circulatory arrest. This energy expenditure is necessary to preserve membrane integrity and maintain transmembrane ionic gradients vital to cellular integrity. Extensive clinical experience using DHCA has shown the duration of a safe circulatory arrest period to be approximately 50 to 60 minutes.[18] A more precise method of predicting safe limits for TCA based on brain metabolism has been described recently.[3] For the brain, the metabolic reduction induced by hypothermia is described by the temperature coefficient (Q_{10}), which is the ratio of brain metabolism measured at two temperatures separated by 10°C. Recent data suggest that hypothermia decreases the cerebral metabolic rate for oxygen by a mean of 3.6 for every 10°C reduction in temperature in children.[3] If one assumes that the brain can tolerate an ischemic period of 3 to 5 minutes at normothermia without causing ischemic brain damage, Q_{10} data means that brain metabolism is sufficiently reduced to allow for a safe circulatory arrest period of 45 to 62 minutes, if the brain is thoroughly cooled to 17°C. Since brain temperature determines the cerebral metabolic rate, complete cerebral cooling is essential.

The increased metabolic suppression for younger patients may be due to a greater susceptibility of the immature neurons and glial elements to hypothermia or may reflect reduced brain mass and more efficient brain cooling. Inter- and intraspecies variability for Q_{10} may explain why variables other than temperature have been implicated as major contributors to cerebral protection during CPB. If one used adult-derived Q_{10} data, temperature-induced metabolic suppression would appear insufficient to explain clinically acceptable safe circulatory arrest periods, and other variables would need to be sought.

Recent studies, however, suggest that hypothermia alone can account for the majority of the protection seen during deep hypothermic circulatory arrest.[3,19] Other variables, such as anesthetic agents, provide much smaller contributions to cerebral protection, once deep hypothermic temperatures (15° to 20°C) are reached.[4] At more moderate temperatures, anesthetic agents and other cerebroprotective agents, such as calcium channel blockers, barbiturates, and N-methyl-D-aspartate antagonists, may be more important because cerebral metabolism is higher. If deep hypothermia is the only cerebroprotective agent employed, then factors such as CO_2 that modify cerebral blood flow may be important adjuncts to achieving uniform brain cooling and thereby to improving global cerebral protection.[17]

How rapidly and effectively the brain is cooled is variable and appears to be dependent on several factors. These include length of cooling time, biological variability within the patient population, characteristics of aortic cannula flow, and institutional differences in CPB management.

Bellinger and associates demonstrated that accelerated rates of cooling (>1°C/min) during CPB using alpha-stat regulation is associated with a lower developmental quotient in neonates undergoing deep hypothermic circulatory arrest.[20] A recent study describes 4 patients who, despite having achieved nasopharyngeal and rectal temperatures of 18°C, had significantly higher cerebral oxygen extraction and cerebral metabolic rates than their co-horts.[3] Three of these patients went on to have significant neurologic dysfunction despite a relatively short period of circulatory arrest. Unexpectedly high jugular venous O_2 extraction and brain metabolism, despite hypothermic temperatures, were noted. The most likely explanation is inadequate cerebral perfusion resulting in inefficient brain cooling and the existence of temperature gradients throughout the brain.

In a recent study of 17 infants, jugular venous saturation measurements were used to monitor oxygen extraction across the brain.[21] Six infants had a significantly lower jugular venous saturation despite similar cooling times and tympanic and rectal temperatures of between 15° and 17°C. This suggests that conventional temperature monitoring may not be an effective method for assuring thorough and complete brain cooling. Speculating on the mechanisms for the variability in cooling time required for minimal jugular venous oxygen extraction is difficult. Saturation differences may simply reflect biological differences between patients. However, it is noteworthy that jugular venous desaturation was more likely to occur in neonates and particularly in patients with modified aortic cannula placement. Neonates have a smaller ascending aorta. When the conventional aortic cannulation site is moved, as occurs in TGA and hypoplastic left heart syndrome (HLHS), the distribution of cold perfusate may be preferentially directed away from the brain.

In the arterial switch procedure for TGA, the coronary arteries are translocated to the aortic root. To facilitate coronary transfer, the aortic cannula is placed as far from the aortic root as possible. In this position, the tip of the aortic cannula may promote preferential flow down the aorta or induce a Venturi effect to steal flow from the cerebral circulation. This would also help explain the reverse cooling pattern observed in 4 of our patients with TGA. In the stage I repair of HLHS, the aorta cannot be cannulated due to the extreme hypoplasia of the ascending aorta. Instead, the arterial cannula is placed in the main pulmonary artery. The head vessels are perfused in a retrograde fashion through the ductus. This type of arterial perfusion may result in poor distribution of cold perfusate to the cerebral circulation.

Institutional variability in CPB management may be an additional factor in jugular venous bulb saturation differences. In our study mentioned above, the two institutions studied had differing cooling kinetics based on different cooling techniques.

After circulatory arrest, cerebral metabolism ($CMRO_2$) is depressed. This is in marked contrast to continuous moderate and deep hypothermic cardiopulmonary bypass, in which cerebral metabolism measured after bypass is equal to or greater than metabolic measurements made prior to the initiation of CPB.[3,22] After circulatory arrest, the degree of $CMRO_2$ depression is a function of the length of the circulatory arrest period. With a shorter arrest period, cerebral metabolic recovery is improved. Therefore, metabolic recovery appears to be a marker of cerebral injury after circulatory arrest. In addition, experimental data from our lab suggest that if a 60-minute arrest period is interrupted after 30 minutes and the animal is perfused for 5 minutes at 100 mL/kg/min, metabolic recovery measured after 60 minutes of combined arrest and reperfusion is much better than after a 60-minute arrest period without a period of reperfusion.[23] This suggests that longer periods of circulatory arrest may be tolerated if ATP stores are replenished through brief periods of intermittent perfusion.

Near-infrared spectroscopy (NIRS) has been demonstrated to be sensitive to trends in oxidative metabolism, both experimentally and clinically in intact brain tissues.[22,24,25] Using this noninvasive technique, relative changes in brain oxyhemoglobin (HbO$_2$), deoxyhemoglobin (Hb), tissue blood volume (tBV), and the oxidation state of cytochrome C oxidase (cyt aa3) can be assessed continuously. Cyt aa3, the terminal enzyme of the intramitochondrial respiratory chain, reduces oxygen during electron transport for production of high-energy phosphates by oxidative phosphorylation. When oxygen availability is limited, the reduction/oxidation of cyt aa3 (redox state) decreases, eventually decreasing oxidative metabolism. For this reason, monitoring the redox states of cyt aa3, as well as tissue HbO$_2$ and Hb, provides important indices of brain oxygenation during CPB and DHCA. The importance of assessing the redox state of cyt aa3 becomes apparent when one views its function in the mitochondrial respiratory chain. Mitochondrial electron transport is the primary means of producing high-energy phosphates for cellular function. Cyt aa3, the terminal enzyme of the electron transport chain, reduces oxygen to water in a 4-electron process during aerobic respiration. Tissue ischemia or hypoxia decreases the oxygen available to cyt aa3, causing it to be become reduced and ultimately to decrease oxidative metabolism. Therefore, monitoring the redox state of cyt aa3 is potentially of great importance in assessing impaired oxygen delivery during deep hypothermic cardiopulmonary bypass.

We used CMRO$_2$ and NIRS to determine how CPB, with and without circulatory arrest, altered intracellular brain oxygenation and O$_2$ utilization in neonates, infants, and children during cardiac surgery.[22] We noted that the CMRO$_2$ in the nonarrested, continuous-flow patients returned to control during rewarming on CPB and was above baseline level after bypass. The latter finding may represent a hypermetabolic response to deep hypothermia, implying restoration from an oxygen debt or possibly a heightened response to accelerated brain rewarming. The elevated CMRO$_2$ after CPB was a direct result of both increased cerebral blood flow and oxygen extraction as evidenced by the widening CaO$_2$–CvO$_2$ difference after separation from CPB. The increased flow and extraction presumably represent a normal physiologic compensatory response to the increased metabolic demand during and after rewarming. In the DHCA patients, cerebral metabolism was significantly lower during rewarming and after separation from CPB compared to baseline, prebypass levels. We also observed that CBF and CaO$_2$–CvO$_2$ differences were reduced in the DHCA patients during rewarming and after CPB, accounting for the reduced $CMRO_2$.[22] Our observation of reduced oxygen extraction after DHCA is an abnormal response in support of $CMRO_2$ where blood flow is low. The expected compensatory response in the setting of low CBF would have been an increase in oxygen extraction. These findings suggest that a distributive defect in oxygen delivery or utilization has occurred after DHCA.

The NIRS optical responses in the brain compliment the changes in cerebral metabolism ($CMRO_2$) measured simultaneously during cardiac surgery. In the patients undergoing deep hypothermic bypass (18°C) with continuous flow (CF), oxyhemoglobin (HbO_2) and deoxyhemoglobin (Hb) did not decline significantly from baseline conditions, suggesting adequacy of oxygen delivery during these conditions. However, tissue blood volume (tBV) did decrease in this group of patients, probably due to the effects of hemodilution. During CPB, cytochrome oxidase (cyt aa3) gradually decreased and was significantly reduced from baseline after CPB. This finding probably represents a decrease in intracellular oxygen concentration due to insufficient delivery of oxygen to the mitochondria, perhaps related to a distributive or diffusive defect in oxygen delivery or to altered affinity of the enzyme for oxygen. Since the hemoglobin parameters (HbO_2, Hb, and tBV) were normal after CPB and because $CMRO_2$ returned to normal in these patients, the compensatory response of the brain to a decreased oxidation level of cyt aa3 was probably adequate.

In the patients undergoing deep hypothermic bypass with DHCA, HbO_2, Hb, and tBV were unchanged from baseline during CPB except during circulatory arrest. At the termination of circulatory arrest and prior to rewarming on CPB, HbO_2 was significantly reduced from baseline, reflecting ongoing metabolic activity in the absence of blood flow and resultant tissue hypoxia. After CPB, the HbO_2, Hb, and tBV showed relative increases compared to control, consistent with a heightened compensatory response of brain metabolism to an oxygen debt. Importantly, cyt aa3 redox level and $CMRO_2$ both remained reduced after bypass in these patients, indicating a defect due to either impaired delivery or utilization of oxygen by the mitochondria. Because $CMRO_2$ was reduced after bypass in these patients and excess compensatory responses in the NIR hemoglobin signals occurred in the presence of an altered redox state after DHCA, we conclude that DHCA impaired recovery of oxidative metabolism postoperatively. This impairment may be due to an increased diffusion barrier of oxygen to the mitochondria, possibly due to such factors as increased intracranial water or, alternatively, to mitochondrial damage resulting in a decreased ability of the enzyme to bind oxygen during electron transport.

The temporal sequence of infant cardiac surgery is designed so that the actual cardiac repair occurs *during* DHCA or continuous flow CPB. This is a high risk period for injury due to the conditions of total circulatory arrest or low flow. This phase of surgery is *preceded* by a preparation period design to maximize protection by cooling and is *followed* by rewarming and post-operative periods designed to allow recovery from the effects of deep hypothermia and ischemic arrest. Because the causes of brain injury appear to be multifactorial and are not limited solely to the DHCA period, strategies for brain protection should be more comprehensive and specifically directed at each period, where the mechanisms for injury differ. Accordingly, mechanisms for brain injury, as well as potential methods of brain protection strategies, need to be assessed for each of these different periods of infant cardiac surgery.

In conclusion, moderate hypothermic CPB in children has similar cerebral effects as have been reported in adults. However, deep hypothermia differs considerably. During deep hypothermic CPB, cerebral metabolism decreases in an exponential fashion while CBF decreases linearly. This divergence in flow/metabolism coupling may be used to predict safe minimal perfusion flow limits for continuous flow CPB in neonates, infants, and children. If DHCA is selected it is important to maximize neurologic outcome. Complete cerebral cooling is paramount and jugular venous saturation monitoring should be considered. If DHCA is to be chosen, intermittent reperfusion may improve substrate availability to the brain and, it is hoped, will result in better postoperative neuropsychologic function.

References

1. Ferry PC. Neurologic sequelae of cardiac surgery in children. *Am J Dis Child* 1987;141:309–312.
2. Ferry PC. Neurologic sequelae of open-heart surgery in children. An "irritating question." *Am J Dis Child* 1990;144:369–373.
3. Greeley WJ, Kern F-I, Ungerleider RM, Boyd JL, Quill T, Smith LR, Baldwin B, Reves JG. The effect of hypothermic cardiopulmonary bypass and total circulatory arrest on cerebral metabolism in neonates, infants, and children. *J Thorac Cardiovasc Surg* 1991;101:783–794.
4. Michenfelder JD. *Anesthesia and the brain.* New York, Edinburgh, London, Melbourne: Churchill Livingstone, 1988, pp. 23–34.
5. Swain JA, McDonald TJ, Griffith PK, Balaban RS, Clark RE, Ceckler T. Low flow hypothermic cardiopulmonary bypass protects the brain. *J Thorac Cardiovasc Surg* 1991;102:76–84.
6. Norwood WI, Norwood CR, Castaneda AR. Factors influencing survival and successful weaning from clinical ventricular bypass with local heparinization and blood filtration: An analysis in 21 consecutive patients. *Trans Am Soc Artif Intern Organs* 1979;25:176–181.
7. Govier AV, Reves JG, McKay RD, Karp RB, Zorn GL, Morawetz RB, Smith LR, Adams M, Freeman AM. Factors and their influence on regional cerebral blood flow during nonpulsatile cardiopulmonary bypass. *Ann Thorac Surg* 1984;38:592–600.
8. Fox L, Blackstone E, Kirklin J, Bishop S, Bergdahl L, Bradley E. Relationship of brain blood flow and oxygen consumption to perfusion flow rate during pro-

foundly hypothermic cardiopulmonary bypass. *J Thorac Cardiovasc Surg* 1984; 87:658–664.

9. Greeley WJ, Ungerleider RM, Smith LR, Reves JG. The effects of deep hypothermic cardiopulmonary bypass and total circulatory arrest on cerebral blood flow in infants and children. *J Thorac Cardiovasc Surg* 1989;97:737–745.

10. Tanaka J, Shiki K, Asou T, Yasui H, Tokunaga K. Carbon dioxide, brain damage, and cardiac surgery (letter). *Lancet* 1988;1:353.

11. Kety S. Human cerebral blood flow and oxygen consumption as related to aging. *J Chron Dis* 1956;3:478–486.

12. Scheinberg P, Stead EA. The cerebral blood flow in male subjects as measured by the nitrous technique: Normal values for blood flow, oxygen utilization, glucose utilization, and peripheral resistance with observations on the effect of tilting and anxiety. *J Clin Invest* 1949;28:

13. Stullken EH Jr., Michenfenlder JD, et al. The non-linear responses of cerebral metabolism to low concentrations of halothane, enflurane, isoflurane and thiopental. *Anesthesiology* 1977;46:28.

14. Rosenberg AA, Jones MD, Traystman RJ, Simmons MA, Molteni RA. Response of cerebral blood flow to changes in $paCO_2$ in fetal, newborn and adult sheep. *Am J Physiol* 1982;242:H862–H866.

15. Prough DS, Stump DA, Roy RC, Gravlee GP, Williams T, Mills SA, Hinshelwood L, Howard G. Response of cerebral blood flow to changes in carbon dioxide tension during hypothermic cardiopulmonary bypass. *Anesthesiology* 1986; 64:576–581.

16. Murkin JM, Farrar JK, Tweed WA, McKenzie FN, Guiraudon G. Cerebral autoregulation and flow/metabolism coupling during cardiopulmonary bypass: The influence of $paCO_2$. *Anesth Analg* 1987;66:825–832.

17. Kern FH, Ungerleider RM, Quill TJ, Baldwin B, White WD, Reves JG, Greeley WJ. Cerebral blood flow response to changes in arterial carbon dioxide tension during hypothermic cardiopulmonary bypass in children. *J Thorac Cardiovasc Surg* 1991;101:618–622.

18. Kirklin JW, Barratt-Boyes BG (eds.). *Cardiac surgery.* New York: John Wiley & Sons, 1986, pp. 29–82.

19. Sutton LN, Clark BJ, Norwood CR, Woodford EJ, Welsh FA. Global cerebral ischemia in piglets under conditions of mild and deep hypothermia. *Stroke* 1991;22:1567–1573.

20. Bellinger DC, Wernovsky G, Rappaport LA, Mayer JE, Castaneda AR, Farrell DM, Lang P, Hickey PR, Jonas RA, Newburger JW. Cognitive development following repair as neonates of transposition of the great arteries using deep hypothermic circulatory arrest. *Pediatrics* 1991;87:701–707.

21. Kern FH, Jonas RA, Mayer JE, Hanley FL, Castaneda AR, Hickey PR. Temperature monitoring during infant CPB: Does it predict efficient brain cooling? *Ann Thor Surg* 1992;54:749–754.

22. Greeley WJ, Bracey VA, Ungerleider RM, Greibel JA, Kern FH, Boyd JL, Reves JG, Piantadosi CA. Recovery of cerebral metabolism and mitochondrial oxidation state is delayed after hypothermic circulatory arrest. *Circulation* 1991; 84 III:400–415.

23. Mault JR, Whitaker EG, Heinle JS, Lodge AJ, Greeley WJ, Ungerleider RM. Intermittent perfusion during hypothermic circulatory arrest: A new and effective technique for cerebral protection. *Surg Forum* 1992;44:314–316.

24. Jobsis A, vander Vliet FF. Niroscopy: Noninvasive near infrared monitoring of cellular oxygen sufficiency in vivo. *Adv Exp Med Biol* 1986;191:833–836.
25. Brazy JE, Lewis DV, Mitnick MH, Jobsis A, vander Vliet FF. Noninvasive monitoring of cerebral oxygenation in preterm infants: Preliminary observations. *Pediatrics* 1985;75:217–225.

CHAPTER 19

Assessment by Nuclear Magnetic Resonance Spectroscopy of the Effects of Cardiopulmonary Bypass, Hypothermia, and Circulatory Arrest on the Brain

Julie A. Swain

A series of investigations were undertaken to determine the effects of cardiopulmonary bypass, hypothermia, hyperglycemia, and barbiturates on cerebral high-energy content and intracellular pH, as measured by nuclear magnetic resonance spectroscopy (NMR) in an adolescent sheep model. These experiments were designed to determine an optimal cerebral protection protocol.

Cardiopulmonary Bypass

The effect of nonpulsatile cardiopulmonary bypass on cerebral metabolism was investigated. Adolescent sheep were placed on cardiopulmonary bypass and had NMR measurements of cerebral phosphocreatine (PCr), ATP, and intracellular pH made before and after the initiation of nonpulsatile cardiopulmonary bypass. There was no change in high-energy phosphates or intracellular pH with normothermic cardiopulmonary bypass.[1]

Hypothermia

Hypothermia is the mainstay of cerebral protection because it increases ischemic tolerance. The change in metabolic rate per 10°C change in temperature is called the Q_{10}. Michenfelder[2] showed that, when the temperature is decreased from 37°C to 27°C, the Q_{10} is 2.2, but when temperature is decreased very low, to the temperatures that we usually associate with circulatory arrest, the Q_{10} is much higher. Therefore, the predicted ischemic tolerance time at 15°C with a Q_{10} of 4.5 is 69 minutes, compared to the 34 minutes predicted for a Q_{10} of 2.2. Clinical experience confirms this increase in ischemic protection at deep hypothermia. Our research group has spent several years trying to determine why hypothermia is more cerebroprotective than predicted by metabolic calculations alone. We used phosphorus-31 nuclear magnetic resonance spectroscopy to look at cerebral high-energy phosphate levels and intracellular pH in a sheep model.

In the first study, sheep were placed in a magnet and baseline studies were performed on cardiopulmonary bypass at 37°C. The animals were slowly cooled to 15°C. A 10% increase in brain high-energy phosphate content occurred with hypothermia.[3] Increasing the basal energy state of the brain would be predicted to increase the cerebral ischemic tolerance; this is a partial explanation of the cerebroprotective effect of hypothermia.

The effect of hypothermia on intracellular pH relative to blood pH also was investigated.[3] Alpha-stat and pH-stat blood acid-base regulation during hypothermia were compared by measuring the effect of these two pH strategies on the intracellular pH of the brain. Figure 19–1 demonstrates that regardless of the blood pH level, the brain intracellular pH increased parallel to the neutral pH of water and the alpha-stat curve. This was the first demonstration in warm-blooded animals that the brain intracellular pH is defended along the alpha-stat curve regardless of the blood pH. If one postulates that the final mechanism of tissue damage is acidosis, then by starting at a more alkalotic pH, one gets increased protective time during circulatory arrest. The mechanism that creates a pH gradient between the blood and the intracellular pH of the brain is unknown.

Therefore, it has been shown that, besides metabolic rate suppression, hypothermia is protective by two other mechanisms: an increase in the basal tissue energy state and an increase in intracellular pH. These two mechanisms are enough to explain the increased protective effects of hypothermia that have been known clinically for years.

Hyperglycemia

Previous experimental work has shown that animals pretreated with glucose prior to cerebral ischemia have a poor neurologic outcome.[4] Diabetic patients with hyperglycemia who have strokes have a worse outcome than

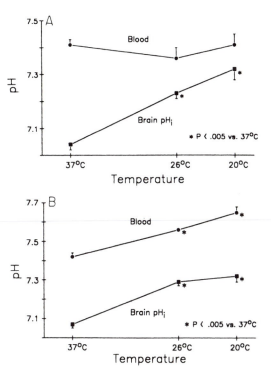

FIGURE 19–1. Relationship between blood pH and brain intracellular pH (pH$_i$) during pH-stat (A) and alpha-stat (B) blood pH management strategies. (Reprinted with permission from Swain, et. al., *Am J Physiol* 1991;260: H1640–H1644.)

normoglycemic patients.[5] The mechanism postulated for these findings is that hyperglycemia supplies additional substrate for anaerobic metabolism during ischemia. With acidosis, there is disruption of the energetics of homeostasis. Ion pump dysfunction and the subsequent abolishment of ion gradients changes membrane permeability and leads to the irreversible processes of lipolysis and proteolysis.

A previous study has shown a linear relationship between intracellular pH and cellular lactate levels,[6] which is consistent with the hypothesis that anaerobic glycolysis produces cellular lactate. Thus phosphorus-31 NMR can be used to measure intracellular pH indirectly as a correlation to anaerobic glycolysis.

Hyperglycemia is common during cardiopulmonary bypass. During hypothermia, there is impaired insulin production and action, decreased glucose utilization, and increased production of gluconeogenic hormones

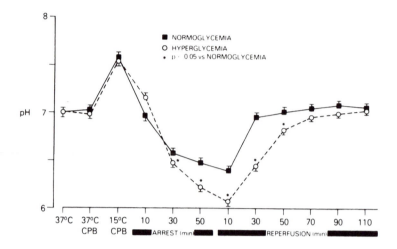

FIGURE 19–2.   Cerebral intracellular pH. (CPB = cardiopulmonary bypass.) (Reprinted with permission from Anderson RV, Siegman MG, Balaban RS, Ceckler TL, Swain JA. Hyperglycemia exacerbates cerebral intracellular acidosis during hypothermic circulatory arrest and reperfusion. *Ann Thor Surg* 1992;54:1126–1130.)

(epinephrine, norepinephrine).[7] Exogenous glucose administration during cardiopulmonary bypass and in intravenous fluids add to the glucose load.

Our hypothesis was that animals with high glucose levels prior to circulatory arrest would develop greater intracellular acidosis than normoglycemic animals. The sheep were cooled to 15°C, subjected to one hour of circulatory arrest, which was followed by two hours of reperfusion. There were two groups of sheep: normoglycemic animals with a blood glucose averaging 75 mg/dL and a hyperglycemic group (glucose 250 to 300 mg/dL). As predicted, there was a significant decrease in intracellular pH in the hyperglycemic animals. The pH differences were substantial by the end of circulatory arrest and persisted during much of the reperfusion period (Figure 19–2).[8]

On the basis of these experiments, we recommend that one avoid hyperglycemia during all cardiopulmonary bypass procedures to avoid exacerbation of the inevitable cerebral ischemia produced by microemboli during bypass.

Barbiturates

Barbiturates have been advocated for cerebroprotection during cardiac surgical procedures.[9] Barbiturates may be beneficial because of anticonvulsant

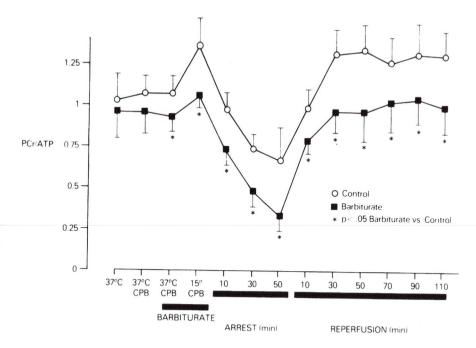

FIGURE 19–3. Changes in the phosphocreatine/adenosine triphosphate (PCr/ATP) ratio for both the barbiturate-treated animals and controls at selected periods throughout the course of the experiment. (Reprinted with permission from Siegman MG, Anderson RV, Balaban RS, Ceckler TL, Clark RE, Swain JA. Barbiturates impair cerebral metabolism during hypothermic circulatory arrest. *Ann Thorac Surg* 1992;54:1131–1136.

and antioxidant properties and because they decrease brain oxygen consumption. The effect on brain ischemia of pretreatment with barbiturates prior to hypothermic circulatory arrest was studied.[10] When barbiturates were given prior to instituting hypothermic bypass, the normal increase in high-energy phosphate levels associated with hypothermia was prevented. Therefore, at the beginning of circulatory arrest, there are significantly lower levels of high-energy phosphates in the barbiturate-treated animals; these lower levels persist during circulatory arrest and throughout the reperfusion period (Figure 19–3).

High-energy phosphate content is related to ischemic tolerance; therefore, by decreasing high-energy phosphates, barbiturates may be deleterious. Therefore, there is some concern about the use of barbiturates in patients who are going to undergo circulatory arrest. The beneficial effects of barbiturates, such as antioxidant and antiseizure properties, can be produced with other drugs.

References

1. Swain JA, Robbins RC, Balaban RS, McDonald TJ, Schneider B, Groom RC. The effect of cardiopulmonary bypass on brain and heart metabolism: A ^{31}P NMR study. *Magn Reson Med* 1990;15(3):446–455.
2. Michenfelder JD, Milde JH. The relationship among canine brain temperature, metabolism, and function during hypothermia. *Anesthesiology* 1991;75: 130–136.
3. Swain JA, McDonald TJ, Balaban RS, Robbins RC. Metabolism of the heart and brain during hypothermic cardiopulmonary bypass. *Ann Thorac Surg* 1991; 51(1):105–109.
4. Gardiner M, Smith M, Kagstrom E, Shohami E, Siesjo BK. Influence of blood glucose concentration on brain lactate accumulation during severe hypoxia and subsequent recovery of brain energy metabolism. *J Cereb Blood Flow Metab* 1982;2:429–438.
5. Pulsinelli WA, Levy DE, Sigsbee B, Scherer P, Plum F. Increased damage after ischemic stroke in patients with hyperglycemia with or without established diabetes mellitus. *Am J Med* 1983;74:540–544.
6. Corbett RJT, Laptook AR, Nunnally RL, Hassan A, Jackson J. Intracellular pH lactate, and energy metabolism in neonatal brain during partial ischemia measured *in vivo* by ^{31}P and ^{1}H nuclear magnetic resonance spectroscopy. *J Neurochem* 1988; 51:1501–1509.
7. Weiland AP, Walker WE. Physiologic principles and clinical sequelae of cardiopulmonary bypass. *Heart Lung* 1986;15:34–39.
8. Anderson RV, Siegman MG, Balaban RS, Ceckler TL, Swain JA. Hyperglycemia exacerbates cerebral intracellular acidosis during hypothermic circulatory arrest and reperfusion. *Ann Thor Surg* 1992;54:1126–1130.
9. Nussmeier NA, Arlund C, Slogoff S. Neuropsychiatric complications after cardiopulmonary bypass: Cerebral protection by a barbiturate. *Anesthesiology* 1986;64:165–170.
10. Siegman MG, Anderson RV, Balaban RS, Ceckler TL, Clark RE, Swain JA. Barbiturates impair cerebral metabolism during hypothermic circulatory arrest. *Ann Thorac Surg* 1992;54,1131–1136.

CHAPTER 20

pH Management During Hypothermic Cardiopulmonary Bypass with Circulatory Arrest

Richard A. Jonas

Introduction

pH management during cardiopulmonary bypass remains controversial. Both clinical and laboratory studies from Children's Hospital have addressed this problem as it applies specifically to infants and neonates undergoing cardiopulmonary bypass and circulatory arrest. Although no clear answers have emerged, these studies provide some insights into the advantages and disadvantages of these alternative strategies.

Rationales for the Alternative pH Strategies

Cooling is associated with an alkaline shift in the pH of neutrality of water and blood in a closed system. In cooling from 37°C to 15°C the pH of neutrality of water shifts from approximately 6.8 to 7.2 as defined by the Rosenthal factor.[1] This shift is parallel to the shift in the pK of the major buffering system of the body, namely, the imidazole moiety of the amino acid histidine, which is present in most proteins.

Two strategies have been used in response to the pH shift during hypothermic bypass. From the 1960s to the late 1970s, the more popular strategy was the *pH-stat strategy*, in which carbon dioxide is added to the gas mixture in the oxygenator to compensate for the alkaline shift. The resulting respiratory acidosis causes the pH to remain constant at 7.40 as determined at the patient's hypothermic body temperature. As measured at 37°C—as is standard in blood-gas analyzers, which warm the cold blood sample to 37°C to perform the analysis—there will appear to be an increasing respiratory acidosis as the temperature decreases. The alternative *alpha-stat strategy* does not compensate for the natural shift in pH. With the alpha-stat strategy the pH remains at 7.40 as measured at 37°C. Generally, pure oxygen is used as the gas mixture in the oxygenator.[2]

When the pH-stat strategy was first introduced, its principle advantage was thought to be the increased cerebral blood flow resulting from the cerebral vasodilation secondary to the added carbon dioxide.[3] The additional cerebral blood flow was thought to provide a useful reserve when low-flow bypass was required. Additional advantages of the pH-stat strategy are possible. For example, hypothermia is associated with a leftward shift in the oxyhemoglobin dissociation curve. The respiratory acidosis of the pH-stat strategy results in a rightward shift of the oxyhemoglobin curve which counteracts the leftward shift induced by hypothermia.[4] This will increase oxygen availability, which may be particularly important when hypothermic blood must deliver adequate oxygen to warm tissues during the early phase of cooling. Increased blood flow will theoretically improve the efficiency, and perhaps the homogeneity, of cooling of the brain before circulatory arrest. Finally, evidence from neuronal cell culture studies and brain slices suggests that extracellular acidosis following reperfusion after cerebral ischemia may reduce reperfusion injury. This is most likely related to competition between protons and calcium ions for cell entry during reperfusion. An increased number of protons in the extracellular milieu during reperfusion results in less calcium entry and therefore less reperfusion injury.

Advantages of the alpha-stat strategy include the preservation of flow/metabolism coupling, i.e., cerebral blood flow is appropriate for the degree of cerebral metabolism.[5] The lesser blood flow relative to the pH-stat strategy reduces the potential for embolism. Furthermore, intracellular enzyme function is optimized with the alpha-stat strategy.[6]

Clinical Experience with Alternative pH Strategies at Children's Hospital

At Boston Children's Hospital, the pH-stat strategy was the standard method of pH management during hypothermic bypass until 1985 (Figure 20–1). At that time, based on comparative physiological studies of cold-blooded vertebrates reported by Rahn, et al.[7] and Swan,[2] the strategy was changed to the alpha-stat strategy. These studies had demonstrated that many cold-blooded vertebrates follow an alpha-stat strategy when their body temperature decreases as ambient temperature decreases. Of note, however, was the observation that, in contrast to animals that remain active when their body

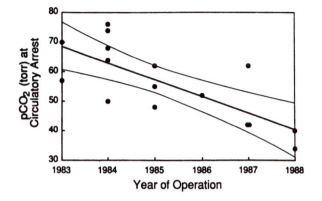

FIGURE 20–1. Arterial pCO_2 (as measured at 37°C) before deep hypothermic circulatory arrest, according to year of operation, for 16 patients undergoing Senning operation. Change from a more acidotic strategy (pH-stat) to a more alkalotic strategy (alpha-stat) is apparent.

temperature is hypothermic, animals that become inactive during hypothermia (i.e., animals that hibernate) generally employ the pH-stat strategy; they hypoventilate even relative to the decreased rate of CO_2 production, secondary to their decreased rate of metabolism.

There were few, if any, clinical trials between 1975 and 1985—when many centers including our own changed from the pH-stat to the alpha-stat strategy—to confirm the efficacy of either strategy in providing optimal protection, either for the brain or for the heart. However, in 1987 Nevin and colleagues [8] described a study in the *Lancet* in which they had undertaken psychometric studies of adult patients undergoing coronary artery bypass grafting. They found that the pCO_2 *before* bypass was an important determinant of the incidence of postoperative psychometric deficits. Patients who were more alkalotic, with a CO_2 less than 35mm, had a 71% incidence of deficits whereas patients with a more normal CO_2 had a lesser incidence of deficits. Subsequent to this study we were stimulated to review the influence of carbon dioxide management before bypass, as well as pH strategy during hypothermic bypass, on developmental outcome.

Retrospective Clinical Study of pH
Strategy and Developmental Outcome
after Hypothermic Circulatory Arrest

As stated above, in 1985, the routine management of arterial pCO_2 at Boston Children's Hospital was changed from pH-stat to alpha-stat, with a shift toward a progressively more alkaline strategy over time. Thus, infants in the period between 1983 and 1988 underwent cardiac repair over a wide range of arterial pCO_2. The purpose of this retrospective study [9] was to examine the influence of arterial pCO_2 management during corrective cardiac surgery in infancy on later cognitive function.

Patients were selected according to the following criteria: (1) diagnosis of d-transposition of the great arteries, with intact ventricular septum (dTGA,IVS); (2) repair by Senning procedure at Children's Hospital, Boston, between 1983 and 1988; (3) age at repair less than six months; (4) residence in New England; and (5) informed consent by parents. We attempted to enroll all eligible children, regardless of prior or intercurrent medical history or operative course.

Perfusion and monitoring techniques were as follows. Infants were not actively cooled, but they underwent spontaneous surface cooling during the induction of general anesthesia and introduction of arterial and venous catheters to a rectal temperature at the commencement of bypass of 32° to 34°C. Esophageal and tympanic temperatures were also monitored. Subsequently, core cooling was performed on cardiopulmonary bypass to a rectal temperature of 20°C or less.

The perfusate was a pH-balanced crystalloid solution (Normosol-R), with addition of citrated blood to achieve a hematocrit of 20 on bypass. The ionized calcium was not corrected and, therefore, was low. The activated clotting time was maintained at greater than 400 seconds. During the period of the study, an arterial filter was not used. The perfusate temperature was 20°C before beginning bypass. Following the onset of bypass, the chilled wall water was turned on to the heat exchanger. The perfusion flow rate during cooling for patients weighing between 2.5 and 10 kg was 150 mL/kg. Within the first minute of bypass, the following drugs were given: phentolamine (Regitine) 0.2 mg/kg, furosemide 0.25 mg/kg, and methylprednisolone (Solu-Medrol) 30 mg/kg. Pentothal, 10 mg/kg, was given approximately ten minutes after initiation of bypass. Before 1987, the Bentley infant bubble oxygenator was used. Subsequently, the Cobe variable prime membrane oxygenator was used.

Before 1985, the pH-stat method of pH management was applied. The pH, as read from a blood-gas analyzer at 37°C, was corrected to the patient's esophageal temperature using a nomogram, aiming to achieve a pH of 7.40 corrected to the patient's temperature. This required adding carbon dioxide to the gas mixture. After 1985, the alpha-stat strategy was used.

At the end of the arrest period, the heart was filled with saline to exclude air, and the single venous cannula was reinserted. Bypass was recommenced with the perfusate at 18°C. Water temperature was maintained 10° to 12°C higher than the venous blood return, to a maximum water temperature of 42°C. In general, the cross clamp was removed shortly after recommencing bypass. Mannitol, 0.5 g/kg, was given at the time of cross clamp removal. At a rectal temperature of 30°C, calcium gluconate was given in a dose of 1.0 g for the first unit of whole blood used in the prime and 0.5 g for each additional unit. Thereafter, calcium gluconate was given as needed to maintain normal ionized calcium levels.

Information about preoperative health status (birth weight, 5-minute Apgar score, lowest documented arterial oxygen tension, and pH) was obtained from the medical record. The operative reports and perfusion records were reviewed for the following information: (1) temperatures (rectal, tympanic, esophageal) prior to initiation of cardiopulmonary bypass; (2) temperatures at the onset of total circulatory arrest; (3) minutes of cardiopulmonary bypass prior to total circulatory arrest (duration of core cooling); (4) minutes of total circulatory arrest; (5) temperatures at reinstitution of cardiopulmonary bypass; (6) degrees (C) of ambient rewarming during total circulatory arrest; (7) minutes of cardiopulmonary bypass until rectal temperature reached 34° to 36°C (core rewarming); (8) minutes of cardiopulmonary bypass at greater than 35°C; (9) aortic cross clamp time; (10) total minutes of cardiopulmonary bypass (i.e., total bypass time); and (11) total support time (time on cardiopulmonary bypass plus total circulatory arrest).

The following information was recorded regarding the postoperative period: (1) hours of mechanical ventilation; (2) days in the intensive care unit; (3) days of hospitalization; and (4) presence or absence of seizures noted during routine clinical care by nurses, cardiovascular surgeons, or cardiologists.

The Bayley Scales of Infant Development were administered to children younger than 30 months of age (n = 4).[10] This instrument yields two scores, the Mental Development Index and the Psychomotor Development Index. The McCarthy Scales of Children's Abilities were administered to children who were at least 30 months of age (n = 12).[11] This instrument yields a General Cognitive Index and five scale scores: Verbal, Perceptual-Performance, Quantitative, Memory, and Motor. In this retrospective study we focused on global indices of early cognitive function, namely, the Mental Development Index of the Bayley Scales and the General Cognitive Index of the McCarthy Scales. Both were originally age-normed to have a mean of 100 and a standard deviation of 16. Recent data suggests that the population mean has drifted upward to approximately 110.

At the time of the developmental assessment, we recorded the occupation and education of parents (social class), as well as the birth order of the patients.

Results of the Retrospective Study of pH Strategy

Of 35 children who met eligibility criteria for the study, 16 (46.5%) were tested. The median age of study subjects at the time of operation was 32 days (range, 2 to 156 days). Ten (62.5%) were male. Developmental testing was performed at a median age of 47.5 months (range, 11 to 79 months). The median developmental IQ score was 109.0 (range, 74 to 129); 4 of 16 patients (25%) were tested with the Bayley Scales of Infant Development, and 12

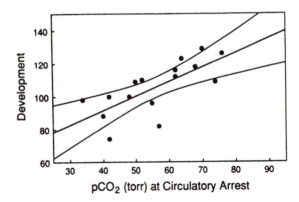

FIGURE 20–2. Association between cognitive function and arterial pCO_2 (as measured at 37°C) before deep hypothermic arrest (r=.71, p=.002).

(75%) were tested with the McCarthy Scales of Children's Abilities. The socioeconomic status of the sample was high.

We evaluated the association between arterial pCO_2 at the onset of circulatory arrest and cognitive function (Figure 20–2). There was a strong positive correlation between arterial pCO_2 and developmental score. Over the arterial pCO_2 range of approximately 30 to 80 torr, developmental score increased 0.88 points for every 1-torr increase in pCO_2 (r = .71, p = .002).

To investigate whether this association could be attributed to confounding by other intraoperative or sociodemographic variables, we examined the impact of adjusting for certain of these variables on the pCO_2 coefficient (i.e., the change in developmental score for each change of 1 torr in pCO_2). When we controlled for intraoperative variables including cooling duration, duration of circulatory arrest, and total bypass time, the coefficient of pCO_2 remained stable, with a statistically significant p value. In the regression model including social class index, the pCO_2 coefficient decreased by 25%; however, the association between arterial pCO_2 and development remained statistically significant (p = .037). Adjustment for other patient variables, such as sex and birth order, did not affect the pCO_2 coefficient. Similarly, the association between pCO_2 and development was not explained by either preoperative variables (e.g., birth weight, intubation, age at surgery, lowest pO_2, lowest pH) or postoperative variables (length of stay in the ICU, days of hospitalization, presence of seizures).

The relationship between intraoperative variables other than pCO_2 and developmental score is shown in Table 20–1. Higher pH at the onset of total circulatory arrest was significantly associated with a worse developmental outcome (r = −.51, p = .05), as expected from the observed association between development and pCO_2. The duration of total circulatory arrest among study subjects ranged from 35 to 60 minutes (median, 43 min-

TABLE 20-1.
Correlations Between Development and Other Intraoperative and Postoperative Variables

	Correlation	p Value
Age at operation	.08	.76
Temperature before CPB		
Esophageal	.12	.66
Rectal	.26	.33
Tympanic	.20	.47
pCO$_2$ before CPB	.26	.39
pH before CPB	−.15	.63
Duration of core cooling	−.43	.10
Temperature before DHCA		
Esophageal	.36	.17
Rectal	.41	.12
Tympanic	.33	.22
pH before DHCA	−.51	.05
Duration of DHCA	−.19	.49
Temperature rise during DHCA		
Esophageal	−.45	.08
Rectal	.08	.77
Tympanic	−.11	.69
Temperature after DHCA		
Esophageal	−.10	.72
Rectal	.58	.02
Tympanic	.33	.21
Duration of core rewarming	−.39	.14
Time on CPB after warming	.27	.32
Duration of CPB	−.38	.15
Duration of crossclamping	−.42	.11
Lowest pO$_2$	−.40	.22
Lowest pH	.14	.72
ICU stay	.10	.72
Mechanical ventilation	−.09	.74
Time to discharge	−.11	.68

DHCA, Deep hypothermia and circulatory arrest; *ICU,* intensive care unit.

utes) and was not significantly associated with development in this cohort. Similarly, development was not significantly associated with total bypass time, total support time, temperature at the onset of circulatory arrest, the extent of ambient rewarming during total circulatory arrest, or the duration of cross clamping.

There are several limitations to this study. Data were collected retrospectively and were subject to incomplete and inconsistent recording. In addition many other aspects of surgical and support procedures, other than acid-base management, changed over the same period. For example, the oxygenator was changed from bubble to membrane in this time frame. This was associated with a change in the tubing circuit design in that a recirculation line was added to allow continuous recirculation during the period of circulatory arrest. Recirculation was also used prebypass. Even with minimal gas flow there was often a very alkaline pH of the perfusate at the onset of bypass. The patient population may have also changed importantly over this time frame of 1983 to 1988, which was the period of introduction of the arterial switch for transposition. Early in the time frame, the study patients were likely to have been representative of the spectrum of transposition, but this is not likely to have been the case late in the series when children having the Senning procedure had to have been rejected from the arterial switch protocol, perhaps because of complex coronary artery anatomy. In addition the surgeons' recent familiarity with the Senning procedure decreased later in the series.

Another limitation of this study is the variable follow-up interval so that the age of the children varied widely at the time of their developmental assessment, necessitating different age-appropriate tests of cognitive function. This problem is exacerbated by the fact that age at follow-up (and thus, specific test administered) is strongly confounded by pCO_2 before circulatory arrest owing to the shift from pH-stat to alpha-stat in 1985. Children who were youngest at testing had the lowest pCO_2 values and achieved among the lowest developmental scores. A possible explanation for the findings of the study is that the time elapsed since operation, not pCO_2, is the key factor affecting development. If a recovery or compensatory process is operative, the children assessed at the youngest ages should show improvement over time. Arguing against this proposition is the recent finding from our prospective study of development after either circulatory arrest or low-flow bypass that the developmental scores achieved at 4 years of age are lower than those achieved in the same patient population at 1 year of age (preliminary unpublished data).

Another aspect of this study which warrants discussion is its apparent discrepancy relative to an earlier *retrospective* study of development after circulatory arrest in patients undergoing the arterial switch procedure at Boston Children's Hospital.[12] In that retrospective study, a significant association was found between duration of core cooling and developmental outcome, which was not identified in the second study of patients undergoing Senning procedures as described above. In the arterial switch retrospective study, for cooling periods less than 20 minutes, each additional minute of cooling was associated with a 5-point increase in developmental score ($r = .85$, $p < .001$). In that study the mean circulatory arrest time was relatively long (64.5 + 9.8 minutes), there was a wide range of cooling times, and the alpha-stat strategy was used in most patients. Under these circumstances a longer cooling duration might be required to achieve adequate homogenous brain cooling. In the Senning study the duration of circulatory arrest and of cooling were shorter than in the previous study (43.4 + 6.6 minutes and 14.5 + 6.2 minutes, respectively), and different pH strategies were used. No relationship was found between cooling duration and cognitive function. It is possible that when a uniform alpha-stat pH strategy is used, the associated lesser cerebral blood flow results in the duration of cooling being critical with respect to the homogeneity and completeness of brain cooling. However, when the cooling time is uniform, the pH strategy becomes the determining factor with respect to homogeneity of brain cooling.

In summary, these two retrospective studies suggest that a more alkaline pH strategy during the cooling phase of cardiopulmonary bypass, before circulatory arrest, may be associated with a worse developmental outcome. These data conflict with other studies of neuropsychometric outcome, predominantly in adults who have undergone moderately hypothermic bypass without circulatory arrest. These studies have found no important differences between pH-stat and alpha-stat or have favored alpha-stat. These results are consistent with the view that cerebral morbidity associated with continuous cardiopulmonary bypass is predominantly secondary to microembolic load, which is increased with the pH-stat strategy.

*Prospective Clinical Study of pH Strategy
and Developmental Outcome*

To further analyze the unexpected result of the retrospective clinical study, we began a prospective clinical study in which neonates and infants less than nine months of age undergoing cardiac repair under deep hypothermia are enrolled in a study of neurological and developmental outcome. Patients are randomized to either the alpha-stat or pH-stat strategy. They are assessed at 1 year of age by a neurologist and developmental psychologists. Additional secondary end points are the same as those used in the prospective study (see Part V) of development of infants who were randomized between circulatory arrest and low-flow bypass with a uniform alpha-stat strategy. These secondary end points are perioperative and include continuous EEG monitoring intraoperatively and for 48 hours postoperatively.

Laboratory Studies of pH Strategy

In an attempt to better understand the basic mechanisms underlying the advantages and disadvantages of the alternative pH strategies, we have applied our juvenile piglet model of deep hypothermic circulatory arrest.[13]

Direct Comparison of Alpha-stat and pH-stat

In the initial study,[14] four week old Yucatan piglets weighing mean 3.8 kg underwent one hour of hypothermic circulatory arrest at a nasopharyngeal temperature of 15°C. Half the animals underwent alpha-stat pH management during cooling and rewarming, and the remainder underwent the

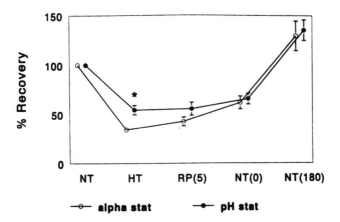

FIGURE 20–3.   Cerebral blood flow and metabolism by microsphere study. Acute percent recovery of cerebral blood flow after 1 hour of circulatory arrest determined by microsphere injection. NT(0) = after 45 minutes of rewarming, when normothermia (nasopharyngeal temperature > 35°C) was achieved; NT(180) = after 180 minutes of reperfusion at normothermia; RP(5) = 5 minutes after initiation of reperfusion and rewarming after 1 hour of total circulatory arrest. (Reprinted with permission from Aoki M, Nomura F, Stromski ME, Tsuji MK, Fackler JC, Hickey PR, Holtzman DH, Jonas RA. Effects of pH on brain energetics after hypothermic circulatory arrest. *Ann Thorac Surg* 1993;55:1092–1103.)

pH-stat strategy. The end points studied were cerebral blood flow by microspheres, cerebral oxygen consumption estimated by jugular venous oxygen extraction, cerebral edema determined by brain water content after sacrifice, and cerebral high-energy phosphate and intracellular pH determined by magnetic resonance spectroscopy.

As anticipated, this study demonstrated that cerebral blood flow during cooling is greater with pH-stat than with alpha-stat (Figure 20–3). This is secondary to the cerebral vasodilation resulting from the carbon dioxide added to the gas mixture as part of the pH-stat strategy. A particularly interesting and probably important finding of the study was the regional distribution of cerebral blood flow. Absolute flow was greater with pH-stat relative to alpha-stat in all regions during hypothermia. However, there was a decrease in the proportion of the total cerebral flow to the basal ganglia with alpha-stat and an increase in the proportion of the total flow going to the basal ganglia, cerebellum, pons, and medulla oblongata with pH-stat during cooling (Figure 20–4). The cerebral metabolic rate determined by both oxygen and glucose consumption indicates continuing metabolic activity during hypothermia to 15°C with both strategies.

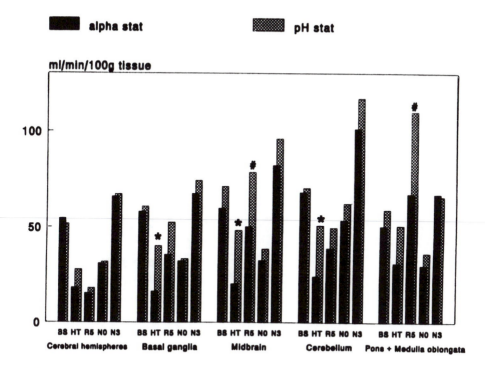

FIGURE 20–4.   Intracerebral distribution of blood flow. +p < .05 for the within-group increase by paired t-test; −p < .05 for the within-group decrease by paired t-test).

The magnetic resonance spectroscopy studies demonstrated that the pH-stat strategy is associated with faster recovery of cerebral high-energy phosphates and intracellular pH than is the alpha-stat strategy (Figure 20–5). In the alpha-stat animals there was a continuing decrease in pH for the first 40 minutes after circulatory arrest, while the pH-stat animals demonstrated an immediate return toward baseline. Both groups demonstrated an increase in both phosphocreatine and ATP during the cooling phase before circulatory arrest. We had observed this in a previous laboratory study in which we compared circulatory arrest and continuous low-flow bypass. This effect had previously been described by Swain,[15] who suggested that this may be one of the mechanisms by which hypothermia is protective. Presumably, cooling decreases the rate of utilization of high-energy phosphates faster than it decreases production.

An interesting observation was also made regarding the intracellular pH during cooling. Although we anticipated that animals undergoing the alpha-stat strategy would demonstrate an alkaline shift in pH during cooling, we thought that pH would remain stable in the pH-stat animals since, by definition, blood pH remains stable as measured at body temperature (MRS

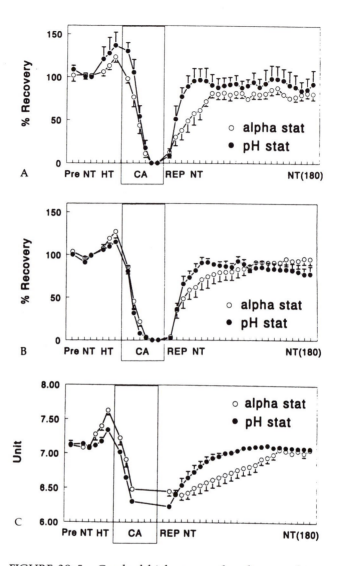

FIGURE 20–5. Cerebral high-energy phosphates and intracellular pH by magnetic resonance spectroscopy. (A) Percent recovery of cerebral adenosine triphosphate after 1 hour of circulatory arrest (CA). Baseline (100%) is taken at 20 minutes of normothermic cardiopulmonary bypass (NT) before cooling to a nasopharyngeal temperature of 15°C (HT). (B) Percent recovery of phosphocreatine after 1 hour of circulatory arrest. (C) Recovery of intracellular pH after 1 hour of circulatory arrest. (NT(180) = after 180 minutes of reperfusion at normothermia; REP = reperfusion and rewarming). (Reprinted with permission from Aoki M, Nomura F, Stromski ME, Tsuji MK, Fackler JC, Hickey PR, Holtzman DH, Jonas RA. Effects of pH on brain energetics after hypothermic circulatory arrest. *Ann Thorac Surg* 1993;55:1092–1103.)

measures at body temperature). However, a significant alkaline shift was also observed in the pH-stat animals, suggesting that cells regulate their intracellular pH independent of blood pH during hypothermia and, furthermore, that they regulate with an alpha-stat strategy (Figure 20.5).[15]

The significance of the findings of this study are limited by two main issues. First, although recovery of pH and high-energy phosphates was delayed with alpha-stat, ultimate recovery after more than 3 hours of reperfusion was similar in the two groups. Although delayed recovery of EEG and somatosensory potentials has been correlated with a worse outcome after circulatory arrest,[16,17] a direct demonstration of delayed recovery of MRS-determined pH and ATP and a worse neurological and developmental outcome has not been documented to date. Second, this study failed to differentiate whether the mechanisms resulting in more rapid recovery with pH-stat were primarily operative during the cooling phase or the rewarming phase. Accordingly, a second study of pH strategy using the piglet model was devised to examine this issue more closely.[18]

Mechanisms of Cerebral Protection According to pH Strategy

Possible mechanisms for the differences observed between alpha-stat and pH-stat in our initial laboratory study include (1) improved oxygen delivery and homogeneity of brain cooling in effect *before* deep hypothermic circulatory arrest and (2) greater cerebral blood flow and reduced reperfusion injury, secondary to extracellular acidosis during the rewarming phase *after* circulatory arrest.[19] To identify whether mechanisms in effect *before* versus those in effect *after* circulatory arrest were more important, we studied 49 4-week old piglets undergoing one hour of deep hypothermic circulatory arrest. Four groups were defined according to pH strategy during cooling and rewarming periods. In one group, animals underwent cooling with the alpha-stat strategy and rewarming with the alpha-stat strategy and were termed alpha/alpha (group A-A). A second group underwent alpha-stat during the cooling phase and pH-stat during rewarming and were termed alpha/pH (group A-P). The third and fourth groups were termed pH/alpha (group P-A) and pH/pH (group P-P). In approximately half the animals, cerebral high-energy phosphates and intracellular pH were measured by magnetic resonance spectroscopy (A-A 7, A-P 5, P-A 7, P-P 5). In the remaining animals, cerebral blood flow was measured by labeled microspheres, and cerebral metabolic rate was determined by oxygen and glucose extraction using samples drawn from a jugular venous catheter. In addition, near-infrared spectroscopy (NIRS) was used to assess the level of cerebral hemoglobin oxygenation and redox state of cytochrome aa3.[20] (Cytochrome aa3 is the terminal cytochrome of the oxidative phosphorylation chain. Therefore the redox state of this cytochrome is a measure of oxygen availability at mitochondrial level).

This study confirmed the findings of the previous study in that cerebral blood flow was greater with pH-stat than alpha-stat during cooling ($p < .001$).

Cytochrome aa3 became more reduced during cooling with alpha-stat than with pH-stat (p = .049). This finding is consistent with the hypothesis that an important advantage of the pH-stat strategy is that it counteracts the leftward shift in the oxyhemoglobin dissociation curve induced by hypothermia. This may be particularly important in the early phase of cooling when the brain temperature is relatively high in comparison with blood temperature. This observation however should be interpreted with care because the NIRS assessment of cytochrome has not been fully validated.

There was more rapid recovery of cerebral ATP when the pH-stat strategy was employed both before and after DHCA compared to use of alpha-stat during the cooling and/or rewarming phases. Cerebral intracellular pH decreased during the first 40 minutes of rewarming reperfusion only when alpha-stat was applied during both the cooling and rewarming phases. Global and regional cerebral blood flow was greater with pH-stat during cooling and also was greater during rewarming with pH-stat, irrespective of the strategy used during cooling.

We concluded from this study that there are mechanisms in effect during both the cooling and rewarming phases, before and after deep hypothermic circulatory arrest, which could contribute to an improved cerebral outcome with pH-stat relative to more alkaline strategies.

Myocardial Protection versus Cerebral Protection[21]

Studies of myocardial protection have suggested that the alpha-stat strategy provides more effective myocardial protection than the pH-stat strategy. It may be necessary to choose a pH strategy that is least compromising to both cerebral and myocardial protection. It is hoped that the current prospective study of pH strategy at Boston Children's Hospital will help to answer this question.

Conclusions

Evidence from both retrospective clinical studies and laboratory studies suggests that in the specific setting of infants undergoing deep hypothermic circulatory arrest with core cooling, the pH-stat strategy may provide more effective cerebral protection than the alpha-stat strategy. It should be emphasized that these findings should not be extrapolated to the older patient undergoing continuous moderate to full flow, mildly to moderately hypothermic bypass where the bulk of evidence currently favors the alpha-stat strategy. The prospective study of pH strategy should help to better define the optimal strategy for the infant undergoing cardiac repair under deep hypothermia.

References

1. Swan H. The hydroxyl-hydrogen ion concentration ratio during hypothermia. *Surg Gynecol Obstet* 1982;155:897–912.
2. Swan H. The importance of acid base management for cardiac and cerebral preservation during open heart operations. *Surg Gynecol Obstet* 1984;158: 391–414.
3. Belsey RHR, Dowlatshahi K, Keen G, Skinner DB. Profound hypothermia in cardiac surgery. *J Thorac Cardiovasc Surg* 1968;56:497–509.
4. Severinghaus JW. Respiration and hypothermia. *Ann NY Acad Sci* 1959;80: 384–394.
5. Murkin JM, Farrar JK, Tweed WA, McKenzie FN, Guiraudon G. Cerebral autoregulation and flow/metabolism coupling during cardiopulmonary bypass: The influence of $PaCO_2$. *Anesth Analg* 1987;66:825–832.
6. Reeves RB. An imidazole alphastat hypothesis for vertebrate acid-base regulation: Tissue carbon dioxide content and body temperature in bullfrogs. *Respir Physiol* 1972;14:219–236.
7. Rahn H, Reeves BR, Howell BJ. Hydrogen ion regulation, temperature, and evolution. The 1975 J. Burns Amberson Lecture. *Am Rev Respir Dis* 1975;112: 165–172.
8. Nevin M, Colchester AC, Adams S, Pepper JR. Evidence for involvement of hypocapnia and hypoperfusion in aetiology of neurologic deficit after cardiopulmonary bypass. *Lancet* 1987;2:1493–1495.
9. Jonas RA, Bellinger DC, Rappaport LA, Wernovsky G, Hickey PR, Farrell DM, Newburger JW. Relation of pH strategy and developmental outcome after hypothermic circulatory arrest. *J Thorac Cardiovasc Surg* 1993;106:362–368.
10. Bayley N. *Bayley scales of infant development.* New York: The Psychological Corporation, 1969.
11. McCarthy D. *McCarthy scales of children's abilities.* New York: The Psychological Corporation, 1969.
12. Bellinger DC, Wernovsky G, Rappaport LA, et al. Cognitive development of children following early repair of transposition of the great arteries using deep hypothermic circulatory arrest. *Pediatrics* 1991;87:701–707.
13. Kawata H, Fackler JC, Aoki M, et al. Recovery of cerebral blood flow and energy state after hypothermic circulatory arrest versus low-flow-bypass in piglets. *J Thorac Cardiovasc Surg* 1993;106:671–685.
14. Aoki M, Nomura F, Stromski ME, Tsuji MK, Fackler JC, Hickey PR, Holtzman DH, Jonas RA. Effects of pH on brain energetics after hypothermic circulatory arrest. *Ann Thorac Surg* 1993;55:1092–1103.
15. Swain JA, McDonald TJ, Robbins RC, Balaban RS. Relationship of cerebral and myocardial intracellular pH to blood pH during hypothermia. *Am J Physiol* 1991; 260:H1640–1644.
16. Robbins RC, Balaban RS, Swain JA. Intermittent hypothermic asanguineous cerebral perfusion (cerebroplegia) protects the brain during prolonged circulatory arrest. *J Thorac Cardiovasc Surg* 1990;99:878–884.
17. Coles JG, Taylor MJ, Pearce JM, et al. Cerebral monitoring of somatosensory evoked potentials during profoundly hypothermic circulatory arrest. *Circulation* 1984;70 (suppl 1):96–102.

18. Hiramatsu T, Miura T, Forbess JM, Du Plessis A, Aoki M, Walter G, Holtzman D, Jonas RA. pH strategies and cerebral energetics before and after circulatory arrest. *J Thorac Cardiovasc Surg* 1995;948–957.
19. Matsuda N, Kuroda H, Mori T. Beneficial actions of acidotic initial reperfusate in stunned myocardium of rat hearts. *Basic Res Cardiol* 1991;86:317–326.
20. Jobsis-vanderVliet FF, Piantadosi CA, Sylvia AL, Lucas SK, Keizer HH. Near infrared monitoring of cerebral oxygen sufficiency: I, Spectra of cytochrome C oxidase. *Neurol Res* 1988;10:7–17.
21. Jonas RA. Myocardial protection or cerebral protection: A potential conflict. *J Thorac Cardiovasc Surg* 1992;104:533–534.

PART **V**

A Prospective Clinical Study of Circulatory Arrest at Children's Hospital, Boston

CHAPTER 21

Methods and Procedures

Jane W. Newburger
David Wypij

Congenital heart lesions are among the most common birth defects.[1] Indeed, children with structural heart disease now constitute the largest single patient population in many pediatric in-patient services. Of the 30,000 infants born annually with congenital heart disease, more than one-third will require cardiac surgery early in life.[2] Recent dramatic reductions in surgical mortality have been accompanied by the recognition that the survivors frequently suffer adverse neurologic sequelae, including mental retardation, seizures, cerebral palsy, and lifelong language and learning disorders. The majority of such brain injury may be attributable to operative events, particularly the support techniques used to protect vital organs during cardiac repair.[2]

The two major support techniques used in repair of complex congenital heart lesions in infancy are (1) deep hypothermia with total circulatory arrest (circulatory arrest) and (2) deep hypothermia with continuous low-flow cardiopulmonary bypass (low-flow bypass). Since its introduction in the early 1960s,[3,4] circulatory arrest has been widely used in centers with expertise in infant open heart surgery. A great advantage of this technique is the absence of perfusion cannulae and of blood from the operative field. The use of circulatory arrest for open heart surgery assumes that there is a safe duration of total circulatory arrest, which is inversely related to body temperature and is characterized by the absence of detectable structural or functional organ derangements in the early or late postoperative period.[5] The organ with the shortest safe circulatory arrest time is the brain. Conflicting reports of transient cerebral dysfunction and late neurologic and developmental adverse effects after circulatory arrest have generated considerable controversy about its use. An alternative support method, low-flow bypass, maintains continuous cerebral circulation during repair and has been advocated as preferable to circulatory arrest, with respect to neurologic outcome.[6–8] However, low-flow bypass may increase exposure to other sources of brain injury.

In 1988, we began a multidisciplinary trial (i.e., the Boston Circulatory Arrest Study) to compare the occurrence of brain injury after use of deep hypothermia with total circulatory arrest (circulatory arrest) versus deep hypothermia with continuous low-flow cardiopulmonary bypass (low-flow bypass) for repair of critical congenital heart disease in infancy. Our goals were pursued in a prospective, randomized, single-center trial using a homogeneous population of infants with d-transposition of the great arteries requiring surgery within the first month of life. The two support techniques were compared specifically with respect to neurologic and developmental function during the perioperative period, at age 1 year, and at age 4 years, with the latter phase of the study ongoing at the time of this report. The purpose of this chapter is to give a detailed description of the methods used during the perioperative and 1-year follow-up phases of the Boston Circulatory Arrest Study. This research was supported by the National Institute of Health (HL41786).

Study Population

Eligibility criteria included (1) a diagnosis of d-transposition of the great arteries (dTGA) with intact ventricular septum (IVS) or ventricular septal defect (VSD), (2) scheduled repair by 3 months of age, and (3) coronary artery anatomy thought to be suitable for the arterial switch operation. Exclusion criteria included (1) birth weight less than 2.5 kg, (2) recognizable syndrome of congenital anomalies, (3) associated extracardiac anomalies of greater than minor severity, (4) previous cardiac surgery, or (5) associated cardiovascular anomalies requiring aortic arch reconstruction or additional open surgical procedures. Informed consent was obtained from the parents of all subjects according to the guidelines of the institutional Human Investigation Committee.

The homogeneous patient population enrolled in this trial travelled from a wide geographical area to one clinical center because of the center's expertise in the arterial switch operation, thus providing the statistical power necessary for comparison of treatment groups. The arterial switch procedure requires minimal intracardiac exposure, so either support technique can be employed with equal facility. This unique aspect of the repair of dTGA by arterial switch allowed randomization of patients to either support technique without generating concomitant changes in surgical methods that might alter the outcome. Additional advantages of this study population included its low incidence of associated cardiac or extracardiac anomalies, relatively uniform age at repair, and low incidence of significant postoperative hemodynamic problems.

We enrolled patients from January 1989 through February 1992 at a single center, Children's Hospital, Boston. Of 174 eligible infants, 166 (95.4%) were enrolled. The arterial switch operation was performed in 157 infants (94.6% of those enrolled); the remaining 9 patients were found at operation to have coronary artery anatomy unsuitable for the arterial switch operation and thus were ineligible for the study. Fourteen additional infants met eligibility criteria, were enrolled, and were randomized according to the study protocol between February 1988 and October 1988 (prior to the onset of the funded enrollment phase of the trial); all underwent the arterial switch operation. Inclusion of these infants was approved by the Safety and Data Monitoring Board, yielding a total of 171 study subjects.

Of the 171 infants enrolled in the original trial, 168 were alive at age one year. Of these, 155 (92.3%) returned for evaluation. Among the 13 remaining infants, 9 (5.4%) declined participation, 2 (1.2%) could not be located, and 2 (1.2%) declined because of residence outside of the country. Children who did not return did not differ significantly from those who were tested with respect to sociodemographic features, intraoperative perfusion variables, hospital course, or occurrence of seizure activity.

Randomization and Blinding of Treatment Assignment and Outcome Analyses

We randomly assigned participating patients to receive either predominantly total circulatory arrest or predominantly low-flow bypass, with stratification according to diagnosis and surgeon. Randomization schemes were developed using a permuted blocks design; the support method was assigned immediately prior to surgery.

Treatment assignment was directly observed by the surgeons, anesthesiologists, perfusionists, study nurse, and EEG technician, as well as, occasionally, by the intensivist. However, these individuals did not have access to interim results during the study. The neurologist, psychologist, developmental pediatrician, and neuroradiologist were blinded to the treatment assignment of the patient.

Perfusion Methods

Perfusion methods, including the extracorporeal circuit and apparatus, perfusate, adjunctive drugs, and use of the alpha-stat method of acid-base management, were identical for both groups except as defined below. Surface cooling was instituted with low ambient room temperature, a cooling mattress, and ice packs to the head; the mean tympanic membrane temperature at the onset of bypass was 32.7 ± 1.3°C (mean ± S.D.). An ascending aorta arterial cannula and a single right atrial venous cannula were used. Cardiopulmonary bypass and core cooling were begun as soon as the cannulae were in place. When the rectal temperature reached 18°C or lower and the necessary preliminary surgical dissection had been completed, low-flow bypass or circulatory arrest was begun. In the group randomized to circulatory arrest, there was usually a period of low-flow bypass before perfusion was discontinued and the body was exsanguinated through the venous cannula into the oxygenator reservoir. During circulatory arrest, hypothermic temperatures were maintained by using ice bags applied to the head and by using a cooling mattress. Circulatory arrest was continued until left ventricular-to-aortic continuity was established, the coronary arteries were reimplanted, and the atrial septal defect or ventricular septal defect was repaired. In the low-flow bypass group, perfusion was reduced to 50 mL/kg/min (approximately 0.7 L/m²/min) for the duration of the aortic and coronary repairs. A brief period of circulatory arrest was used during closure of the atrial septal defect. Longer periods of circulatory arrest were necessary in infants with moderate or large ventricular septal defects. After the period of circulatory arrest in both groups, rewarming on bypass was carried out as continuity between the right ventricle and pulmonary artery was established. Perfusion pressures and flow rates during rewarming were the same in both groups.

Detailed Protocol Administered by Perfusionists

Before the patient entered the room, the blanket was kept warm at 42°C. When the patient entered the room, the Blanketrol pump was turned off, and the cold water bath was precooled to 4°C. While the patient was being prepped, ice bags were placed on the head and the Blanketrol was turned on at 3 to 4°C. The perfusate was heparinized to 2.5 units/mL and was recirculated at room temperature. When bypass was initiated, the heat exchanger water was turned on at 5°C. Blood flows for patients of 2.5 to 10.0 kg was 150 mL/kg during both the cooling and rewarming phases. Within the first minute of bypass, the following drugs were administered: Regitine 0.2 mg/kg, Lasix 0.25 mg/kg, Solumedrol 30.0 mg/kg, and Ketzol 25 mg/kg. For patients randomized to circulatory arrest, maximum cooling took place during the entire cooling phase. For patients randomized to low-flow bypass, patients were cooled to a rectal temperature of 18°C. Periodic cooling occurred to maintain a rectal temperature of 18°C. During low-flow bypass, blood flows were maintained at 50 mL/kg/min (0.75 L/m²/min). During circulatory arrest, the perfusate recirculated at 18°C. Upon rewarming, another dose of Regitine (0.2 mg/kg) was administered. During the rewarming phase, the water temperature was maintained 10 to 12°C higher than the esophageal or venous blood temperature, whichever was available. Mannitol (0.5 g/kg) was administered at the time of cross-clamp removal. Calcium gluconate was administered when the rectal temperature reached 28°C. For a crystalloid prime, we administered 500 mg of calcium gluconate. For a blood prime, 1.0 g of calcium gluconate was administered for the first unit of blood, and 500 mg more was given for each additional unit of blood used. Regitine (0.2 mg/kg) was used for hypertension >70 mmHg. Neosynephrine was administered for hypotension <30 mmHg during rewarming.

Anesthesia Methods

Anesthetic management was standardized for all patients. Intravenous fluids given intraoperatively were restricted to Lactated Ringers solution at 10 to 20 mL/kg/h unless blood glucose was less than 50 mg%. Anesthesia was induced with Fentanyl 50 μg/kg and Pancuronium 100 μg/kg. After the patient was placed on bypass, plasma levels of Fentanyl and Pancuronium were maintained using an additional 25 μg/kg of Fentanyl and 100 μg/kg of Pancuronium. Thiopental, 10 μg/kg, was given when the tympanic temperature reached 18°C. Upon rewarming, an additional 25 μg/kg of Fentanyl and 100 μg/kg of Pancuronium were given to maintain anesthesia. A Thiopental level was obtained when the rectal temperature reached 32°C. Other drugs given intraoperatively are detailed below.

After bypass, filling pressures and perfusion pressures were maintained within the limits defined in the protocols. Thus, anesthetic drugs and muscle relaxants—which have substantial effects on whole body and cerebral oxygen consumption and metabolic rate, as well as on EEG activity—were standardized for both groups. Likewise, levels of perfusion and filling pressures known to affect the cerebral circulation were controlled intraoperatively. We monitored preischemic levels of glucose and postischemic levels of calcium, both of which are known to influence recovery of brain function after ischemic insults.

Detailed Anesthesia and Perfusion Protocol

Anesthetic induction and maintenance

No premedication was used. Anesthesia was induced with Pancuronium 100 μg/kg, IV and Fentanyl 25 μg/kg, IV. Subsequently, the patients underwent intubation of trachea and placement of intravenous and intra-arterial catheters. We then obtained baseline levels of arterial blood gases, blood glucose electrolytes (including ionized calcium), serum osmolarity, hematocrit, and baseline activated clotting time (ACT) and CPK-isoenzyme levels. Anesthesia was maintained with Fentanyl 25 μg/kg, given prior to incision. Fluid balance was maintained with Lactated Ringers at 10 to 20 mL/kg/h until the commencement of bypass, unless serum glucose was less than 50 μg/dL. If this occurred, 5% dextrose in water was substituted, and blood glucose was carefully monitored. Surface cooling was accomplished with ice packs to head, cooling mattress at 5°C, an ambient temperature in the operating room of 20°C, and unheated dry gas supply to the ventilator circuit. We monitored esophageal, rectal, and tympanic temperatures.

Cardiopulmonary bypass

We used a prime comprised of varying amounts of Normosol-R and whole blood depending on the patient's estimated blood volume, hematocrit, and the total priming volume used. The Cobe Variable Prime Membrane Oxygenator was used. Heparin (3 mg/kg) was given into the right atrium. We measured the activated clotting time two minutes after heparin was administered before cardiopulmonary bypass. Drugs given at the beginning of cardiopulmonary bypass were Fentanyl 25 μg/kg, Pancuronium 100 μg/kg, Solumedrol 30 mg/kg, Regitine 0.2 mg/kg, and Lasix 0.25 mg/kg. Activated clotting time was measured two minutes after bypass started and every 20 minutes thereafter. ACT was maintained over 400 seconds. Perfusion flow rates during cooling were 150 mL/kg/min. The alpha-stat method of acid-base management was used by maintaining uncorrected arterial pH at 7.40 (measured at 37°C) and arterial pCO_2 at 40 mmHg (measured at 37°C) regardless of patient temperature. We made the following measurements five minutes after the start of bypass: arterial and venous blood gases, calcium, electrolytes, hematocrit, glucose, and serum osmolarity (serum osmolarity not available weekends or late nights). Thereafter, arterial and venous gases, hematocrit, glucose, and osmolarity were drawn every 30 minutes while the patient was on bypass.

Cooling

Patients were cooled to a rectal temperature of 18°C. If tympanic temperatures were higher than 18°C at this point, cooling was continued until this tympanic temperature was reached. At this point, circulatory arrest or low flow was begun depending upon treatment assignment. Prior to commencement of low-flow bypass or circulatory arrest, blood was again sampled for all parameters including arterial and venous gases, calcium, hematocrit, glucose, serum osmolarity, and electrolytes. Pentothal 10 mg/kg was given approximately 10 minutes after initiation of cardiopulmonary bypass.

Low-flow bypass and circulatory arrest techniques

The low-flow perfusion rate was 50 mL/kg/min. Five minutes after resumption of bypass following circulatory arrest, we measured arterial gases, electrolytes, hematocrit, glucose, calcium, and osmolarity. CPK samples were drawn when the rectal temperature reached 32°C, during the rewarming phase. Mannitol 0.5 g/kg was administered at the time of cross-clamp removal.

Rewarming

Water temperature was maintained 10 to 12°C higher than esophageal or venous blood return temperature, whichever was available, to a maximum of 42°C. At rectal temperatures of 28°C, calcium gluconate was administered in a dose of 1.0 g for the first unit of whole blood prime used and 0.5 g for each additional unit. Thereafter, calcium gluconate was given as needed to maintain normal ionized calcium levels. Fentanyl 25 µg/kg and Pancuronium 100 µg/kg were administered at a temperature of 30°C on rewarming. Mean perfusion pressures were maintained between 30 and 70 mmHg during rewarming after arrest using Regitine 0.2 mg/kg or phenylnephrine 5 µg/kg as needed. At rectal temperatures of 32°C, arterial gases, electrolytes, calcium, glucose, and osmolarity were measured and adjusted to normal.

Termination of cardiopulmonary bypass

Cardiopulmonary bypass was terminated at a rectal temperature of 36°C after a dopamine infusion of 5 µg/kg/min was started and satisfactory perfusion pressures were achieved. When necessary, higher dopamine infusion rates were used. Our clinical experience with neonates undergoing low-flow bypass had revealed that patients who rewarm rapidly to this temperature have a marked tendency to drop their body temperature to as low as 32°C within 10 to 15 minutes of weaning from bypass. Our practice, therefore, was to have a minimum rewarming period of 30 minutes. The surgeon must also have believed that satisfactory myocardial function had been regained and that all aspects of the procedure had been completed. Cardiac filling pressures were maintained at levels necessary to give arterial systolic perfusion pressures of at least 60 mmHg. We administered Lactated Ringers solution at 10 mL/kg/h, as well as blood and blood products as indicated to maintain filling pressures. Calcium and other electrolytes were administered to maintain serum values within the normal ranges. We measured arterial blood gases, hematocrit, electrolytes, glucose, and osmolarity within 15 minutes after cessation of bypass and additionally as needed. CPK levels were measured 1.5 hours after resumption of bypass if the patient was still in the operating room. No other anesthetic drugs were administered. Additional doses of Fentanyl or Pancuronium were administered only if clinically indicated.

Miscellaneous

The weight of the infant was measured upon arrival to the operating room, prior to transfer to the operating table. The weight was obtained without diapers or clothing. However, by necessity, the weight included any equipment already accompanying the child (e.g., endotracheal tubes, intravenous tubing, EEG electrodes). The infant's weight was again measured upon completion of the operation, prior to transfer to the transport bed. Equipment already attached to the child was not removed, although tubing was suspended so as to exert as little influence on the weight as possible.

The EEG camera was trained on the monitor, rather than on the child, to record hemodynamic parameters in the operating room that may have influence on brain wave activity.

Standardization of Surgical Care

The development of the surgical techniques used in the neonatal arterial switch operation during the time that Drs. Castaneda, Jonas, and Mayer were colleagues led to a uniformity of approach that is unusual to find even at a single institution. When our fourth cardiovascular surgeon, Dr. Hanley, joined the staff in 1989, his technique for the arterial switch operation was standardized with that of the other surgeons, and his first three arterial switch operations on study subjects were performed with Dr. Jonas' assistance.

Repair of dTGA, IVS, and dTGA, VSD

Surgical repair of dTGA by arterial switch procedure using circulatory arrest was performed as previously described.[9,10] The use of low-flow bypass required no modification of surgical technique, e.g., single venous cannulation was used. The pump was simply allowed to keep turning through the procedure at a flow rate of 50 mL/kg/min. The four surgeons—Drs. Jonas, Mayer, Castaneda, and Hanley—performed in a similar fashion all aspects of the procedure, including cannulation; cardioplegia solution used; coronary mobilization; Lecompte maneuver; aortic, coronary, and pulmonary anastomoses; and atrial septal defect (ASD) closure.

For patients with VSD who were randomized to circulatory arrest, an assessment was made preoperatively as to the size of the VSD. A reasonably accurate estimate could usually be made as to how many minutes would be required to close the VSD. If the VSD was large, its closure generally required at least 30 minutes of circulatory arrest. An additional 5 to 10 minutes were required for ASD closure and closure of the right atriotomy. Therefore, for a patient with a large VSD, the preliminary part of the arterial switch operation was done on low-flow cardiopulmonary bypass, that is, division of the ascending aorta, excision of the coronary arteries, Lecompte maneuver, and reimplantation of the coronary arteries. At this stage, bypass was ceased, the right atrium was opened, and the VSD and ASD were closed. The right atriotomy was closed and the venous cannula was reinserted. The arterial switch procedure could then be continued under circulatory arrest. Bypass was recommenced at any point in the procedure at the surgeon's discretion. The additional steps still required were aortic anastomosis (approximately 10 minutes), pericardial patch insertion in the coronary donor areas (approximately 10 minutes), and pulmonary anastomosis (approximately 10 minutes). The surgeons expressly avoided, if at all possible, extension of the circulatory arrest time beyond 70 minutes. If the VSD was small, then the arrest period was begun at an earlier point during the procedure, for example, after excision of the coronary arteries but before coronary reimplantation.

For patients with VSD randomized to low-flow cardiopulmonary bypass, the entire arterial switch procedure was performed on low-flow bypass.

In general, the intracardiac part of the procedure was done following the aortic anastomosis or implantation of the pericardial patch. The surgeon worked as expeditiously as possible to minimize the circulatory arrest time in this group. Nevertheless, with a large VSD, it was customary for the arrest time to be at least 30 to 40 minutes.

Cardioplegia Solution

The cardioplegia solution used was Plegisol, which is St. Thomas' cardioplegia solution manufactured by Abbott Laboratories. This solution was buffered with sodium bicarbonate (10 mL of 8.4% sodium bicarbonate, specifically Abbott list 4900). Filtered 100% oxygen (250 mL) was injected directly into the plastic bag containing the cardioplegia solution.

Standardization of ICU Care

In the first 24 hours, when frequent assessments of myocardial performance required uniform management, medications for hemodynamic support were standardized as described below. After 24 hours, the acute effects of aortic cross-clamping, cardioplegia, and cardiopulmonary bypass had resolved, and management decisions were made according to our routine practice.[11] Detailed protocol for ICU management in the first 24 postoperative hours was as follows:

1. All patients arriving in the Intensive Care Unit received Dopamine at a minimum of 5 μg/kg/min.
2. There was a standardized infusion of Fentanyl at 5 to 10 μg/kg/h for at least 12 hours following cessation of cardiopulmonary bypass. Patients also received neuromuscular blockade.
3. Determinations of cardiac index and systemic vascular resistance were made using intracardiac catheters (pulmonary artery, right atrium, left atrium) placed during surgery. Cardiac index was determined by thermodilution.
4. Standardized treatments assumed that the clinical assessment of the patient correlated with the measured values of cardiac index and calculated systemic vascular resistance. Deviations from standardized treatment could occur at the discretion of the responsible physician.

Hemodynamic and Metabolic Assessment

During the first 24 hours after surgery, hemodynamic status was determined at specified intervals following removal of the aortic cross-clamp. Measurements include cardiac index, systemic and pulmonary resistance, and calculated oxygen consumption. Myocardial and brain isoenzymes of creatine kinase (CK-MB and CK-BB) were measured upon induction of anesthesia; upon reaching 32°C (rectal) during the rewarming phase; and then 1.5, 3, and 6 hours following resumption of bypass. Measurements of CK-BB (in IU/L) were performed by International Immunoassay Laboratories Inc., Santa Clara, California. The study nurse recorded daily medications, respiratory status, laboratory studies, fluid balance, blood and blood product requirements, and significant medical events until hospital discharge.

Recognition of Seizures

Definite or suspected seizures were recorded by the nurses and physicians caring for the infant. Training sessions in recognition and description of seizures were held for intensive care unit nurses, and characteristics of seizures were recorded on a form designed for this purpose. Definite or suspected seizures were manifested by a single or recurrent motor event, with tonic or clonic extremity or cranial muscle movements that were associated with alteration of consciousness and were not interruptable by manipulation of the body part involved. Most often, such events were associated with tachycardia and respiratory irregularities.

Electroencephalography (EEG)

We monitored the EEG continuously for at least two hours prior to surgery, during surgery, and for 48 hours following surgery by video-EEG (Telefactor, Modac) with a 15-channel EEG covering all head regions and 1-channel pneumocardiogram. On the occasions when two infants underwent surgery on consecutive days, we maintained full 48-hour continuous postoperative monitoring on the first infant and waived such monitoring on the second infant. A 16-channel EEG was performed at the time of hospital discharge. The EEGs were recorded using filter settings of 1 to 70 Hz. During the intraoperative period, EEG sensitivity was as high as 1.5 μV/mm and paper speed was 15 mm/s; for the preoperative and postoperative periods, the sensitivity was 5 to 7 μV/mm and paper speed was 30 mm/s. The electroencephalographic data were interpreted by one of four pediatric electroencephalographers according to predetermined criteria. To represent a consensus view, the data were reviewed in a weekly EEG conference devoted to EEG standardization.

Reappearance latencies were assessed as the time in minutes from the onset of rewarming as follows: (a) *first EEG activity* was the time until reappearance of EEG activity in channels F_z-C_z, F_3-C_3, or F_4-C_4; (b) *close bursts* was the time until the first 60-second period at which the interburst (measured mid-burst to mid-burst) interval was less than 15 seconds; (c) *relative continuous* was the time until the first 60-second period in which interburst intervals (less than 15 microvolts in voltage) were less than 6 seconds in duration; (d) *continuous pattern* was the time until EEG activity contained no interburst intervals longer than 1 second and was continuous for a minimum of 60 seconds.

Rhythmic paroxysmal activity on continuous video-EEG during the first 48 hours postoperatively was classified as ictal (i.e., EEG seizure activity) if the duration of the discharge was longer than 5 seconds.

Cranial Ultrasound

Early in the study, cranial ultrasound examinations were performed on the day before surgery and again one week postoperatively to provide information about brain structural injury in the perioperative period. On September 17, 1990, investigators and members of the Safety and Data Monitoring Committee appointed by the National Heart, Lung, and Blood Institute (NHLBI) agreed that the scarcity of abnormalities detected at this time (halfway through the enrollment period) suggested that cranial ultrasound findings could not significantly contribute to the inferences from the study. Therefore, this test was discontinued.

Magnetic Resonance (MR)

At age 1 year, patients underwent magnetic resonance imaging (MRI) of the brain using a 1.5 Tesla MRI system (General Electric Medical Corporation, Milwaukee, Wisconsin). Conventional spin-echo techniques were used as follows: Sagittal T1-weighted images (TR 600 msec/TE 15 msec/NSA 2) and axial proton density and T2-weighted images (TR 2000 msec/TE 20, 90 msec/NSA 2). Five millimeter slice thickness with 1.0 to 2.5 mm interslice spacing was used with a 24-cm field of view. Gadolinium enhancement was not employed. In all cases, sedation was achieved using chloral hydrate 50 to 75 mg/kg, orally. Monitoring included pulse oximetry.

Two experienced pediatric neuroradiologists, blinded to infants' treatment assignments, independently assessed structural and intensity abnormalities. Findings were classified as normal, possibly abnormal, or definitely abnormal (mild, moderate, or severe). More specific descriptions of abnormalities were provided, including ventricular dilatation, abnormal mineralization (e.g., calcification), focal or diffuse atrophy (e.g., postinfarction), and undermyelination. Judgments of the anatomic distribution of abnormalities was also provided. Disagreements were resolved by a third consensus reading by the two examiners. A consensus reading was required for 14% of studies.

Neurologic Examination

Systematic neurologic examinations[12-15] were performed by a child neu-rologist according to a predetermined, uniform protocol on three occasions: (1) within 24 hours prior to surgery; (2) 1 week (range 7 to 10 days) after surgery or before hospital discharge, by which time transient metabolic-based abnormalities should have subsided; and (3) at 1 year of life. The neu-rologist was blinded to the treatment assignment and clinical course (e.g., occurrence of seizures) of the infant. We classified the neurologic examina-tion as normal, possibly abnormal, or definitely abnormal.

In addition to the overall classification, we subclassified patients with respect to specific types of abnormality. In the perioperative period, these in-cluded abnormalities of mental status, head circumference, anterior fontanelle, cranial nerves, and the motor system and were subclassified as diffuse/generalized, lateralized, focal, neck flexion/extension discrepancy (a measure of the degree of tendency toward extensor posture), or other. At age 1 year, patients were classified with respect to the following specific types of abnormality: (1) cerebral palsy, (2) tone alteration but not cerebral palsy (hypotonia, hypertonia), (3) ataxia/dysmetria, (4) focal abnormalities apart from those related to cerebral palsy, (5) special senses, and (6) development delayed greater than 2 months.

Developmental Testing

We administered the Bayley Scales of Infant Development,[16] which yield two scores: the Mental Development Index (MDI), which reflects sensori-motor skills and emerging cognitive skills, and the Psychomotor Development In-dex (PDI), which reflects a child's progress in large muscle activities (e.g., sit-ting, crawling, walking, climbing) and in eye-hand coordination. The Fagan Test of Infant Intelligence (FTII)[17] was also administered. This test of an in-fant's information processing abilities (perception, recognition, retention) consists of 10 trials. Each trial involves presentation of a target stimulus (a human face) for a familiarization period of approximately 20 seconds, fol-lowed by paired presentation of the target and a similar but novel stimulus. A mean novelty preference score (% fixation of the novel stimulus) is com-puted for the 10 trials. Considerable experience has accumulated in the use of this paradigm in studies of high-risk infants.[17-21]

The Bayley Scales were administered by one of two investigators. Based on a group of 13 infants, the percentage agreement between examiners on an item-by-item basis was 98.7% for the MDI and 99.5% for the PDI. The cor-relation between the raw scores assigned by examiners to the 13 infants was greater than .99 for both the MDI and the PDI. Both examiners were certi-fied as competent in the administration of the FTII by the test developers. All developmental assessments were videotaped, permitting review of the session when questions arose concerning a child's performance. All assessments were conducted at 8 a.m. in a testing suite in the Child Development Unit of The Children's Hospital.

Data were also collected on important correlates or determinants of infant development, including sociodemographic factors, such as family social class,[22] maternal age, birth order, and infant gender; prenatal and perinatal factors, such as length of gestation, birth weight, and size for gestational age; and quality of the rearing environment.[23,24] A test of verbal intelligence, the Peabody Picture Vocabulary Test,[25] was administered to one parent (in nearly all cases the mother). We evaluated the impact of a child's illness and recovery on family members using the following instruments: the Family Adaptability and Cohesion Evaluation Scales,[26] the Social Readjustment Rating Scale,[25] the Social Support Network Inventory,[27] and the Parenting Stress Index.[28]

The first 10 infants who returned for 1-year examinations were considered to be a pilot group. Prior to data analysis, the decision was made not to include the developmental test scores of these infants due to the suboptimal conditions under which testing was conducted (a lack of standardization with respect to infant state).

Timing of Evaluations

The timing of all evaluations was as follows:

1. *Preoperative* evaluations included demographic information, medical history, neurologic examination, and EEG. (See Figure 21–1)
2. *Intraoperative* evaluations included recording of variables concerning surgery, anesthesia, and support techniques; continuous electroen-

Timing of Evaluations

Evaluations performed indicated with an X	Preoperative	Intraoperative	Postoperative					
			≤24 hrs	1-2 d	2-6 d	7-10d (once)	1 yr old	4 yr old
History	X						X	X
Daily Medical Events/ Clinical Assessment			X	X	X	X		
Hemodyamic Measurements			X					
Neurologic Examination	X						X	X	X
Electroencephalogram (EEG)	X	X	X	X		X		
Creatine Phosphokinase-Brain Isoenzyme (CK-BB)		X	X					
Magnetic Resonance Imaging (MR)							X	
Psychometric Testing							X	X

FIGURE 21–1. Timing of Evaluations

cephalography; and measurement of serial CK-BB and metabolic studies (arterial blood gases, osmolality, glucose, electrolytes, calcium, and thiopental levels).

3. During the *first postoperative 24 hours,* we measured EEG (recorded continuously for the first postoperative 48 hours); obtained serial serum CK-BB levels; measured hemodynamic variables; and recorded medical events, medications, and clinical status, and collected 24 hour urine for creatinine clearance. During *each postoperative day in the Intensive Care Unit,* we recorded medical events, medications, and clinical status. *Seven to 10 days postoperatively* or prior to hospital discharge, we repeated the neurologic examination and electroencephalogram. We also summarized all medical events, use of medications, clinical status, and information regarding discharge medications and disposition on a discharge assessment form. At *1 year of age,* we obtained interim history, psychometric testing, neurologic examination, and MRI scan. At *4 years of age,* we are obtaining interim history, psychometric testing, and neurologic examination. This phase of the study is ongoing at the time of this report.

Statistical Analysis

Treatment group comparisons were made in intent-to-treat analyses, comparing a predominant total circulatory arrest strategy versus a predominant low-flow bypass strategy. Secondary analyses examined the effect of duration (minutes) of circulatory arrest on outcome. Except where noted, all hypothesis tests and regression analyses were adjusted for diagnosis (dTGA–IVS vs. dTGA–VSD). All hypothesis tests were 2-sided, and a p-value less than .05 was considered statistically significant. Except where noted, estimated treatment effects within each diagnostic group were similar to those in the study population as a whole.

Major outcome variables in the early postoperative period for this trial were the occurrence of clinical seizures in the first postoperative week; the occurrence of ictal activity by EEG in the first 48 hours postoperatively; reappearance latency times by EEG; CK-BB release integrated over the first six hours postoperatively; and status on neurologic examination, cranial ultrasound, and EEG prior to hospital discharge.

Primary outcome variables at age 1 year included developmental scores on the Bayley Scales of Infant Development and Fagan Test of Infant Intelligence, presence of abnormalities on neurologic examination, and detection of structural brain abnormalities on Magnetic Resonance Imaging.

Outcomes included continuous and categorical variables. We used a natural logarithm transform (ln) of serum CK-BB levels integrated over 6 hours and of EEG reappearance latency times to normalize their distributions before analysis. Multiple linear regression was used to analyze measured outcome variables. Stratified exact tests[29] and logistic regression methods were used to analyze binary outcome variables. Ordered categorical outcome variables were analyzed using exact Wilcoxon tests.[29] For outcome variables with preoperative and postoperative measurements, such as EEG and neurologic examination, we first adjusted for baseline status by including preoperative status as a covariate; however, our inferences concerning treatment differences were not influenced by such adjustments and so the unadjusted results are presented.

Time Sequence of Study

Planning Phase

During this period (3 months—December 1, 1988 through February 28, 1989), we finalized methodology and study protocol, completed the design and printing of data forms, completed a Manual of Operations for the protocol, and held standardization sessions within appropriate subspecialty domains. These tasks could be accomplished within the relatively short interval of three months with intensive efforts of the key investigators at a single center. (Figure 21–2)

Admission and Data Collection

In this time interval (3 years—March 1, 1989 through February 29, 1992), we admitted subjects to the study, processed data, and performed preliminary data analysis.

Completion of One-Year Evaluations

During this period (1 year—March 1, 1992 through February 28, 1993), follow-up visits were completed on subjects enrolled near the end of the admission period.

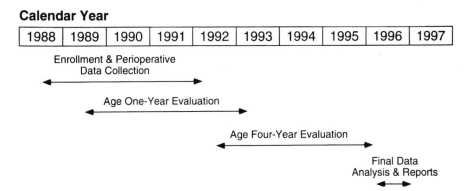

FIGURE 21–2. Time Sequence of Study

One-Year Evaluation Data Analysis and Inference

Since data were periodically analyzed and summarized during the previous phases of the study, the edited and corrected data set was available for final analysis during the early part of this phase. During this phase (9 months—March 1, 1993 through November 30, 1993), we wrote the archives of the project, reported the results of the study, and formulated recommendations warranted by the data concerning optimal perfusion techniques during open heart surgery in infants.

Completion of Four-Year Evaluations,
Data Analysis, and Inference

During this period (4 years and 1 month—December 1, 1993 through December 31, 1997), follow-up visits are being completed on subjects at age 4 years, to be followed by final analysis of the data, reporting of the results, and formulation of recommendations.

Organizational Structure

The organization of the study reflected the multidisciplinary approach necessary in the care and evaluation of children with congenital heart disease. In those subspecialties in which more than one physician may be caring for study subjects, we designated subspecialty co-chairs. The study was administered by an *Executive Committee* comprised of the principal investigator (Dr. Newburger), co-principal investigator (Dr. Jonas), statistician (Dr. Ware), anesthesiology co-chair (Dr. Hickey), neurology co-chair (Dr. Kuban), intensive care co-chair (Dr. Wessel), psychologist (Dr. Bellinger), developmental pediatrician (Dr. Rappaport), and physician-coordinator (Dr. Wernovsky).

The *Safety and Data Monitoring Committee* was comprised of eight members, each of whom is eminent in one of the specific areas at issue in the study: Pediatric Cardiology, Cardiovascular Surgery, Cardiac Anesthesia, Neurology, Developmental Psychology, and Biostatistics. Members of the Safety and Data Monitoring Committee included Julien I.E. Hoffman, M.D. (Chair); John W. Kirklin, M.D.; Barry M. Lester, Ph.D.; Robert J. Levine, M.D.; Eli M. Mizrahi, M.D.; Joseph G. Reves, M.D.; George W. Williams, Ph.D.; and Joel I. Verter, Ph.D. The function of the Safety and Data Monitoring Committee was to advise the National Heart, Lung, and Blood Institute, the Executive Committee, and the Coordinating Center on (1) final study design and protocol prior to the beginning of data collection, (2) problems with protocol implementation, (3) frequency of occurrence of adverse effects of perfusion techniques, (4) withdrawals and losses to follow-up, (5) data interpretation and ethical issues, and (6) recommendations arising from the study. The Safety and Data Monitoring Committee met initially during the Planning Phase to review the final protocol, Manual of Operations, and data forms. Thereafter, the Committee met at intervals no longer than 6 months. Members reviewed whether patient accrual was progressing as projected, the incidence of adverse effects in the two treatment groups, and results of preliminary data analyses.

The *Coordinating Center* was located in the Children's Hospital and had the following functions: (1) implementation of the policies determined by the Executive Committee; (2) ensuring adherence to protocol within the various subspecialty domains; (3) conducting data management activities; (4) monitoring the quality of data submitted by each project investigator; (5) cooperating with the Executive Committee in administrative matters, such as preparing reports or scheduling meetings; and (6) directing data analysis. The Coordinating Center was under the co-direction of the Principal Investigator (Dr. Newburger) and Associate Statistician (Dr. Wypij).

The *Physician-Coordinator*, Dr. Wernovsky, coordinated patient care, data acquisition, adherence to protocol, and supervision of the study nurse. He assisted the nurse in case ascertainment and evaluation of study eligibility and was responsible for obtaining informed consent. Dr. Wernovsky acted as the physician liaison between the subjects' families, primary physicians, and study personnel and was available on a daily basis to answer their questions about matters pertaining to the study. He performed daily evaluations on hospitalized patients, as well as the follow-up evaluations. The *Project Coordinator*, Ms. O'Brien, executed the administrative details of the study. She was responsible for handling the accounting, scheduling and arranging meetings, establishing appropriate record-keeping procedures, and assisting in preparation of reports. The *Associate Statistician*, Dr. Wypij, conducted statistical analyses together with Dr. Ware. The *Data Managers*, Ms. Donati and Ms. Duva, were responsible for seeing that data forms were correctly completed and promptly transmitted between the Coordinating Center and study investigators in the case of errors and omissions. Other members of the Coordinating Center included a *Programmer*, Ms. Kyn, and *Secretary-Data Entry Clerk*, Ms. Buckley.

Description of Study Cohort

Perioperative Period

Subjects

Among the 171 infants with d-transposition of the great arteries, 129 (75%) were in the intact ventricular septum group, and 42 (25%) were in the ventricular septal defect group (Table 21–1). As anticipated, infants with ventricular septal defect, compared to those with intact ventricular septum, were older and less acutely ill at the time of enrollment. Treatment assignment was balanced within the randomization strata of diagnostic group and surgeon. Infants randomized to the two support methods, within

TABLE 21–1.
Preoperative Characteristics According to Ventricular Septal Status and Treatment Group

Variable	Intact Ventricular Septum		Ventricular Septal Defect	
	Circulatory Arrest (N = 66)	*Low-flow Bypass (N = 63)*	*Circulatory Arrest (N = 21)*	*Low-flow Bypass (N = 21)*
	Mean ± S.D.			
Birth weight (g)	3601 ± 466	3485 ± 403	3345 ± 372	3656 ± 385
Age at surgery (days)	7.5 ± 5.5	6.7 ± 3.9	22.0 ± 20.5	14.9 ± 17.0
Gestational age (wk)	39.8 ± 1.3	39.7 ± 1.1	39.9 ± 1.3	39.6 ± 1.0
Apgar score				
1 min	7.3 ± 1.6	7.6 ± 1.1	7.7 ± 1.1	7.8 ± 0.9
5 min	8.1 ± 1.0	8.4 ± 0.7	8.8 ± 0.4	8.7 ± 0.7
Lowest pH	7.27 ± 0.09	7.26 ± 0.11	7.34 ± 0.07	7.29 ± 0.08
Lowest partial pressure of oxygen (mmHg)	24.5 ± 6.8	24.1 ± 5.5	31.3 ± 16.4	30.8 ± 10.5
No. (%) intubated	50 (76)	46 (73)	7 (33)	12 (57)

each diagnostic group, were similar at enrollment in preoperative variables that might influence neurologic outcome and in preoperative neurologic assessments.

Intraoperative data

In accordance with the randomized assignments, the treatment groups differed significantly in the durations of total circulatory arrest and low-flow bypass, as well as in total bypass time (Table 21–2). Surgical circumstances sometimes required use of a predominant circulatory arrest strategy in infants randomized to a predominant low-flow bypass strategy. There were no significant differences between the treatment groups in total support time (i.e., total bypass time plus circulatory arrest time) or cross-clamp time, demonstrating that the choice of support method did not affect the difficulty of the surgery.

Postoperative course

Infants in the two treatment groups were similar in surgical mortality and non-neurologic hospital course and events. Three infants (2%) died within one month of surgery, two in the early postoperative period and one shortly after hospital discharge; one was assigned to circulatory arrest and two to low-flow bypass. In the combined groups, infants were intubated for a me-

TABLE 21–2.
Intraoperative Data According to Ventricular Septal Status and Treatment Group

Variable	Intact Ventricular Septum		Ventricular Septal Defect		p-Value[1]
	Circulatory Arrest (N = 66)	Low-flow Bypass (N = 63)	Circulatory Arrest (N = 21)	Low-flow Bypass (N = 21)	
	Mean ± S.D.				
Low-flow (min)	21 ± 15	64 ± 15	40 ± 20	66 ± 18	<.001[2] .002
Circulatory arrest (min)	52 ± 13	14 ± 11	55 ± 8	33 ± 16	<.001[2] <.001
Total bypass time (min)	82 ± 27	127 ± 25	111 ± 27	139 ± 49	<.001
Total Support time (min)	134 ± 30	141 ± 30	166 ± 27	172 ± 54	.52
Cross-clamping time (min)	76 ± 11	75 ± 10	99 ± 9	99 ± 20	.82
Fluid balance (mL)[3]	625 ± 247	773 ± 318	591 ± 295	828 ± 497	.001
No. (%) of subjects with >30 min of circulatory arrest	64 (97)	4 (6)	21 (100)	13 (62)	<.001[4]

[1]p-Values were calculated by linear regression for the effect of treatment, with adjustment for diagnosis
[2]Upper p-Value is for patients with an intact ventricular septum, and lower value is for patients with a ventricular septal defect
[3]Calculated as the intake of fluid minus the output
[4]Exact p-Value is shown for the effect of treatment, with adjustment for diagnosis

dian of 3 days (range 1 to 61 days) and were discharged from the hospital at a median of 9 days (range 5 to 71 days) after surgery.

One-Year Evaluation

Of the 171 infants enrolled in the original trial, 168 were alive at age 1 year and of these 155 (92%) returned for evaluation. Of the 13 infants who did not return for the 1-year evaluation (7 assigned to circulatory arrest, 6 to low-flow bypass), the parents of nine declined participation, two children could not be located, and two resided outside of the country. Children who returned did not differ significantly from those who did not return with respect to sociodemographic factors, intraoperative perfusion variables, or preoperative or postoperative neurologic status. Aspects of the hospital course did differ, however. Infants who did not return had a longer median period of intubation (3.4 vs. 2.9 days, Wilcoxon test, p = .02) and a longer median hospital stay (11 vs. 9 days, Wilcoxon test, p = .08).

Of the children who returned for evaluation, 120 (77%) had intact ventricular septum and 35 (23%) a ventricular septal defect. Treatment groups, within each diagnosis, were similar with respect to preoperative variables, sociodemographic variables, and interim medical history. However, infants with a diagnosis of ventricular septal defect were older at time of surgery, making it difficult to distinguish the independent contributions of age at surgery and diagnosis to 1-year status. Neither age-adjusted weight nor length at 1 year differed by treatment group. Between the neonatal arterial switch operation and the 1-year evaluation, 78 children (51%) underwent cardiac catheterization, and one child (intact ventricular septum, assigned to low-flow bypass) underwent repeat cardiac surgery. Eleven children (7%) were on digoxin and two (1%) were on diuretics at the time of the 1-year evaluation. No child experienced nonfebrile seizures after hospital discharge. Two children (1%) had febrile seizures; neither had seizures detected clinically or by EEG in the perioperative period.

Four-Year Evaluation

Follow-up of subjects at age 4 years is ongoing at the time of this report. Neurologic examinations are being categorized as normal, minor abnormalities, and major abnormalities, with specific types of dysfunction also classified. Developmental status is being assessed using standardized measures of cognition, behavior, language, attention, and motor skills. Follow-up of this study cohort will help to elucidate the long-term neurologic and developmental outcomes of enrolled subjects.

References

1. Fyler DC. Report of the New England Regional Infant Cardiac Program. *Pediatrics* 1980;65:S375–S461.
2. Ferry PC. Neurologic sequelae of cardiac surgery in children. *Am J Dis Child* 1987;141:309–312.
3. Weiss M, Piwnica A, Lenfant C, Sprovieri L, Laurent D. Deep hypothermia with total circulatory arrest. *Trans Am Soc Artif Intern Organs* 1960;6:227–239.
4. Kirklin JW, Dawson B, Devloo RA, Theye RA. Open intracardiac operations: Use of circulatory arrest during hypothermia induced by blood cooling. *Ann Surg* 1961;154:769–775.
5. Kirklin JW, Barratt-Boyes BG. Hypothermia and total circulatory arrest. In *Cardiac surgery*. New York: John Wiley and Sons, 1986, pp. 30–82.
6. Rebeyka IM, Coles JG, Wilson GJ. The effect of low-flow cardiopulmonary bypass on cerebral function: An experimental and clinical study. *Ann Thorac Surg* 1987;43:391–396.

7. Wilson GJ, Rebeyka IM, Coles JG, et al. Loss of the somatosensory evoked response as an indicator of reversible cerebral ischemia during hypothermic, low-flow cardiopulmonary bypass. *Ann Thorac Surg* 1988;45:206–209.

8. Swain JA, McDonald TJ Jr, Griffith PK, Balaban RS, Clark RE, Ceckler T. Low-flow hypothermic cardiopulmonary bypass protects the brain. *J Thorac Cardiovasc Surg* 1991;102:76–83.

9. Castaneda AR, Norwood WI, Jonas RA, Colan SD, Sanders SP, Lang P. Transposition of the great arteries and intact ventricular septum: Anatomical repair in the neonate. *Ann Thorac Surg* 1984;38:438–443.

10. Mayer JE Jr, Jonas RA, Castaneda AR. Arterial switch operation for transposition of the great arteries with intact ventricular septum. *J Card Surg* 1986; 1:97–104.

11. Lang P, Gordon D. Intensive care of the infant after cardiac surgery. In Vidyasagar D, Sarniak AP (eds.), *Neonatal and pediatric intensive care.* PSG Publishing Co., Inc., 1985.

12. O'Doherty N. *Neurological exam of the newborn: A routine for all.* Boston: MTP Press, 1986.

13. Dubowitz L, Dubowitz V. *The neurological assessment of the preterm and full-term newborn infant.* London: Spastics Society in association with Heinemann Medical, 1981.

14. Prechtl HFR. *The neurological examination of the full term newborn infant: A manual for clinical use,* 2nd ed. Oxford, England: Blackwell Scientific, 1977.

15. Paine RS, Oppe TE. *Neurological examination of children.* London: Spastics Society in association with Heinemann Medical, 1966.

16. Bayley N. *Bayley scales of infant development.* New York: The Psychological Corporation, 1969.

17. Fagan J, Singer L, Montie J, Shepherd P. Selective screening device for the early detection of normal or delayed cognitive development in infants at risk for later mental retardation. *Pediatrics* 1986;78:1021–1026.

18. Rose S. Enhancing visual recognition memory in preterm infants. *Dev Psych* 1980;16:85–92.

19. Shepherd P, Fagan J. Visual pattern detection and recognition memory in children with profound mental retardation. In *International review of research in mental retardation,* 10th ed. New York: Academic Press, 1981, pp., 31–130.

20. Fagan JF III, Singer LT, Montie JE, Shepherd PA. Selective screening device for the early detection of normal or delayed cognitive development in infants at risk for later mental retardation. *Pediatrics* 1986;78:1021–1026.

21. Shepherd P, Fagan J, Kleiner K. Visual pattern detection in pre-term neonates. *Infant Behavior and Dev* 1985;8:47–63.

22. Hollingshead A. Four factor index of social status, Unpublished manual, 1975.

23. Bradley R, Caldwell B. Early home environment and changes in mental test performances in children 6–36 months. *Child Dev* 1976;12:93–97.

24. Bradley R, Caldwell B. The relation of infants' home environments to achievement test performance in first grade: A follow-up study. *Child Dev* 1984;55:803–809.

25. Dunn L. *The Peabody Picture Vocabulary Test,* rev. ed. Circles Pines, MN: American Guidance Service, 1981.

26. Olson D, Portner J. Family adaptability and cohesion evaluation scales. In Filsinger E (ed.), *Marriage and family assessment.* Beverly Hills: Sage, 1983, pp. 299–315.

27. Flaherty J, Gaviria M, Pathak D. The measurement of social support. The Social Support Network Inventory. *Comprehen Psych* 1983;24:521–529.

28. Abidin R. *Parenting stress index—Manual, 2nd ed.* Charlotteville, VA: Pediatric Psychology Press, 1986.

29. StatXact. Statistical software for exact nonparametric inference, user manual, StatXact-Turbo. Cambridge, MA: CYTEL Software Corporation, 1992.

CHAPTER 22

EEG Findings

Gregory L. Holmes
David Wypij
Sandra L. Helmers

Although it is one of the older neurophysiologic tests available, the EEG remains an important diagnostic tool in disorders of the central nervous system despite recent advances in diagnostic technology. It is an essential tool in the assessment and detection of seizures. This is especially true when seizures might be clinically unsuspected, and conversely the EEG may prevent the incorrect diagnosis of non-seizure behaviors. When appropriately used, the EEG supports the diagnosis of seizures, can localize the onset of the seizure, delineate an epileptic syndrome, and even aid in choosing appropriate therapy. In addition, the EEG is a useful window for assessing the neurological status in infants who need to be paralyzed. However, the main value of the EEG in young children is its powerful contribution to the assessment of short- and long-term prognosis. Studies have demonstrated that the EEG is a better predictor of outcome than the neurological examination. In effect, this noninvasive test is singularly more valuable in this respect during the first few months of life than at other ages.

In the context of ictal disorders, the EEG has been shown to be an excellent predictor of outcome by the vast majority of prospective or retrospective investigations performed.[1,2] Since the EEG has previously been demonstrated to be useful in predicting outcome from a variety of insults, we elected to employ EEG monitoring prior to, during, and following hypothermic arrest for transposition of the great arteries.

Relation of EEG Outcome Variables to Support Strategy

In the Boston Circulatory Arrest Study, the incidence of perioperative seizures after deep hypothermia, with support consisting predominantly of total circulatory arrest was compared with the incidence after deep hypothermia with support consisting predominantly of low-flow cardiopulmonary bypass, in children undergoing surgical correction of d-transposition of the great arteries. A total of 171 infants were eligible and underwent the randomized protocol of deep hypothermia with either circulatory arrest (DHCA) or predominantly low-flow bypass (LFB).[3] The group was further classified as to whether there was an intact ventricular septum (IVS) or a ventricular septal defect (VSD). One hundred twenty-nine infants (75%) had an intact ventricular septum, and 42 infants (25%) had a ventricular septal defect. Preoperative demographic characteristics within each diagnostic group were similar in the infants assigned to the two support techniques. The infants from each diagnostic group were approximately the same gestational age, but infants with a ventricular septal defect were slightly older and less acutely ill at the time of enrollment than those with an intact ventricular septum.

Intraoperatively, there were no significant differences between the treatment of groups in total support time (circulatory arrest plus total bypass time).[3] As expected from the randomized treatment assignment, there were significant differences in the total duration of circulatory arrest, low-flow bypass, and total bypass time between the DHCA and LFB groups, and the number of patients with a circulatory arrest duration of more than 30 minutes was significantly higher in the DHCA group.

The EEG was monitored continuously for at least two hours prior to surgery, during surgery, and for 48 hours following surgery by video-EEG. A full EEG was also repeated at 7 to 10 days after the surgical procedure. The EEG data were interpreted by one of four blinded pediatric electroencephalographers according to predetermined criteria and then reviewed by the group to develop a consensus on the final interpretation. The video-EEG studies were usually analyzed weeks following the procedure and results of the monitoring were not used to influence treatment decisions.

The preoperative EEGs were analyzed with regard to age-appropriate background continuity, symmetry, and paroxysmal features (Table 22–1). Infants in the IVS group had more EEG abnormalities preoperatively, most of which were defined as dysmature features. This group also had a small, but higher, proportion of infants with an abnormal background or paroxysmal features. Abnormalities in the preoperative EEG were similar in both treatment groups due to the randomization, and the small differences between the two diagnostic groups most likely reflect the fact that infants with an intact ventricular septum were more acutely ill preoperatively.

The EEG from the intraoperative and first 48 perioperative hours were assessed for reappearance latencies of EEG activity and paroxysmal activity. Reappearance latencies were defined as the time in minutes from the onset of rewarming until the appearance of various EEG patterns as follows: (a) *first activity* was the time until reappearance of activity in three channels; (b) *close bursts* was the time until the first 60-second period at which the in-

TABLE 22–1
Preoperative EEG Status, According to Ventricular Septal Status and Treatment Group

	Intact Ventricular Septum		Ventricular Septal Defect	
Variable	Circulatory Arrest	Low-Flow Bypass	Circulatory Arrest	Low-Flow Bypass
	No. with abnormality/total no. (%)			
EEG Abnormalities	26/56 (46)	23/51 (45)	2/13 (15)	8/14 (57)
Paroxysmal activity	5/56 (9)	8/51 (16)	0/13	1/14 (7)
Dysmature	23/56 (41)	18/51 (35)	2/13 (15)	7/14 (50)
Background abnormal	9/56 (16)	5/51 (10)	0/13	0/14

terburst interval (measured mid-burst to mid-burst) was less than 15 seconds; (c) *relative continuous* was the time until the first 60-second period in which interburst intervals (less than 15 microvolts in voltage) were less than 6 seconds in duration; and (d) *continuous pattern* was the time until EEG activity contained no interburst intervals longer than 1 second and was continuous for a minimum of 60 seconds.

Rhythmic paroxysmal activity on continuous video-EEG during the first 48 postoperative hours was classified as ictal (i.e., EEG seizure activity) if the duration of the discharge was longer than 5 seconds. Figure 22–1 is an example of an EEG seizure recorded from an infant during the postoperative monitoring period. There were no clinical changes. Note that there is a migration of the ictal discharge from the left hemisphere to the right as the seizure progresses.

Infants assigned to the circulatory arrest group had significantly longer recovery times to first EEG activity, close bursts, and relative continuous activity (Table 22–2). Using the number of minutes as a continuous variable, it was found that longer periods of arrest were associated with longer recovery times to first EEG activity (Figure 22–2), close bursts (Figure 22–3), and relative continuous activity.

Epileptiform activity on continuous EEG monitoring during the first 48 hours postoperatively occurred in 27 out of 136 patients (20%) who were monitored. This contrasts with 11 out of 170 patients (6%) who had clinical seizures detected within the first week after surgery. Electroencephalographic seizures tended to be more frequent in the children assigned to the circulatory arrest group (odds ratio 2.5, p = .07, Table 22–2). Assignment to the circulatory arrest group was significantly associated with the occurrence of clinical seizures (odds ratio 11.4, p = .009).

Additionally, the risk of EEG seizures increased as a function of duration of circulatory arrest (Figure 22–4). The effect of circulatory arrest on

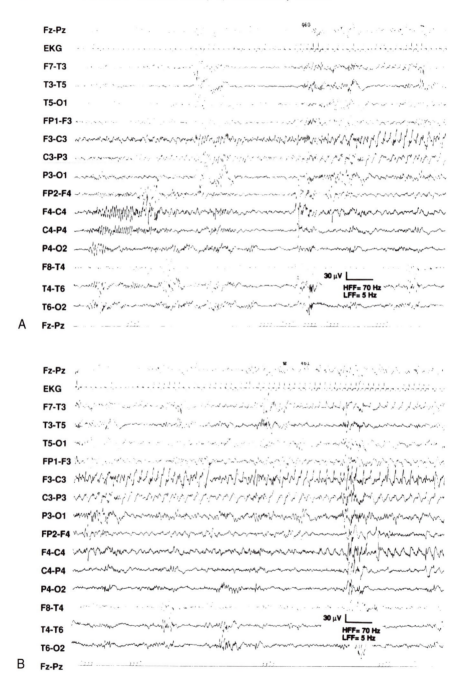

FIGURE 22–1.   16-channel EEG recording from an infant during the first 48 postoperative hours. Note ictal discharge beginning in C3 (A) and eventually spreading to right hemisphere (F). There was no clinical accompaniment.

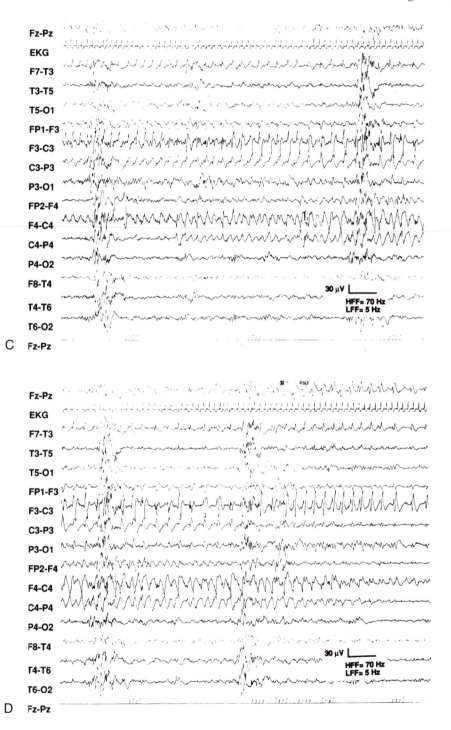

FIGURE 22–1.   (*continued*)

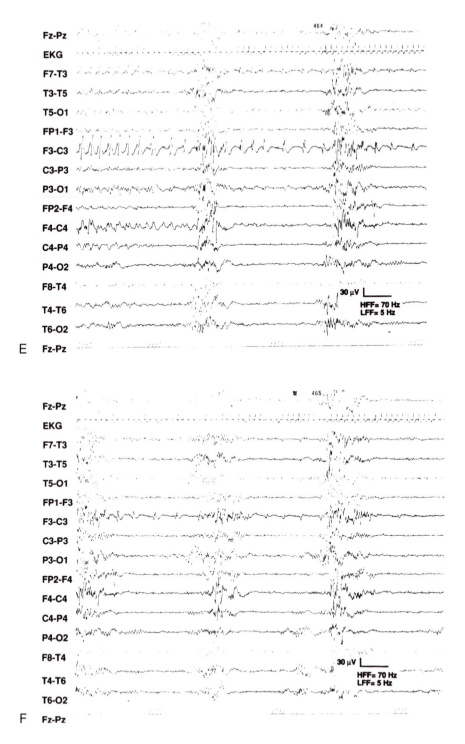

FIGURE 22–1. (continued)

TABLE 22–2
EEG Outcomes after Surgery, According to Ventricular Septal Status and Treatment Group

Variable	Intact Ventricular Septum		Ventricular Septal Defect		p-Value[1]
	Circulatory Arrest	Low-Flow Bypass	Circulatory Arrest	Low-Flow Bypass	
	No. with abnormality/total no. (%)				
48-hr continuous EEG[2]					
Ictal activity[3]	9/58 (16)	6/49 (12)	10/16 (63)	2/13 (15)	.07
	Median (interquartile range)				
Recovery time (min)					
First activity	21 (15,45)	13 (4,18)	19 (11,25)	27 (16,30)	<.001[4] .75
Close bursts	139 (72,227)	57 (32,85)	221 (175,238)	204 (83,303)	<.001[5]
Relative continuous	288 (143,366)	181 (66,309)	250 (236,411)	289 (75,481)	.02[5]
Continuous	1140 (541,1740)	1079 (602,1626)	840 (106,1435)	1137 (469,1680)	.94[5]
	No. with abnormality/total no. (%)				
At hospital discharge					
EEG abnormalities	30/58 (52)	22/53 (42)	8/14 (57)	7/14 (50)	.31
Paroxysmal activity	9/58 (16)	5/53 (9)	3/14 (21)	1/14 (7)	.21
Dysmature	27/58 (47)	19/53 (36)	6/14 (43)	6/14 (43)	.39
Background abnormal	9/58 (16)	8/53 (15)	2/14 (14)	0/14	.63

[1] Exact p-Values are shown for the effect of treatment, with adjustment for diagnosis
[2] Denotes continuous video EEG during the first 48 hours after surgery
[3] Denotes rhythmic epileptiform activity continuing for more than five seconds
[4] Upper p-Value is for patients with an intact ventricular septum, and lower value is for patients with a ventricular septal defect, for the natural logarithm of the total number of minutes of EEG recovery time plus 1, because of the interaction of treatment with diagnostic group
[5] p-Value was calculated by linear regression for the effect of treatment, with adjustment for diagnosis, for the natural logarithm of the total number of minutes of EEG recovery time plus 1

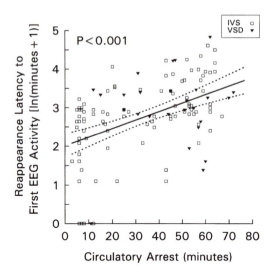

FIGURE 22–2. Time to the recovery of first EEG activity as a function of the duration of total circulatory arrest. In the scatterplot, open squares denote infants with an intact ventricular septum, and filled triangles those with a ventricular septal defect. The solid line was derived by linear regression of the data, and the dashed lines delimit the 95% percent confidence interval. Diagnosis was not predictive of this outcome. Time to the recovery of first EEG activity was expressed as the natural logarithm of the number of minutes to the recovery of first activity plus 1. The linear regression p-Value shown is for the effect of duration of circulatory arrest on outcome.

EEG seizure activity was not modified by potentially predictive preoperative variables, though both the associated diagnosis of ventricular septal defect and older age at surgery were independent risk factors for the occurrence of EEG seizures. Three of the infants had onset of seizure activity within the first 12 hours postoperatively, while 24 of 27 infants had the onset of ictal activity between 13 and 36 hours after surgery. No patient had the onset of EEG activity after 36 hours. Duration of the ictal activity ranged from 6 seconds to 980 minutes.

During the continuous 48 postoperative hours of video-EEG monitoring there were a total of 16 patients who had EEG seizures without clinical accompaniment. Twelve of these patients were in the intact ventricular septum group, and nine were assigned to the circulatory arrest group. Eleven patients had both EEG and definite or suspected clinical seizures. Ten of the

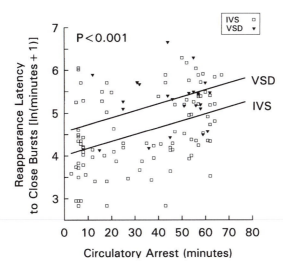

FIGURE 22–3. Time to the recovery of close bursts as a function of the duration of total circulatory arrest. In the scatterplot, open squares denote infants with an intact ventricular septum, and filled triangles those with a ventricular septal defect. Separate linear regression curves are shown for infants with intact ventricular septum (IVS) and ventricular septal defect (VSD). Time to the recovery of close bursts was expressed as the natural logarithm of the number of minutes to the recovery of close bursts plus 1. The linear regression p-Value shown is for the effect of duration of total circulatory arrest on outcome, with adjustment for diagnosis.

11 patients in this group underwent deep hypothermic circulatory arrest, with only one undergoing low-flow bypass. Continuous EEG monitoring was able to identify ictal events before clinical signs were noted, with the ictal events on the EEG being detected from a few hours up to more than 20 hours before clinical seizures were noted. Since the physicians caring for these infants were blinded to the EEG findings, patients were treated with anticonvulsants (diazepam, lorazepam, midazolam, phenobarbitol) only after the onset of definite or possible clinical seizures, hours after the EEG seizures had begun.

In addition to time of onset and duration of ictal activity in these 27 patients, EEG localization of the seizure onset was surveyed. There were over 1000 discrete EEG seizures in this group, and the regions of onset for each seizure were recorded. Twenty-five of these 27 infants had multiple seizures, accounting for the large number of sites of onset. The majority of seizures

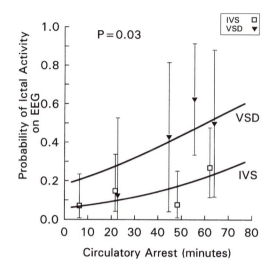

FIGURE 22–4.   Estimated probabilities of an ictal activity on continuous video-EEG in the first 48 hours after surgery as a function of the duration of total circulatory arrest. Separate logistic regression curves are shown for children with an intact ventricular septum (IVS; open squares) and for those with a ventricular septal defect (VSD; filled triangles). Point estimates and exact 95% confidence intervals for outcome probabilities are plotted for the mean of each quartile of duration of circulatory arrest. The logistic regression p-Value shown is for the effect of the duration of total circulatory arrest on outcome, with adjustment for diagnosis.

had an onset in the central and frontal regions. There were no significant differences between left and right hemisphere onset.

Follow-up results from EEG studies at the time of hospital discharge did not correlate with the type of support rendered during the cardiac surgery (Table 22–2). Follow-up EEGs showed normal or dysmature features in most of these patients.

Relation of EEG Seizure Activity and One-Year Outcomes

Of the 171 infants enrolled in the original trial, 155 returned for evaluation at age 1 year.[4] In the combined treatment groups, the Psychomotor Development Index (PDI) score was 95.1 ± 15.5 (mean ± S.D.) and the Mental Development Index (MDI) score was 105.1 ± 15.0. The PDI and MDI scores were lower in the circulatory arrest group, and there was a significant association between PDI score and the duration of circulatory arrest. In the combined treatment groups, 33 out of 142 patients (23%) had possible or definite abnormalities on magnetic resonance imaging. The prevalence of these abnormalities was not related to treatment assignment, duration of circulatory arrest, or associated diagnosis of ventricular septal defect.

In regression analyses adjusting for diagnosis and treatment group, the occurrence of EEG seizure activity in the early postoperative period was associated with a mean reduction of 11.2 points on the PDI (p = .002) and with a significantly greater risk of possible or definite magnetic resonance imaging abnormalities (odds ratio 9.4, p <.001).

Discussion

In summary, a strategy consisting predominantly of circulatory arrest is associated with greater central nervous system perturbation, as measured by EEG in the early postoperative period, than is a strategy consisting predominantly of low-flow bypass. Perioperative EEG epileptiform activity was associated with poorer prognosis at age 1 year.

EEG seizures were common in this study, occurring in 20% of infants, while clinical seizures occurred in only 6% of infants. EEG ictal discharges without clinical seizures are a common occurrence in neonatal electroencephalography and can be seen in a variety of settings. As with the patients in this study, one of the situations occurs when the neonate is purposefully paralyzed, a context in which the EEG proves invaluable as the main tool available to assess the neurological status of these infants.[5–9] However, sustained electroencephalographic seizures also occur without peripherally discernable manifestations in nonparalyzed infants.[7,10–19] This dissociation may be seen in neonates whose clinical seizures have been controlled by antiepileptic drugs (AEDs),[12,20–22] in infants following a bout of seizures, or in neonates with severe brain or spinal cord compromises that may impede the discharges from reaching the effector structures. Dissociation may also be seen when the discharges arise from apparently silent areas.[14,22–28] EEG seizures without clinical changes are relatively common. Clancy et al.[13] studied 41 infants with electroencephalographic seizures and found that only 21% of 393 such EEG seizures were associated with clinical activity.

This study also demonstrates that, in this patient population, the EEG is a safe and noninvasive technique for assessing prognosis. A worse developmental outcome and greater frequency of MRI abnormalities were more common in children with EEG seizures compared to children without seizures. The value of the EEG in predicting outcome has been noted by other authors. Rowe et al.,[26] in a prospective study of 74 neonates with clinical seizures, found that the EEG background patterns were highly correlated with outcome. The EEG discharges, interictally, were not as highly significant. However, ictal discharges, when evaluated independently of interictal discharges, were clearly correlated with generally poor outcomes.

Similar conclusions were reached by Holmes et al.[29] for a group of 38 infants who had suffered perinatal asphyxia. In this study, besides confirming that the background EEG activity was the important determining factor in the correlation with clinical follow-up, the authors also established that the efficiency of using the EEG as a predictive test was significantly higher than that of using the initial neurological examination. This is an important finding since the clinical repertoire of behavior in the neonate is narrow, making the neurological and developmental examination of rather limited value in the newborn. While more sophisticated techniques have been developed and shown to be effective for the neurological assessment of newborns, these unfortunately are time consuming and are rarely used in clinical practice. Furthermore, Saint-Anne Dargassies,[30] as a pioneer in neonatal neurology, wrote in 1979: "Unfortunately, one cannot always ascertain, (in neonates), the location or extent of a lesion, or even its pathology, by clinical examination alone. Thus the goal becomes one of recognizing general CNS dysfunction, either transient or permanent."

It is not clear whether seizures—either electroencephalographic, clinical, or both—are associated with a poor prognosis because they are reflective of severe underlying brain pathology or because they actually add to the damage. This study was not designed to investigate treatment of EEG seizures, and for that reason we cannot answer this important question.

There is little doubt that prolonged seizures in the mature animal can cause brain damage.[31-36] However, whether seizures lead to brain damage in the immature brain is more controversial. Wasterlain and Plum[37] separated rats into three age groups and subjected the animals to daily seizures for nine days. Reductions in cell numbers in brains of newborn rats shocked between the ages of 2 and 11 days, and decreases in cell size in rats between days 9 and 18 were found. However, daily seizures in older rats (age 19 to 28 days) did not affect the cell size or weight. This study suggests that the immature brain is more prone to the adverse effects of seizures than the mature brain.

However, other investigators have challenged the concept that seizures in the immature brain are more detrimental than in older animals.[38,39] The kainic acid (KA) model has been used to investigate the chronic cognitive and behavioral effects of epilepsy on the developing brain. KA is a potent analogue of the excitatory amino acid (EAA) glutamate, the most prevalent excitatory neurotransmitter in the CNS. After systemic or intracerebral administration in rats, KA causes a seizure syndrome that resembles human temporal lobe epilepsy.[40,41] Weeks to months later, rats develop brief spontaneous recurrent seizures (SRS).[42,43] Histologic examination of brains of KA-treated animals show widespread neuronal necrosis, most notably in hippocampal subfield CA3. In addition, adult animals receiving KA have profound behavioral deficits with impairment in learning and memory in a variety of tests. However, when KA is given to rats below age 20 days, no histological lesions or behavioral changes are noted, despite the fact that the seizures are as severe, if not more severe, than in older animals.[44,45] Other animal models have produced similar results. Status epilepticus, produced by continuous electrical hippocampal stimulation in the immature animal, has been associated with fewer histological lesions and behavioral abnormalities in immature animals than mature animals.[46] Likewise, pilocarpine administration, which produces severe seizures in both immature and mature animals, results in fewer behavioral abnormalities and less histological damage in the immature animal than the mature animal.[47,48] This experimental data challenges the clinical dictum that seizures in the young child or infant are more detrimental than in the older child.

One possible reason the immature brain is less vulnerable to prolonged seizures is that the immature brain has fewer, or functionally immature, EAA receptors. However, there are studies demonstrating that KA and NMDA receptors are present at birth and increase dramatically during the first few weeks of life. Miller and colleagues[49] studied the ontogeny of KA binding sites in the rat forebrain using *in vitro* receptor autoradiography. Specific binding was detectable in the hippocampus by postnatal day 1. In the CA3 region binding increased progressively with age, peaking at postnatal day 21. Insel et al.[50] also found that specific binding to NMDA and quisqualic acid receptors occurred at postnatal day 1 in the hippocampus and striatum, with the adult pattern of binding of NMDA receptors emerging by postnatal day 14. Physiological development of EAAs parallels the biochemical maturation. The population spike elicited by NMDA application to CA1 cells of the hippocampus peaks at 10 days, with long-term potentiation peaking around 15 days of age in the rat.[51-53]

Furthermore, some EAAs produce greater neurotoxicity in the immature brain than in the mature brain.[54-57] McDonald and colleagues[54] found that NMDA neurotoxicity is greater following injection in the corpus striatum in 7-day-old rats than in adults. NMDA toxicity *in vivo* transiently peaks near postnatal day 7 in rats, with the severity (of the developing brain to direct intrastriatal infusion of equimolar NMDA) approximately 60 times greater at this age compared to adults. The severity of brain injury produced by infusion of NMDA at age 1, 14, 21, and 28 days was comparable to that produced by NMDA in adults, whereas intermediate levels of injury are present at 4 and 10 days and peak levels are present at 7 days. Likewise, when given by a single injection, AMPA and quisqualic acid have greater toxicity in immature animals than mature animals.[56,57] In unpublished data from our laboratory, we show that KA, when infused by osmotic pump, also causes lesions similar in size to those of the mature brain.

Therefore, though it appears that the immature brain is as sensitive as, if not more sensitive than, the mature brain to the direct effects of

EAAs, brain damage following prolonged seizures is significantly less in immature animals than mature animals. One possible reason for this apparent discrepancy is that less glutamate is released from presynaptic terminals during prolonged seizures in the immature brain than in the mature brain. This hypothesis is supported by the finding that glutamate concentrations in the immature rat brain are low,[58] as are concentrations of glutamaterelated enzymes.[58-61] Hippocampal slices from immature rats have low presynaptic release of EAAs[62] and low sodium-dependent high-affinity uptake of glutamate and aspartate into presynaptic terminals and into glial cells.[63] In addition, Ribak and Navetta[64] found that mossy fiber synapse development in the subgranular layer of the hilus did not reach adult levels until age 21 days and in the deep hilus until age 30 days. They suggested that immaturity of the mossy fibers, with subsequent decreased release of glutamate, in rats less than 20 days could explain the lack of cell loss following prolonged seizures.

Future prospective studies randomizing infants undergoing open heart surgery to prophylactic anticonvulsants versus no prophylactic treatment may provide insight as to whether EEG seizures are detrimental and require intervention. Such studies will help elucidate whether EEG seizures are merely a marker for underlying brain pathology or are an independent cause of such injury. Until such studies are done, EEG seizures should be viewed as a marker for brain injury with prognostic significance.

References

1. Lombroso CT, Holmes GL. Value of EEG in neonatal seizures. *J Epilepsy* 1993; 6:39–70.
2. Holmes GL, Lombroso CT. Prognostic value of background patterns in the neonatal EEG. *J Clin Neurophysiol* 1993;10:323–352.
3. Newburger JW, Jonas RA, Wernovsky G, et al. A comparison of the perioperative neurologic effects of hypothermic circulatory arrest versus low-flow cardiopulmonary bypass in infant heart surgery. *N Engl J Med* 1993;329: 1057–1064.
4. Bellinger DC, Jonas RA, Rappaport LA, et al. Developmental and neurologic status of children after heart surgery with hypothermic circulatory arrest or low-flow cardiopulmonary bypass. *N Engl J Med* 1995; 332:549–555.
5. Tharp BR, Laboyrie PM. The incidence of EEG abnormalities and outcome of infants paralyzed with neuromuscular blocking agents. *Crit Care Med* 1983;11: 926–929.
6. Bridgers SL, Ebersole JS, Ment LR, Ehrenkranz RA, Silva CG. Cassette electroencephalography in the evaluation of neonatal seizures. *Arch Neurol* 1986;43: 49–51.
7. Lombroso CT. Neonatal electroencephalography. In Niedermeyer E, Lopes da Silva F (eds.), *Electroencephalography. Basic principles, clinical applications and related fields.* Baltimore: Urban & Schwarzenberg, 1982, pp. 599–637.

8. Goldberg RN, Goldman SL, Ramsay RE, Feller R. Detection of seizure activity in the paralyzed neonate using continuous monitoring. *Pediatrics* 1982;69:583–586.
9. Scher MS, Painter MJ, Bergman I, Barmada MA, Brunberg J. EEG diagnoses of neonatal seizures: Clinical correlations and outcome. *Pediatr Neurol* 1989; 5:17–24.
10. Lombroso CT. Seizures in the newborn period. In Vinken PJ, Bruyn GW (eds.), *Handbook of clinical neurology*, Vol. 15. *The epilepsies*. Amsterdam: North-Holland, 1974, pp. 189–218.
11. Lombroso CT. Neonatal polygraphy in full-term and premature infants: A review of normal and abnormal findings. *J Clin Neurophysiol* 1985;2:105–153.
12. Mizrahi EM, Kellaway P. Characterization and classification of neonatal seizures. *Neurology* 1987;37:1837–1844.
13. Clancy RR, Legido A, Lewis D. Occult neonatal seizures. *Epilepsia* 1988;29: 256–261.
14. Shewmon DA. What is a neonatal seizure? Problems in definition and quantification for investigative and clinical purposes. *J Clin Neurophysiol* 1990; 7:315–368.
15. Hellström-Westas L, Rosen I, Svenningsen NW. Cerebral complications detected by EEG-monitoring during neonatal intensive care. *Acta Paediatr Scand* 1989;360 (Suppl):83–86.
16. Clancy R, Legido A, Newell R, Bruce D, Baumgart S, Fox WW. Continuous intracranial pressure monitoring and serial electroencephalographic recordings in severely asphyxiated term neonate. *Am J Dis Child* 1988;142:740–747.
17. Connell J, Oozeer R, de Vries L, Dubowitz LMS, Dubowitz V. Continuous EEG monitoring of neonatal seizures: Diagnostic and prognostic considerations. *Arch Dis Child* 1989;64:452–458.
18. Fischer-Perroudon C, Loche D, Courjon J. 595 cas de décharges critiques localisées sans traduction clinique. Valeur séméiologique et diagnostique. *Rev Electroenceph Neurophys Clin* 1975;5:56–60.
19. Loche D, Revol M. Définition, études morphologique et topographique des activités critiques localisées, sans traduction clinique apparente. *Rev Electroenceph Neurophys Clin* 1975;5:52–55.
20. Connell J, Oozeer R, de Vries L, Dubowitz LM, Dubowitz V. Clinical and EEG response to anticonvulsants in neonatal seizures. *Arch Dis Child* 1989;64: 459–464.
21. Kellaway P, Mizrahi EM. Neonatal seizures. In Lüders H, Lesser RP (eds.), *Epilepsy: Electroclinical syndromes*. Amsterdam: Springer-Verlag, 1987, pp. 13–47.
22. Lombroso CT. Neonatal seizures. In Browne TR, Feldman RG (eds.), *Epilepsy diagnosis and management*. Boston: Little, Brown, & Co. 1983, pp. 297–313.
23. Monod N, Pajot N, Guidasci S. The Neonatal EEG: Statistical studies and prognostic value in full-term and preterm babies. *Electroenceph Clin Neurophysiol* 1972;32:529–544.
24. Radvanyi-Bouvet MF, Vallecalle MH, Morel-Kahn F, Relier JP, Dreyfus-Brisac C. Seizures and electrical discharges in premature infants. *Neuropediatrics* 1985;16:143–148.
25. Hellström-Westas L, Rosén I, Swenningsen NW. Silent seizures in sick infants in early life. Diagnosis by continuous cerebral function monitoring. *Acta Paediatr Scand* 1985;74(5):741–748.

26. Rowe JC, Holmes GL, Hafford J, Baboval D, Robinson S, Philipps A, Rosenkrantz T, Raye J. Prognostic value of the electroencephalogram in term and preterm infants following neonatal seizures. *Electroenceph Clin Neurophysiol* 1985;60:183–196.

27. Radvanyi-Bouvet MF, Cukier-Hemeury F, Morel-Kahn F. Décharges critiques chez le prématurés et les nouveau-nés à terme. *Rév EEG Neurophysiol Clin* 1981;11:404–411.

28. Dreyfus-Brisac C, Monod N. Neonatal status epilepticus. In Rémond A (ed.), *Handbook of electroencephalography and clinical neurophysiology.* Vol. 15. Amsterdam: Elsevier, 1972, pp. 38–52.

29. Holmes GL, Rowe J, Hafford J, Schmidt R, Testa M, Zimmerman A. Prognostic value of the electroencephalogram in neonatal asphyxia. *Electroenceph Clin Neurophysiol* 1982;53:60–72.

30. Saint-Anne Dargassies S. The normal and abnormal neurological examination of the neonate. In Korbokin R, Guilleminault C (eds.), *Advances in perinatal neurology.* New York: Medical and Scientific Books, 1979, pp. 4–42.

31. Meldrum BS. Metabolic factors during prolonged seizures and their relation to nerve cell death. In Delgado-Escueta AV, Wasterlain CG, Treiman DM, Porter RJ (eds.), *Advances in neurology,* Vol. 34. *Status epilepticus: Mechanisms of brain damage and treatment.* New York: Raven Press, 1983, pp.261–275.

32. Meldrum B. Physiological changes during prolonged seizures and epileptic brain damage. *Neuropaediatrie* 1978;9:203–212.

33. Meldrum BS, Brierley JB. Prolonged epileptic seizures in primates: Ischaemic cell change and its relation to ictal physiological events. *Arch Neurol* 1973; 28:10–17.

34. Meldrum BS, Horton RW, Brierley JB. Epileptic brain damage in adolescent baboons following seizures induced by allylglycine. *Brain Res* 1974;97:417–428.

35. Meldrum BS, Vigouroux RA, Brierley JB. Systemic factors and epileptic brain damage. Prolonged seizures in paralysed artificially ventilated baboons. *Arch Neurol* 1973;29:82–87.

36. Menini C, Meldrum BS, Richie DS, Silva-Comte C, Stutzmann JM. Sustained limbic seizures induced by intra-amygdaloid kainic acid in the baboon: Symptomatology and neuropathological consequences. *Ann Neurol* 1980;8: 501–509.

37. Wasterlain CG, Plum F. Vulnerability of developing rat brain to electroconvulsive seizures. *Arch of Neurol* 1973;29:38–45.

38. Albala BJ, Moshé SL, Okada R. Kainic-acid-induced seizures: A developmental study. *Dev Brain Res* 1984;13:139–148.

39. Sperber EF, Haas KZ, Stanton PK, Moshé SL. Resistance of the immature hippocampus to seizure-induced synaptic reorganization. *Dev Brain Res* 1991; 60:88–93.

40. Tremblay E, Nitecka L, Berger ML, Ben-Ari Y. Maturation of kainic acid seizure-brain damage syndrome in the rat: I, Clinical, electrographic and metabolic observations. *Neuroscience* 1984;13(4):1051–1072.

41. Nadler JV. Kainic acid as a tool for the study of temporal lobe epilepsy. *Life Sci* 1981;29:2031–2042.

42. Pisa M, Sanberg MR, Corcoran ME, Fibiger HC. Spontaneously recurrent seizures after intracerebral injections of kainic acid in rat: A possible model of human temporal lobe epilepsy. *Brain Res* 1980;200:481–487.

43. Cavalheiro EA, Richie DA, Le Gal La Salle G. Long-term effects of intrahippocampal kainic acid injection in rats: A method for inducing spontaneous recurrent seizures. *Electroenceph Clin Neurophysiol* 1982;53:581–589.

44. Stafstrom CE, Thompson JL, Holmes GL. Kainic acid seizures in the developing brain: Status epilepticus and spontaneous recurrent seizures. *Dev Brain Res* 1992;65:237–246.

45. Stafstrom CE, Holmes GL, Chronopoulos A, Thurber S, Thompson JL. Age-dependent cognitive and behavioral deficits following kainic acid-induced seizures. *Epilepsia* 1993;34:420–432.

46. Thurber S, Chronopoulos A, Stafstrom CE, Holmes GL. Behavioral effects of continuous hippocampal stimulation in the developing rat. *Dev Brain Res* 1992;68:35–40.

47. Cavalheiro EA, Silva DF, Turski WA, Calderazzo-Filho LS, Bortolotto ZA, Turski L. The susceptibility of rats to pilocarpine-induced seizures is age-dependent. *Dev Brain Res* 1987;37:43–58.

48. Hirsch E, Baram TZ, Snead OC III. Ontogenic study of lithium-pilocarpine-induced status epilepticus in rats. *Brain Res* 1992;583:120–126.

49. Miller LP, Johnson AE, Gelhard RE, Insel TR. The ontogeny of excitatory amino acid receptors in the rat forebrain: II, Kainic acid receptors. *Neuroscience* 1990;35:45–51.

50. Insel TR, Miller LP, Gelhard RE. The ontogeny of excitatory amino acid receptors in rat forebrain: I, N-methyl-D-aspartate and quisqualate receptors. *Neuroscience* 1990; 35:31–43.

51. Harris KM, Teyler TJ. Developmental onset of long-term potentiation in area CA1 of the rat hippocampus. *J Physiol* 1984;346:27–48.

52. Hammon B, Heinemann U. Developmental changes in neuronal sensitivity to excitatory amino acids in area CA1 of the rat hippocampus. *Dev Brain Res* 1988;38:286–290.

53. Ben-Ari Y, Cherubin E, Krnjevic K. Changes in voltage dependence of NMDA currents during development. *Neurosci Lett* 1988;94:88–92.

54. McDonald JW, Silverstein FS, Johnston MV. Neurotoxicity of N-methyl-D-aspartate is markedly enhanced in developing rat central nervous system. *Brain Res* 1988;459:200–203.

55. McDonald JW, Johnston MV. Pharmacology of N-methyl-D-aspartate-induced brain injury in an in vivo perinatal rat model. *Synapse* 1990;6:179–188.

56. McDonald JW, Trescher WH, Johnston MV. Susceptibility of brain to AMPA induced excitotoxicity transiently peaks during early postnatal development. *Brain Res* 1992;583:54–70.

57. McDonald JW, Trescher WH, Johnston MV. The selective ionotropic-type quisqualate receptor agonist AMPA is a potent neurotoxin in immature rat brain. *Brain Res* 1990;526:165–168.

58. Campochiaro P, Coyle JT. Ontogenic development of kainate neurotoxicity: Correlates with glutamatergic innervation. *Proc Natl Acad Sci USA* 1978;75:2025–2029.

59. Barca MA, Toledano A. Histochemical electron microscopic study of the enzyme glutamate dehydrogenase (GD) in post-natal developing cerebellum. *Cell Mol Biol* 1982;28:187–195.

60. Rothe F, Schmidt W, Wolf G. Postnatal changes in the activity of glutamate dehydrogenase and aspartate aminotransferase in the rat nervous system with

special reference to the glutamate transmitter metabolism. *Dev Brain Res* 1983; 11:67–74.

61. Kvanne E, Svenneby G, Torgner IAA, Drejer J, Schousboe A. Postnatal development of glutamate metabolizing enzymes in hippocampus from mice. *Int J Dev Neurosci* 1985;3:359–364.

62. Minc-Golomb D, Levy Y, Kleinberger N, Schramm M. D-[3H]aspartate release from hippocampus slices studied in a multiwell system: Controlling factors and postnatal development of release. *Brain Res* 1987;402:255–263.

63. Schmidt W, Wolf G. High-affinity uptake of L-[3H]glutamate and D-[3H]aspartate during postnatal development of the hippocampal formation: A quantitative autoradiographic study. *Exp Brain Res* 1988;70:50–54.

64. Ribak CE, Navetta MS. An immature mossy fiber innervation of hilar neurons may explain their resistance to kainate-induced cell death in 15-day-old rats. *Dev Brain Res* 1994;79:47–62.

CHAPTER 23

Neurologic and MRI Findings

Karl C.K. Kuban
David Wypij

In this chapter, we present the findings on neurologic evaluation at hospital discharge and neurologic and magnetic resonance imaging (MRI) evaluations at age 1 year of subjects enrolled in the Boston Circulatory Arrest Study. The neurologic status at age 1 year will be related to the neurologic findings during the perioperative period.[1]

Relation of Electrophysiologic and Biochemical Features to Support Strategy

To review the perioperative findings, among those with intact ventricular septum (IVS), 66 infants were randomly assigned to the circulatory arrest strategy of vital organ support and 63 to the low-flow bypass strategy. Among infants with ventricular septal defect (VSD), 21 were assigned to circulatory arrest and 21 to low-flow bypass. Perioperative electrophysiologic measures are summarized in Table 23–1; both clinical seizures and paroxysmal electroencephalographic (EEG) abnormalities were associated with circulatory arrest support. Definite clinical seizures in the first week after surgery occurred more frequently among infants randomized to the circulatory arrest group (exact $p = .009$; odds ratio = 11.4, 95% C.I. [1.4, 93.0]). All infants with definite clinical seizures had at least 35 minutes of total circulatory arrest. Findings on the perioperative EEG have been summarized by Drs. Holmes, Wypij, and Helmers in Chapter 22. Concerning biochemical measures, creatine kinase BB isoenzyme (CK-BB) levels were measured over the first six hours after resumption of cardiopulmonary bypass. As with the seizure and EEG outcome measures, the integrated release of CK-BB levels over the first six hours following surgery was significantly associated with assignment to the circulatory arrest group ($p = .046$) and with the duration of circulatory arrest ($p = .01$, Figure 23–1).

TABLE 23–1
Neurologic Outcomes According to Ventricular Septal Status and Treatment Group

	Intact Ventricular Septum		Ventricular Septal Defect		p-Value[1]
	Circulatory Arrest	Low-Flow Bypass	Circulatory Arrest	Low-Flow Bypass	
	Number with abnormality/Total number (%)				
Definite clinical seizures	5/66 (8)	0/63 (0)	5/21 (24)	1/20 (5)	.009
	Median (Interquartile Range)				
CK-BB release [IU/L][2]	59 (32, 84)	43 (15, 88)	57 (34, 125)	40 (20, 79)	.046[3]
	Number with abnormality/Total number (%)				
Neurologic abnormalities at hospital discharge					.64[4]
Possibly abnormal	21/65 (32)	20/59 (34)	5/19 (26)	4/17 (24)	
Abnormal	12/65 (18)	9/59 (15)	7/19 (37)	4/17 (24)	

[1] Exact p-Values for the effect of treatment, with adjustment for diagnosis
[2] Six-hour integrated CK-BB release in IU/L
[3] Linear regression p-Value for the effect of treatment, with adjustment for diagnosis, for the natural logarithm of the units of integrated CK-BB released in six hours, plus 1
[4] Exact p-Value for the effect of treatment, with normal examination results compared with possibly or definitely abnormal ones, with adjustment for diagnosis

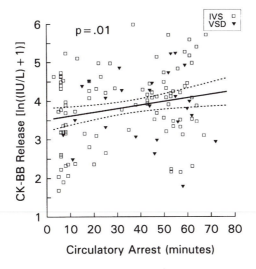

FIGURE 23–1. Estimated regression fit and 95% confidence limits for creatinine phosphokinase brain isoenzyme (CK-BB) released into the serum over the first six hours postoperatively [expressed as ln (six-hour integrated CK-BB release + 1)] as a function of the duration of total circulatory arrest. In the scatterplot, open squares denote infants with an intact ventricular septum, and filled triangles denote those with a ventricular septal defect. Diagnosis was not predictive of this outcome. The linear regression p-Value shown is for the effect of duration of total circulatory arrest on outcome, with adjustment for diagnosis.

The perioperative data suggest that a longer duration of total circulatory arrest was associated with greater neurologic perturbation, as measured by EEG recovery times, EEG seizures, clinical seizures, and release of CK-BB isoenzyme, in the early postoperative period. In addition, older age at surgery and associated diagnosis of VSD were independent risk factors for both clinical and EEG seizures.

Relation of Neurologic Evaluation at Hospital Discharge to Support Strategy

In contrast to the electrophysiologic and biochemical findings demonstrating a worse outcome among infants with circulatory arrest support, the neurologic examination at hospital discharge did not appear to be associated with support strategy (p = .64, Table 23–1). Despite the lack of apparent correlation between neurologic abnormality and mode of support, there were a substantial number of children who had neurologic findings. Twenty percent (32/160) of infants had a definitely abnormal neurologic examination, and 51% (82/160) had a possibly or definitely abnormal neurologic examination in the combined groups.

Analyses of Risk Factors for Neurologic Abnormalities

Since a substantial number of children had neurologic abnormalities that were not associated with assignment to the circulatory arrest or low-flow groups, other risk factors for neurologic examination abnormalities were sought. We organized our analyses of risk factors into those occurring in the prepregnancy, prenatal, perinatal, preoperative, and postoperative epochs.

In univariate analyses, limited to infants with definitely abnormal or normal findings, several risk factors appeared to be significant predictors for neurologic abnormality at hospital discharge (Table 23–2). Some of these risk factors appeared to be surrogates for severity of illness, such as low postoperative arterial pO_2 measurements, prolonged intubation postoperatively, and delay in performing the postoperative neurologic examination beyond the specified 7 to 10 day time period. The usual reason for the delay was that the infant was too ill to be examined, i.e., the infant often was either still intubated or paralyzed.

Abnormalities on postoperative neurologic examination were also associated with the occurrence of clinical seizures in the early postoperative period. In this study, seizures were associated with longer duration of circulatory arrest; however, seizures could have been influenced by other preop-

TABLE 23–2
Univariate Predictors of Definite Abnormalities on Neurologic Examination at Hospital Discharge

Variable	*p-Value[1]*
Preoperative neurologic status	.003
Postoperative pO_2 <50	.04
Hours of intubation >median	.06
Delay to postoperative exam ≥10 days	.02
Definite clinical seizures	.02
Vaginal delivery	.04

[1] Exact p-Values for the association with definitely abnormal vs. normal findings on neurologic examination at hospital discharge.

erative or postoperative factors. Another significant variable associated with abnormal neurologic outcome was vaginal delivery. This association might have been spurious given the number of analyses undertaken or could have reflected a more serious condition (not otherwise captured) of the infant at the time of delivery.

Interestingly, preoperative neurologic status appeared to be the most important clinical predictor of postoperative neurologic abnormality. This finding suggested that the preoperative degree of illness or the presence of some other key factor influenced postoperative neurologic outcome.

Although several pre-, peri-, and postoperative factors were associated with an abnormal neurologic examination, there remains the important question of why the neurologic examination did not show an important correlation with method of support, whereas EEG outcomes and seizure outcomes appeared to be associated with assignment to the predominantly circulatory arrest technique. There are several possible explanations.

First, the neurologic examination in the neonatal period may not be sensitive enough to detect the extant abnormalities. This may be true particularly if infarction, necrosis, or brain dysfunction is either small in size or in a place that is not easily expressed as part of the neurologic examination of infants, the emphasis of which is predominantly the assessment of the motor systems.[2-4]

A second possible explanation relates to the fact that some brain functions normally are not expressed until later in development and therefore may not be recognized until then. Patricia Goldman-Rakic placed prefrontal lesions in a series of newborn monkeys and then allowed them to heal.[5] She then submitted these monkeys and a set of control monkeys to behavioral and neurologic examinations, but was not able to identify a difference between the groups. Yet, when the monkeys were reevaluated at a later time, substantial, clear differences in behavior and neurologic findings were identified in the animals with prefrontal lesions when compared to the controls. Much as the ability to perform algebra cannot be assessed at age 3 years, particular lesions may be undetectable by neurologic examination at certain points of development.

Third, the apparent lack of association between support method and neurologic outcome may be explained by the effects of an unknown confounder. Randomization should minimize the likelihood that unrecognized risk factors or risk modifiers will occur more often in one support strategy group and thereby influence the outcome of the study and the resulting inferences. However, randomization does not ensure that all risk factors or risk modifiers are partitioned equally in the two groups. Extensive analyses with adjustment for measured risk factors, or possible confounding variables, still showed a lack of association between support method and neurologic outcome.

A fourth possible explanation is that clinical and EEG abnormalities are symptoms of the acute cardiovascular alterations but that these perturbations do not cause other short-term or long-term neurologic abnormalities; i.e., the electrophysiologic alterations do not reflect permanent new neuroanatomic and physiologically important alterations.

The possible explanations for the absence of association between support technique and apparent neurologic signs at one week following surgery may be distinguished at the one year postoperative neurologic and developmental evaluations (see next section).

Neurologic Evaluation at One Year

The one year neurologic examination was derived from both the one year National Collaborative Perinatal Project examination and from Richmond Paine's monograph.[4] The examination is an objective, standard, neurologic examination that was administered in almost all instances by a single board-certified neurologist (Dr. Karl Kuban) without knowledge of randomization group, perinatal outcome measures, magnetic resonance imaging results, or developmental testing scores.

The children were classified as either normal, possibly abnormal, or definitely abnormal. The *possibly abnormal* group was comprised of children who had abnormalities that were not clearly neurologically based or neurologically important. These included children who were hypotonic without weakness or other cerebellar signs; children who had isolated cranial nerve abnormalities, such as facial palsy; children with isolated tremor without evidence of other cerebellar or other motor signs; and children with isolated hyperreflexia or with unsustained clonus without evidence of pyramidal signs, such as extensor plantars, weakness, or spasticity. The *abnormal* children were those with microcephaly, cerebral palsy, hypertonia, movement disorders, and/or ataxia or with a greater than 2-month development delay.

The abnormalities were graded as mild, moderate, or severe. We defined as *mild* those neurological abnormalities which still permitted the child to do most tasks expected for age, i.e., there was minimal functional impairment. Children with *severe* abnormalities were those who were completely dependent on caretakers.

Among the 154 children in the combined treatment groups in whom the neurologic examination was performed, 5 (3%) had possible abnormalities and 48 (31%) had definite abnormalities, all of which were judged to be mild in severity (Table 23–3). These abnormalities on neurologic examination tended to be more common among children randomized to the circulatory arrest strategy than to the low-flow bypass strategy (41% vs. 28%; exact $p = .09$). Similarly, possible or definite neurologic abnormalities were significantly associated with longer duration of circulatory arrest ($p = .04$, Figure 23–2). Low five-minute Apgar score and younger gestational age were both independent risk factors for neurologic abnormalities, but adjustment

TABLE 23–3
Outcomes of Neurologic Examination and Magnetic Resonance Imaging at One Year Postoperative Evaluation According to Ventricular Septal Status and Treatment Group.

Variable	Intact Ventricular Septum		Ventricular Septal Defect		p-Value[1]
	Circulatory Arrest	Low-Flow Bypass	Circulatory Arrest	Low-Flow Bypass	
	(N = 60)	(N = 59)	(N = 18)	(N = 17)	
	No. with abnormality (%)				
Overall Neurologic Abnormalities					.09[2]
Possible	2 (3)	1 (2)	2 (11)	0 (0)	
Definite[3]	21 (35)	13 (22)	7 (39)	7 (41)	
Specific Neurologic Abnormalities					
Cerebral Palsy	3 (5)	3 (5)	0 (0)	1 (6)	.72
Tone alteration but not cerebral palsy					
Hypotonia	11 (18)	7 (12)	7 (39)	3 (18)	.14
Hypertonia	5 (8)	3 (5)	0 (0)	4 (24)	.56
Ataxia/dysmetric	1 (2)	0 (0)	0 (0)	0 (0)	1.00
Focal abnormalities apart from those related to cerebral palsy	1 (2)	1 (2)	1 (6)	1 (6)	1.00
Special senses	1 (2)	1 (2)	0 (0)	0 (0)	1.00
Delayed development > 2 months	9 (15)	5 (8)	6 (33)	4 (24)	.26
Overall Magnetic Resonance Imaging Abnormalities	(N = 50)	(N = 58)	(N = 18)	(N = 16)	.84[2]
Possible	5 (10)	4 (7)	1 (6)	1 (6)	
Definite					
Mild	4 (8)	8 (14)	4 (22)	3 (19)	
Moderate	1 (2)	2 (3)	0 (0)	0 (0)	

[1] Exact p-Values for the effect of treatment, with adjustment for diagnosis
[2] Exact p-Value for the effect of treatment, with normal examination results compared with possibly or definitely abnormal ones, with adjustment for diagnosis
[3] All definite abnormalities were judged to be mild in severity

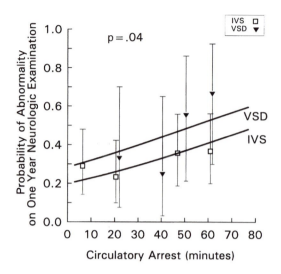

FIGURE 23–2. Estimated probabilities of a possible or definite neurologic abnormality at age one year as a function of the duration of total circulatory arrest. Separate logistic regression curves are shown for children with an intact ventricular septum (IVS; open squares) and for those with a ventricular septal defect (VSD; filled triangles). Point estimates and exact 95% confidence intervals for outcome probabilities are plotted for the mean of each quartile of duration of circulatory arrest. The logistic regression p-Value shown is for the effect of the duration of total circulatory arrest on outcome, with adjustment for diagnosis.

for them did not appreciably affect the estimate of the increased risk associated with assignment to circulatory arrest. Associated diagnosis of ventricular septal defect was not an independent risk factor for neurologic abnormalities.

Among the 48 children with definite neurologic abnormalities were seven with cerebral palsy (5% of the population). There were 28 who were hypotonic (18% of the population), i.e., either with isolated hypotonia or hypotonia and developmental delay, 12 children (8%) who had hypertonia without clear evidence of cerebral palsy, and one who was ataxic. There were four children with focal abnormalities, such as a facial palsy; two with either visual or hearing impairment; and 24 (16% of the population) with delayed development of two months or more. None of the infants had epileptic seizures. The occurrence of specific abnormalities was not associated with treatment group or with duration of circulatory arrest.

Finally, the occurrence of clinical seizures detected by bedside nurses and physicians in the early postoperative period was associated with an increased risk at age 1 year of possible or definite neurologic abnormalities (p = .05, adjusted for diagnosis and treatment group).

Cranial Magnetic Resonance Imaging Evaluation at One Year

The structural correlates of the type of operative support and abnormalities were investigated by performance of cranial MRI when the children were 1 year old. MRI studies were interpreted by two independent, blinded, staff pediatric neuroradiologists. Findings were classified as normal, possibly abnormal, or definitely abnormal. Definite abnormalities were further classified as mild, moderate, or severe. More specific descriptions were provided, including diffuse abnormalities (ventricular dilation, delayed myelination/ maturation, periventricular leukomalacia), focal/multifocal abnormalities (atrophy, intensity abnormality of gray or white matter), and developmental or incidental findings. Disagreements were resolved by a third consensus reading by the two examiners (14% of studies, with 4% frank positive/ negative disagreement).

Among the 142 children in the combined treatment groups in whom MRI was performed, 11 (8%) had possible abnormalities and 22 (15%) had definite abnormalities (Table 23-3). There was no apparent relationship of treatment assignment with MRI abnormalities (p = .84) or with the duration of circulatory arrest (p = .64). Preoperative acidosis was a significant risk factor for presence of possible or definite abnormalities on MRI at age 1 year (p = .05).

Specific abnormalities on MRI were considered to be diffuse in 16 children (i.e., ventricular dilation, delayed myelination/maturation, or periventricular leukomalacia), focal/multifocal in 20 children (i.e., atrophy or intensity abnormality), and developmental/incidental in 3 children (i.e., left temporal lobar hypoplasia, Chiari I malformation, or small left Sylvian arachnoid cyst). Interestingly, there was no apparent relationship between presence or type of MRI abnormality and neurologic examination at age 1 year. Similarly, whereas EEG abnormalities were highly correlated with circulatory arrest support, MRI abnormalities were not. However, there was a significant relationship between MRI and EEG abnormalities; children with EEG seizures were much more likely to have MRI abnormalities (p < .001, Figure 23-3). This association was strongest within the low-flow group. Moreover, the presence of greater release of CK-BB isoenzyme following surgery correlated with the increased likelihood of having an MRI abnormality, adjusting for treatment assignment (p = .03, Figure 23-4). Presumably, CK-BB is released as a result of brain injury such as infarction, although other mechanisms may be at play.

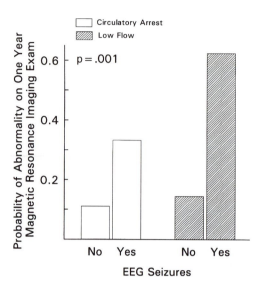

FIGURE 23–3. Probabilities of possible or definite abnormalities on magnetic resonance imaging at age 1 year according to presence or absence of EEG seizures in the perioperative period and according to treatment group. The exact p-Value shown is for the effect of EEG seizures on outcome, with adjustment for treatment group.

Conclusions

Neurologic abnormalities appear to be more strongly associated with assignment to the circulatory arrest strategy and to circulatory arrest duration at the one year assessment than in the perioperative period. This difference suggests that neurologic assessment in the perioperative period may have limited specificity and sensitivity in the determination of long-term neurologic abnormalities associated with circulatory arrest. These limitations may be related either to deficiencies of the neurologic assessment or to incomplete expression of neurologic perturbations at an immature age.

To summarize, we found that (1) abnormal neurologic examination at 1 year was more likely to be identified in infants randomized to circulatory arrest or with longer circulatory arrest times; (2) MRI abnormalities were not associated with circulatory arrest assignment, duration of circulatory arrest, or neurologic abnormalities at 1 year of age; (3) perioperative seizure activity predicted an abnormal MRI and tended to predict abnormalities on neu-

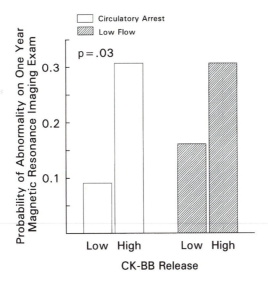

FIGURE 23–4. Probabilities of possible or definite abnormalities on magnetic resonance imaging at 1 year according to the integrated release of serum creatine phosphokinase, brain isoenzyme (CK-BB) over the first six hours postoperatively, classified into values below (low) or above (high) the median, and according to treatment group. The exact p-Value shown is for the effect of CK-BB release on outcome, with adjustment for treatment group.

rologic examination; and (4) the neonatal neurological examination was less specific than the 1-year examination for identifying neurologic abnormalities associated with circulatory arrest.

References

1. Newburger JW, Jonas RA, Wernovsky G, et al. A comparison of the perioperative neurologic effects of hypothermic circulatory arrest versus low-flow cardiopulmonary bypass in infant heart surgery. *N Engl J Med* 1993;329: 1057–1064.
2. Dubowitz L, Dubowitz V. *The neurological assessment of the preterm and full-term newborn infant.* London: Spastics Society International Medical in association with Heinemann Medical, 1981.
3. Prechtl HFR. *The neurological examination of the full-term newborn infant: A manual for clinical use,* 2nd ed. Oxford, England: Blackwell Scientific, 1977.

4. Paine RS, Oppe TE. *Neurological examination of children.* London: Spastics Society in association with Heinemann Medical, 1966.
5. Goldman-Rakic PS. An alternative to developmental plasticity: Heterology of CNS structure in infants and adults. In Stein, DG, Rosen JJ, Butters N (eds.), *Plasticity and recovery of function in the central nervous system.* New York: Academic Press, 1994, pp. 149–174.

CHAPTER 24

Developmental Findings at One Year

Leonard A. Rappaport
David Bellinger
David Wypij

Despite a relatively large number of studies of developmental outcome after circulatory arrest, the developmental impact of this technique remains uncertain. Studies on cognitive, behavioral, and linguistic development of children who underwent circulatory arrest have shown evidence of deficits in these areas, sometimes related to duration of circulatory arrest.[1,2] Wells et al.[3] found that patients who had undergone cardiac surgery with use of circulatory arrest in infancy had scores on the McCarthy scale which were significantly worse than those of their siblings; these differences were positively associated with duration of circulatory arrest. Children with similar cardiac surgery, who were operated upon under moderate hypothermia and continuous cardiopulmonary bypass, had scores comparable to those of their siblings. Other reports have shown no significant differences in children undergoing cardiac surgery with circulatory arrest compared to controls,[4-6] including one study in which patients tested preoperatively acted as their own controls.[7] Most studies focus on intelligence quotient (IQ) or developmental quotient, with a broad definition of normality and with only limited attempts to differentiate the potential impact of the independent variables on important component skills (e.g., attention, visual-motor integration, expressive and receptive language). Methodologic limitations of published investigations include small sample size and limited power, diverse cardiac defects and ages at repair, retrospective study design, comparison of techniques used during different time periods, and follow-up evaluation of children at different ages using different test instruments. In addition, small sample sizes have precluded the use of multivariate techniques to control for potential confounders or effect modifiers.

Inferences concerning the effect of cardiovascular surgical support techniques on neurologic and developmental outcome are further complicated by the presence of other risk factors for brain injury in children with congenital heart disease. An extensive literature on neurologic abnormalities[8,9] suggests a prevalence of central nervous system injury ranging from 5% to 56%, the latter in children with d-transposition of the great arteries (dTGA). While brain injury is thought to result largely from complications during surgery or the early postoperative period, neurologic outcome may also be influenced by preexisting brain abnormalities; severe, chronic hypoxemia or congestive heart failure; episodes of arrhythmia or cardiac arrest; thromboembolic events unrelated to surgery (e.g., at cardiac catheterization); nutritional status; and central nervous system infection. To sort out the contribution to neurologic outcome made by the two support techniques under consideration with the smallest possible number of subjects, it is important to study a patient population in whom potential confounding factors are minimal.

In this report, we compare the developmental status at age 1 year of children assigned to an operative support strategy of either predominantly total circulatory arrest or predominantly low-flow cardiopulmonary bypass. Developmental status was one of the primary outcome variables of the clinical trial.

Methods

Developmental Testing

All assessments were conducted at 8 a.m. in a testing suite in the Child Development Unit of Children's Hospital. Two examiners blinded to treatment assignment and clinical course (e.g., occurrence of seizures) administered the Bayley Scales of Infant Development,[10] which yields two scores: the Psychomotor Development Index and the Mental Development Index. We also calculated the proportion of children whose scores were ≤80, which corresponds to approximately 2 standard deviations below the contemporary mean scores on the 1969 version of the Bayley Scales (Psychomotor Development Index: 110.5 ± 15.3; Mental Development Index: 111.6 ± 17.2).[10,11] We established excellent interexaminer reliability, with 99% agreement on individual items and greater than 0.99 correlations between the raw scores of the examiners. Assessments were videotaped for use in resolving scoring questions.

The Fagan Test of Infant Intelligence,[12] which assesses visual recognition memory, was also administered. A mean novelty preference score (percent fixation on a novel stimulus) was computed, and a score <53% classified as a *failure*.[12] Because we used the version of this test developed for assessing 12 month olds, analyses were restricted to children who were 11 to 13 months old at the time of examination.

Other Data

Information was collected by parental interview on key correlates and determinants of infant development, including family factors such as social class,[13] maternal age, maternal education, birth order, infant gender, quality of the rearing environment,[14,15] parental IQ,[16] family process,[17] social support,[18] and parenting stress;[19] and prenatal and perinatal factors such as length of gestation, birth weight, and size for gestational age.

Statistical Analyses

Treatment group comparisons (predominantly total circulatory arrest versus predominantly low-flow bypass) were conducted by means of intent-to-treat analyses. Secondary analyses examined the effect of duration (minutes) of total circulatory arrest on outcome. All hypothesis tests and regression analyses of outcome variables were adjusted for diagnosis (i.e., intact ventricular septum vs. ventricular septal defect). Adjusting for surgeon or surgeon by treatment interaction did not alter the study conclusions.

One-year outcomes included both continuous and categorical variables. Multiple linear regression methods and Wilcoxon rank tests were used to analyze continuous outcome variables. Stratified exact tests[20] and multiple logistic regression methods were used to analyze categorical outcome variables.

Scores on the Bayley Scales were expressed in two ways. First, standard scores were derived (i.e., Psychomotor Development Index, Mental Development Index). Second, the numbers of items passed on the psychomotor and mental scales were totaled, and these outcomes were adjusted for age at the time of examination. This approach adjusts for slight imbalances between treatment/diagnosis groups in a child's placement within the age span used to derive standard scores.

For some children, not all outcome scores are available. The Bayley Scales could not be administered to one child due to distress, and another child could be administered only the Mental Scale items. Another child, later diagnosed as autistic, was untestable due to reduced social relatedness. In addition, prior to data analysis and without knowledge of treatment assignment, a decision was made to exclude the developmental test scores of the first 10 infants who returned for one-year examinations. The testing of these infants was conducted under suboptimal conditions (physical site and a lack of standardization with respect to infant state). Thus analyses are based on Psychomotor Development Index scores for 142 infants and Mental Development Index scores for 143 infants. Analyses of the Fagan Test are based on the scores of 107 infants. Twenty children had ages outside of the 11 to 13 month range at the time of examination, and the test could not be completed on an additional 17 children due to their failure to cooperate.

Results

Psychomotor Development Index

The Psychomotor Development Index score in the combined treatment groups was 95.1 ± 15.5 (mean ± S.D.). Psychomotor Development Index scores were significantly lower among infants randomly assigned to circulatory arrest (mean difference of 6.5 points; 95% confidence interval, 1.6 to 11.5; p = .01) (Table 24–1). Similarly, lower Psychomotor Development Index scores were associated with longer duration of circulatory arrest (p = .02) (Figure 24–1). None of various nonlinear or "cutpoint" models of the association between Psychomotor Development Index and duration of circulatory arrest fit the data significantly better than the linear model. Adjusting for age at examination, the total number of motor scale items passed was significantly lower for children assigned to the circulatory arrest group (p = .003) and was inversely related to the duration of circulatory arrest (p = .008). Twenty percent of children (28/142) achieved a score on the Psychomotor Development Index of ≤80, i.e., at least 2 SDs below the expected contemporary mean. These low scores were more prevalent among children assigned to the total circulatory arrest group (27% vs. 12%; exact p = .02) and those with a longer duration of circulatory arrest (p = .03) (Figure 24–2).

Using multivariate linear regression techniques, we explored whether perioperative or sociodemographic variables could explain this effect of treatment assignment or duration of circulatory arrest. Lower Psychomotor Development Index scores were significantly associated with lower birth weight, but the inclusion of birth weight in the model increased the magnitude and significance of the effect of assignment to circulatory arrest or the duration of circulatory arrest. Associated diagnosis of ventricular septal defect was an independent risk factor for lower Psychomotor Development Index score (mean difference of 6.6 points; 95% confidence interval, 0.7 to 12.6; p = .03).

Mental Development Index

The Mental Development Index score in the combined treatment groups was 105.1 ± 15.0 (mean ± S.D.). Mental Development Index scores tended to be lower among infants assigned to the circulatory arrest group (mean difference of 4.1 points; 95% confidence interval, −0.7 to 8.8; p = .10) (see Table 24–1), although the association between this score and the duration of circulatory arrest did not achieve statistical significance (p = .33). Adjusting for age at examination, the total number of mental scale items passed was significantly lower among children assigned to the circulatory arrest group (p = .04) but was not significantly related to duration of circulatory arrest (p = .16). Of the eight children in the combined treatment groups with Mental Development Index scores at least 2 SDs below the expected mean (i.e., ≤80), six were assigned to the circulatory arrest group (exact p = .27). In

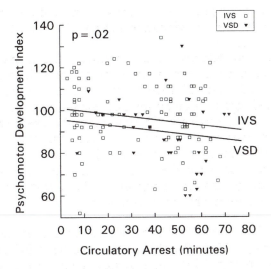

FIGURE 24–1. Psychomotor Development Index Score as a function of the duration of total circulatory arrest. Separate regression lines are shown for infants with intact ventricular septum (IVS; open squares) and those with a ventricular septal defect (VSD; filled triangles). The linear regression p-Value shown is for the effect of duration of total circulatory arrest on Psychomotor Development Index, with adjustment for diagnosis.

multiple regression models, lower Mental Development Index scores were significantly associated with lower maternal education, but adjustment for this variable did not appreciably affect the association between treatment group and score on the Mental Development Index. Associated diagnosis of ventricular septal defect was an independent risk factor for lower Mental Development Index score (mean difference of 8.6 points; 95% confidence interval, 2.8 to 14.4; p = .004).

Fagan Test of Infant Intelligence

In the combined treatment groups, the novelty preference score was 58.8% ± 7.6% (mean ± S.D.), similar to the mean score of 59.5% ± 8.1% observed by Fagan and colleagues in a sample of at-risk infants.[12] Scores were not related to support method, either when examined in terms of treatment assignment (see Table 24–1) or duration of circulatory arrest. Children with an associated diagnosis of ventricular septal defect achieved significantly lower mean novelty scores (3.6%, 95% confidence interval, 0.2% to 7.0%, p = .04).

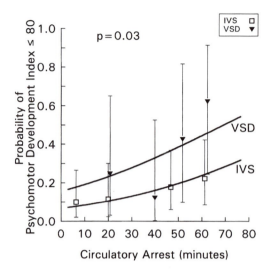

FIGURE 24–2. Estimated probabilities of a Psychomotor Development Index score ≤80 as a function of the duration of total circulatory arrest. Separate logistic regression curves are shown for children with an intact ventricular septum (IVS; open squares) and for those with a ventricular septal defect (VSD; filled triangles). Point estimates and exact 95% confidence intervals for outcome probabilities are plotted for the mean of each quartile of duration of circulatory arrest. The logistic regression p-Value shown is for the effect of the duration of total circulatory arrest on outcome, with adjustment for diagnosis.

Although 21% of infants (23/107) received novelty preference scores less than 53%, the percentage did not differ significantly by treatment group (circulatory arrest, 25%; low-flow bypass, 17%) or diagnosis (intact ventricular septum, 19%; ventricular septal defect, 29%). Furthermore, failure to complete the test was not associated with treatment group.

Relationships Between Perioperative Seizure
Activity and One-Year Status

In the perioperative period, infants assigned to circulatory arrest had been at significantly increased risk of seizure activity as detected with continuous EEG monitoring over the first 48 hours postoperatively.[21] In regression analyses controlling for diagnosis and treatment group, the occurrence of EEG seizure activity in the early postoperative period was associated with a

TABLE 24–1
Developmental Outcomes According to Ventricular Septal Status and Treatment Group

Variable	Intact Ventricular Septum		Ventricular Septal Defect		p-Value[1]
	Circulatory Arrest (N = 58)	Low-Flow Bypass (N = 54)	Circulatory Arrest (N = 16)	Low-flow Bypass (N = 15)	
	Mean ± S.D.				
Psychomotor Development Index	94.1 ± 15.3	99.1 ± 14.2	84.2 ± 18.7	96.0 ± 11.1	.01
Mental Development Index	106.0 ± 15.6	108.0 ± 12.4	92.8 ± 15.7	104.3 ± 15.1	.10
Fagan Test of Infant Intelligence[2]	59.4 ± 7.1	59.8 ± 6.2	54.6 ± 10.7	57.5 ± 9.0	.49
	No. with low score/Total no. (%)				
Psychomotor Development Index ≤ 80	12/57 (21)	5/54 (9)	8/16 (50)	3/15 (20)	.02
Mental Development Index ≤ 80	3/58 (5)	1/54 (2)	3/16 (19)	1/15 (7)	.27
Fagan Test of Infant Intelligence[2] < 53	10/42 (24)	6/41 (15)	4/13 (31)	3/11 (27)	.35

[1]Linear regression p-Values for the effect of treatment, with adjustment for diagnosis, for continuous outcomes or exact p-Values for the effect of treatment, with adjustment for diagnosis, for dichotomous outcomes.
[2]Restricted to infants between 11 and 13 months of age at the time of examination.

mean reduction of 11.2 points on the Psychomotor Development Index (p = .002).

Discussion

We found that a strategy of predominant circulatory arrest, as compared with one of predominant low-flow cardiopulmonary bypass, during open heart surgery in infancy is associated with lower performance on indices of developmental function at 1 year of age. Children who were assigned to the circulatory arrest group had significantly lower scores on the Psychomotor Development Index (motor function) and a tendency to lower Mental Development Index scores (mental function). Similarly, longer duration of circulatory arrest was associated with significantly worse performance on the Psychomotor Development Index. No relationship was found between treatment assignment and findings on the Fagan Test of Infant Intelligence, a test of visual recognition memory. Seizure activity on continuous EEG in the early postoperative period and associated diagnosis of ventricular septal defect were independent risk factors for poor outcome at 1 year of age. This latter finding was surprising given that infants with an associated ventricular septal defect were less acutely ill at the time of surgery.[21] These developmental results at age 1 year are consistent with the greater neurologic morbidity previously reported in the early postoperative period for infants randomized to the circulatory arrest strategy.[21]

The duration of total circulatory arrest is a determinant of severity of brain injury, but the safe duration, i.e., that time within which no irreversible damage occurs, is not known. The safe duration is likely to be affected by factors such as depth of hypothermia, characteristics of the cooling process and of cerebral blood flow during cooling and rewarming, and the biochemical milieu (i.e., pH, pCO_2 during cooling).[22,23] Experimental evidence in animals suggests that circulatory arrest periods less than 30 minutes in duration at brain temperatures of 15° to 20°C do not produce permanent structural or functional damage.[24,25] In analyzing the findings from follow-up studies of children undergoing open heart surgery,[1,3-5,26-29] Kirklin and Barrett-Boyes[23] concluded that arrest times longer than 60 minutes (at 18° to 20°C) are associated with developmental impairment but that the possibility of an increased risk with arrest times as brief as 45 minutes cannot be eliminated. For most outcomes in the present study, risk increased with duration of circulatory arrest. Although we were unable to select a cut-point or threshold duration below which no increase in risk was evident, the data are consistent with the hypothesis that a period of circulatory arrest less than 35 minutes (at 18°C) has minimal adverse impact on 1-year Psychomotor Development Index scores. The occurrence of substantial deficits seemed to be most apparent among children with circulatory arrest periods greater than 45 minutes. Our ability to identify a cut-point was limited by the fact that models including diagnosis, and either treatment group assignment or duration of circulatory arrest, accounted for less than 10% of the variability of developmental indices.

Although the study was designed to compare outcomes between the two treatment strategies and did not include a normal control group, patients in both treatment groups performed at a lower level than expected based on contemporary norms. Many studies have found an upward drift of 10 to 12 points in the mean score of infants on the 1969 version of the Bayley Scales of Infant Development, and a recent restandardization of the Bayley Scales has confirmed that observation.[11] Thus the mean scores of children in this study are approximately 0.5 (Mental Development Index) to 1 standard deviation (Psychomotor Development Index) lower than expected. The reasons for these generally low scores, independent of duration of circulatory arrest, may reside in cyanosis or hemodynamic instability preoperatively, generally deleterious central nervous system effects of cardiopulmonary bypass (e.g., microemboli, hypoperfusion), adverse effects of hemodynamic conditions in the postoperative period, or previously unrecognized underlying central nervous system abnormalities.

Several limitations in the use of infant developmental testing at 1 year of age warrant comment. Although tests such as the Bayley Scales have satisfactory concurrent validity, scores achieved by 1-year-old infants have limited predictive validity.[30,31] Although the relative deficits of the children assigned to circulatory arrest were most prominent in the domain of motor function, assessment at older ages may reveal treatment effects in other domains, such as language or visual-motor integration, that are not easily tested in a 1 year old. In a follow-up study of low-birth-weight infants, for example, infants with deficits in motor function and neurologic status at age 1 year were at increased risk of having lower IQ scores, expressive language delay, and poorer articulation skills at age 3 years.[32]

In summary, the developmental status of children randomized to the predominantly total circulatory arrest method of vital organ support was significantly worse than that of children randomized to the predominantly low-flow bypass method. The findings at age 1 year are consistent with the greater neurologic morbidity previously reported in the early postoperative period for infants randomized to the predominantly circulatory arrest strategy.[21] Ongoing assessments of the children at age 4 will clarify whether these findings portend clinically important differences in the children's neurodevelopmental functioning. In the surgical management of the individual infant, cardiovascular surgeons must continue to balance the technical advantages of total circulatory arrest technique with its potential disadvantages.

References

1. Wright J, Hicks R, Newman D. Deep hypothermic arrest: Observations on later development in children. *J Thorac Cardiovasc Surg* 1979;77:466–469.
2. Settergren G, Ohqvist G, Lundberg S. Cerebral blood flow and cerebral metabolism in children following cardiac surgery with deep hypothermia and

circulatory arrest. Clinical course and follow-up of psychomotor development. *Scand J Thorac Cardiovasc Surg* 1982;16:209–215.

3. Wells F, Coghill S, Caplan H, Lincoln C. Duration of circulatory arrest does influence the psychological development of children after cardiac operation in early life. *J Thorac Cardiovasc Surg* 1983;86:823–831.

4. Clarkson PM, MacArthur BA, Barratt-Boyes BG. Developmental progress following cardiac surgery in infants using profound hypothermia and circulatory arrest. *Circulation* 1980;62:855–861.

5. Dickinson D, Sambrooks J. Intellectual performance in children after circulatory arrest with profound hypothermia in infancy. *Arch Dis Child* 1979;54:1–6.

6. Richter JA. Profound hypothermia and circulatory arrest: Studies on intraoperative metabolic changes and late postoperative development after correction of congenital heart disease. In deLange S, Hennis PJ, Kettler D, Dordrecht D (eds.), *Cardiac anesthesia: Problems, innovations.* New York: Nijhoff, 1986, pp. 121–142.

7. Blackwood M, Haka-Ikse K, Steward D. Developmental outcome in children undergoing surgery with profound hypothermia. *Anesthesia* 1989;65:437–440.

8. Berthrong M, Sabiston DC Jr. Cerebral lesions in congenital heart disease: A review of autopsies on one hundred and sixty-two cases. *Bull Johns Hopkins Hospital* 1951;89:384–401.

9. Newburger JW, Silbert AR, Buckley LP, Fyler DC. Cognitive function and duration of hypoxemia in children with transposition of the great arteries. *N Engl J Med* 1984;310:1495–1499.

10. Bayley N. *Bayley scales of infant development.* New York: The Psychological Corporation, 1969.

11. Bayley N. *Bayley scales of infant development,* 2nd ed. San Antonio, TX: The Psychological Corporation, 1993.

12. Fagan J, Singer L, Montie J, Shepherd P. Selective screening device for the early detection of normal or delayed cognitive development in infants at risk for later mental retardation. *Pediatrics* 1986;78:1021–1026.

13. Hollingshead A. *Four factor index of social status,* Unpublished manual, 1975.

14. Bradley R, Caldwell B. Early home environment and changes in mental test performances in children 6–36 months. *Child Dev* 1976;12:93–97.

15. Bradley R, Caldwell B. The relation of infants' home environments to achievement test performance in first grade: A follow-up study. *Child Dev* 1984;55: 803–809.

16. Dunn L. *The Peabody picture vocabulary test,* rev. ed. Circles Pines, MN: American Guidance Service, 1981.

17. Olson D, Portner J. Family adaptability and cohesion evaluation scales. In Filsinger E (ed.), *Marriage and family assessment.* Beverly Hills: Sage, 1983, pp. 299–315.

18. Flaherty J, Gaviria M, Pathak D. The measurement of social support. The Social Support Network Inventory. *Comprehen Psych* 1983;24:521–529.

19. Abidin R. *Parenting stress index—Manual,* 2nd ed. Charlotteville, VA: Pediatric Psychology Press, 1986.

20. StatXact. Statistical software for exact nonparametric inference, user manual. StatXact-Turbo. Cambridge, MA: CYTEL Software Corporation, 1992.

21. Newburger JW, Jonas RA, Wernovsky G, et al. A comparison of the perioperative neurologic effects of hypothermic circulatory arrest versus low-flow

cardiopulmonary bypass in infant heart surgery. *N Engl J Med* 1993;329: 1057–1064.

22. Jonas RA. Review of current research at Boston Children's Hospital. *Ann Thorac Surg* 1993;56:1467–1472.

23. Kirklin JW, Barratt-Boyes BG. *Cardiac surgery: Morphology, diagnostic criteria, natural history, techniques, results, and indications,* Vol. 1, 2nd ed. New York: Churchill Livingstone, 1993, pp. 72–73.

24. Folkerth TL, Angell WW, Fosburg RG, Oury JH. Effect of deep hypothermia, limited cardiopulmonary bypass, and total arrest on growing puppies. In *Recent advances in studies on cardiac structure,* 10th ed., Baltimore, MD: University Park, 1975, pp. 411–421.

25. Treasure T, Naftel DC, Conger KA, Garcia JH, Kirklin JW, Blackstone EH. The effect of hypothermic circulatory arrest time on cerebral function, morphology, and biochemistry. *J Thorac Cardiovasc Surg* 1983;86:761–770.

26. Subramanian S, Vlad P, Fischer L, Cohen M. Sequelae of profound hypothermia and circulatory arrest in the corrective treatment of congenital heart disease in infants and small children. In Kidd BSL, Rowe RD (eds.), *The child with congenital heart disease at surgery.* Mt. Kiscony: Futura, 1976, pp. 421–431.

27. Haka-Ikse K, Blackwood MJA, Steward DJ. Psychomotor development of infants and children after profound hypothermia during surgery for congenital heart disease. *Dev Med Child Neurol* 1978;20:62–70.

28. Messmer BJ, Schallberger U, Gattiker R, Senning A. Psychomotor and intellectual development after deep hypothermia and circulatory arrest in early infancy. *J Thorac Cardiovasc Surg* 1976;72:495–502.

29. Stevenson J, Stone E, Dillard D, Morgan B. Intellectual development of children subjected to prolonged circulatory arrest during hypothermic open heart surgery in infancy. *Circulation* 1974;49:54–59.

30. Ross G. Some thoughts on the value of infant tests for assessing and predicting mental ability. *J Dev Behav Ped* 1989;10:44–47.

31. Ulvund S. Predictive validity of assessments of early cognitive competence in light of some current issues in developmental psychology. *Human Develop* 1984;27:76–83.

32. Ross G, Lipper EG, Auld PAM. Consistency and change in the development of premature infants weighing less than 1500 grams at birth. *Pediatrics* 1985;76: 885–891.

CHAPTER 25

Choreoathetosis

David L. Wessel
Adre J. du Plessis

The perioperative manifestations of neurologic injury in children with congenital heart disease (CHD) may appear as seizures, delayed recovery of consciousness, focal infarcts, or movement disorders such as choreo-athetosis. For the past 30 years, choreoathetosis following congenital heart surgery has remained a puzzling and sometimes devastating postoperative complication. The first such cases, reported in the 1960s, were noted after cardiac surgery with cardiopulmonary bypass (CPB) and profound hypo-thermia.[1-4] Since then, several reports have described the characteristic postoperative course and neurologic findings.[5-12] The incidence of choreo-athetosis has been estimated between 1% and 12%.[13] Although commonly felt to arise in patients undergoing deep hypothermic circulatory arrest (DHCA),[10] the condition has been noted more recently to occur in in-fants and children undergoing CPB and hypothermia without circulatory arrest.[12] Numerous events during CPB or DHCA have been suggested as etiologies, including hyperglycemia,[5] uneven cooling,[14] the no-reflow phe-nomenon,[15-16] dopaminergic neurotransmitter alterations,[9] and cerebral excitatory amino acid neurotoxicity.[10] Choreoathetosis continues to be reported regularly[9,10,12,17] with no universally accepted single etiology. It is especially frustrating since its appearance is frequently delayed after typi-cally faultless surgery with no apparent hemodynamic or metabolic indica-tors of distress.

Clinical Features

In 1990 we reviewed occurrences of choreoathetosis following car-diac surgery at Children's Hospital, Boston.[18] As our complexity of cases

TABLE 25–1
Patient Characteristics

Transient Form (N = 8)

> Resolved frequently before discharge
> Mild symptoms
> Median age: 3.5 months
> 7/8 had DHCA

Persistent Form (N = 11)

> Persisted > 6 m after surgery
> Severe symptoms
> All had DHCA
> All had cyanotic CHD, 9/11 having a form of pulmonary atresia with systemic-pulmonary collaterals

---

increased and management of pH on CPB evolved, we noted the appearance of choreoathetosis among patients beginning in 1986. We reviewed the hospital course and follow-up of all 19 affected children including 8 younger patients (median age 4.3 months) who developed a mild transient form of choreoathetosis, all of whom survived and had complete resolution of choreoathetosis; 7 of these 8 patients had DHCA. Eleven older patients (median age 16.8 months) developed severe persistent choreoathetosis; 11 had DHCA; 10 were cyanotic; 7 had anatomic pulmonary atresia; and 3 others were physiologically analogous with a systemic-to-pulmonary artery shunt-dependent circulation (Table 25–1). Table 25–2 shows the clinical course of the 11 persistent patients. The severe choreoathetosis made daily management extremely difficult in these patients. A variety of treatment medications were tried in an effort to control the movements. Overall, patients responded poorly to conventional therapy to achieve mild sedation. Recurrent aspiration and respiratory failure were common problems.

TABLE 25–2
Persistent Patients' Clinical Course

> Difficult management
> Refractory to therapy
> Aspiration and respiratory failure common
> CT scans and EEGs not helpful
> 4/11 died prior to discharge
> 4/11 still have choreoathetosis
> 3/11 have no movement disorder (1 normal)

Diagnostic Testing

The electroencephalogram and CT scan were largely unhelpful. The electroencephalogram generally showed diffuse slowing. The CT scans in these patients, who have been in the intensive care unit and quite ill for several days, typically reveal some generalized atrophy. Despite the clinical and pathological indicators implicating basal ganglia injury in children with hyperkinetic movement disorders, we were unable to identify lesions in these structures using cranial CT or MRI. Therefore, we later evaluated regional cerebral perfusion measured by Tc-99m hexamethyl propylene amine oxime single photon emission computed tomography (HMPAO SPECT) as a technique to localize *functional* cerebral abnormalities in 11 children diagnosed with choreoathetosis following cardiac surgery.[19] Of these 11 patients, deep grey matter (basal ganglia) perfusion defects were noted in six patients. Surprisingly, cortical perfusion defects were present in nine patients. For both cortical and subcortical defects, a strong right-sided predilection was present. These findings suggest that functional brain injury may be present but not detectable by conventional cranial CT and MRI in these patients. We speculated that these perfusion defects might relate to the behavioral and developmental sequelae in survivors of this syndrome. SPECT may identify subclinical injury in patients at risk for future neurodevelopmental problems and contribute to our understanding of the mechanisms of cerebral injury in the cardiac patient.

Comparison Patients

We then selected all age- and diagnosis-matched patients from the same time period who were free from neurologic symptoms to use as a comparison group. There were 17 such patients, and we compared their intraoperative profiles to the severely affected, persistent group as shown in Table 25–3.

TABLE 25–3
Intraoperative Profiles: Persistent vs. Comparison

	Persistent	*Comparison*	*p-Value*
CPB elapsed time (minutes)	124	126	NS
DHCA (minutes)	51	41	NS
pH	7.41	7.43	NS
pCO$_2$ (mmHg)	40	37	NS
Hematocrit pre/intraop	43/22	44/22	NS
Rate of cooling (degrees/minute)	11.3	11.8	NS
Time to shut off (minutes)	23	40	.053

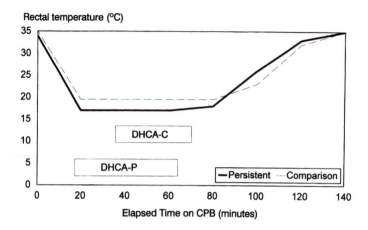

FIGURE 25–1.   Rectal temperature vs. elapsed time on cardiopulmonary bypass (CPB) for patients with (persistent) and without (comparison) development of choreoathetosis. Although
patients with persistent choreoathetosis were cooled to temperatures below 20°C at the same rate as comparison patients
who were matched for age, time of surgery, diagnosis and absence of choreoathetosis, the commencement of circulatory
arrest in the comparison patients (DHCA-C) was delayed while
the first stage of the operation was performed. This additional
time on CPB while the patients were hypothermic may have
allowed more thorough and even cerebral cooling. This may
have conferred some additional protective benefit to these
high-risk patients.

Notice that the two groups cannot be distinguished on the basis of their
time on cardiopulmonary bypass or their deep hypothermic circulatory arrest times. We used an alkaline or alpha-stat strategy for these patients on
CPB, with no significant differences noted in pH or pCO_2 or in preoperative
or intraoperative hematocrits. Although the rate of cooling during the first
10 minutes was no different between groups, the actual time from onset of
cardiopulmonary bypass to onset of deep hypothermic circulatory arrest,
which is the time to shutoff, tended to be shorter in the persistent patients.
This is shown graphically in Figure 25–1, which displays temperature versus
time of the two groups during CPB. Notice that after similar rates of cooling,
comparison patients continued on CPB for another 20 minutes prior to circulatory arrest, shown in the interrupted line.

Collateral Vessels

After reviewing the angiography on all patients, we were impressed with
how often there were significant systemic-pulmonary collateral vessels aris-

TABLE 25-4
Angiography: Systemic-Pulmonary Collaterals

SPCs from Head and Neck	Yes	No	NA	% Yes
Persistent (N = 11)	5	1	5	83%
Comparison (N = 17)	5	7	5	42%
Transient (N = 8)	1	4	3	20%

ing from the head and neck arteries that frequently had stenoses at their origin. Among the persistent patients, six had adequate cine angiography to view the head and neck arteries, and five of these were found to have significant pulmonary blood flow derived from head and neck vessels. The percentage of patients with suitable angiograms who had a head or neck artery supplying the pulmonary arteries was highest in the persistent patients, suggesting the potential for stealing from the cerebral circulation into the pulmonary arteries on CPB (Table 25-4).

pH Strategy

We had no record of a case of choreoathetosis during the first half of the 1980s. It was also noted that we had evolved from a pH-stat strategy in 1984 to a more alkalotic alpha-stat strategy for management of pH and pCO_2 on cardiopulmonary bypass[20] at the beginning of 1985. To confirm this, we examined all of the hospital records from patients between 6 months and 5 years of age who had undergone cardiopulmonary bypass and deep hypothermic circulatory arrest for congenital heart lesions involving pulmonary atresia between January 1, 1980 and June of 1984. According to our analysis these would be patients at high risk for choreoathetosis. There were 24 of these patients whose records were available. The earlier pH strategy was characterized by lower pH and higher pCO_2 compared to that of persistent patients. These are values that are not corrected for the patients' temperatures but are measured at standard temperature of 37°C. There were *no cases* of choreoathetosis among these patients (Table 25-5).

TABLE 25-5
pH Strategy (1980 to 1985)

All patients 6 months to 5 years with pulmonary atresia and DHCA (N=24)
pH: 7.21 vs. 7.41 (after 1985) p<.01
pCO_2:   72 vs. 41 mmHg p<.01
No cases of choreoathetosis 1980 to 1985 compared to observations after 1985

Age Effects

The concept of two different degrees of choreoathetosis, mild and severe, has been alluded to by several authors.[5,9,10,18] However, the potential effect of age has not been previously addressed. We found that seven of eight patients with mild, transient, usually distal choreoathetosis were less than 8 months of age, and all patients with severe, persistent choreoathetosis were older than 6 months of age. These data suggest that choreoathetosis may be an age-related phenomenon, with the most vulnerable period starting at 6 to 9 months and ending after 5 to 6 years. Younger patients, when affected, appear to have a milder form of choreoathetosis, and generally have a better overall prognosis for recovery from the movement disorder, although complete data on other aspects of neurodevelopment are not available. Alternatively this group of younger patients who are mildly affected may represent a different phenomenon related to a response to drugs or critical care treatments, expressed as transient movement disorders.[21] Emergence from prolonged anesthesia in the intensive care unit is commonly associated with self-limited abnormal motor activity.

In contrast, the development of severe choreoathetosis in older children, as described in this series, carries a significantly worse prognosis. The mortality rate in our persistent patients was 36%, compared to an overall surgical mortality rate less than 5% at our institution. Of the seven surviving patients, only one has returned to normal after a follow-up period of five years. The other six survivors have varying degrees of developmental delay, and four patients continue to have choreiform movements.

It remains unclear why the child with cyanotic heart disease who has progressed beyond early infancy appears to be more at risk to develop choreoathetosis. One possibility is increased susceptibility of the basal ganglia to injury after chronic hypoxia. Chaves and Scaltsas-Persson[11] proposed that an acute insult during CPB/DHCA superimposed on chronic hypoxemia results in injury to vulnerable areas of the basal ganglia. Alternatively, time may be required to develop systemic-pulmonary collaterals and a cerebral steal capacity that is not as significant at an earlier age. Neuronal maturational differences might predispose the basal ganglia to increasing susceptibility at this age. Age-specific differences in regional cerebral metabolic rates for glucose have recently been demonstrated by positron emission tomography.[22] It is still unknown why the basal ganglia are so susceptible to injury in this setting, and the exact mechanism of injury is also uncertain although an anoxic ischemic injury is most likely. Wical and Tomasi[10] have suggested that glutamate or other excitatory amino acid neurotoxicity may lead to cellular dysfunction. The potential role of excitatory amino acids in the pathogenesis of anoxic-ischemic brain injury is currently the topic of active investigation,[23,24] and the observation of a transient excessive glutamatergic innervation of the globus pallidus in the human infant is of particular interest in this regard.[25]

Summary of Findings

The severely affected persistent patients in our study were remarkably consistent in the following respects: (1) all patients underwent DHCA; (2) all but one patient had cyanotic congenital heart disease; and (3) preoperatively, all had some type of direct systemic-to-pulmonary artery blood flow, with most patients having collateral vessels arising from the head and neck arteries. When compared to an age-matched group of patients with pulmonary atresia who concurrently underwent DHCA but postoperatively were neurologically normal, there were no differences in CPB time, DHCA time, preoperative or operative hematocrit, or arterial blood gases. Although the rate of cooling during the first 10 minutes was not different between groups, the actual time from onset of CPB to onset of DHCA (time to shutoff) tended to be shorter in the persistent patients. This circumstance arose because either the anatomy or the design of the surgical approach for comparison patients permitted the initial part of the operation to be conducted on CPB. The comparison patients may have benefited from the period of cold (18° to 20°C) while still on CPB before DHCA was commenced. Some studies have suggested that very rapid cooling may fail to provide complete cerebral protection.[4,14] In the persistent patients, this rapid or uneven cerebral cooling, combined with the steal from a systemic-to-pulmonary artery communication, might have predisposed certain areas of the brain to regional ischemia, perhaps during a critical stage of cerebral maturation.

Other Considerations

Pre-1985 patients were maintained at a significantly less alkalotic pH with less hypocarbia than either the persistent or comparison patients, and none of them developed choreoathetosis following DHCA. Our more aggressive attempts to recruit diminutive pulmonary arteries with combined interventional catheterization and surgical approaches in recent years make nonconcurrent comparisons of these patients difficult. Changes in surgical technique and patient complexity offer confounding variables which make it difficult to draw any firm conclusions. Nonetheless, these data and other work[26,27] suggest the possibility that the hypocarbia and alkaline pH, introduced by the more recent extreme alpha-stat strategy, might further diminish cerebral blood flow in a cerebral circuit already compromised by the presence of a systemic-pulmonary shunt. Others[28] reported that an alpha-stat strategy reduces cerebral blood flow, presumably secondary to reduced pCO_2. These observations were made on adult CPB patients with lesser degrees of hypothermia than our patients. It is possible that young children are more vulnerable to the cerebral blood flow effects of low pCO_2. This may be linked to later neurodevelopmental findings.[27]

The neuropathology obtained on two of our patients is unusual.[29] Most reports of basal ganglia pathology following ischemia describe tissue necrosis, often in the globus pallidus, but sometimes in other regions of the basal ganglia.[30-32] Focal areas of myelin loss can also be seen. Our patients showed pallidal neuronal depletion and gliosis but not tissue necrosis. The incomplete destruction of tissue elements suggests that anoxic-ischemic injury is mitigated or altered by hypothermia. Only a few reports have described the neuropathologic changes seen in this condition. In four patients who developed choreoathetosis following cardiac surgery with DHCA, Bjork and Hultquist[1] noted extensive ganglion cell loss in the globus pallidus, along with marked gliosis. Less extensive changes were also seen in the parietal cortex and hippocampus.[3] Chaves and Scaltsas-Persson[11] reported hypoxic neuronal degeneration and capillary proliferation in one patient. Robinson et al.[9] found no abnormal neuropathology in one patient who died after movements had subsided.

DeLeon and associates[12] recently reported choreoathetosis among patients following CPB without DHCA and suggested that prolongation of cooling times >1 hour and temperatures <25°C at high flow rates were risk factors. These observations differ from our experience and undoubtedly reflect the multifactorial nature of risk factors and institutional variation.

After studying these initial 19 patients and while analyzing and reporting the data, we continued to see patients develop choreoathetosis. The total number of cases in this institution reached 37 (0.5% of surgical cases). Many of the more recent cases were milder forms of choreoathetosis that we may not have identified in the past, which we are more sensitive to now. In response to these observations, we changed several aspects of our technique, and after regularly seeing six to seven cases per year, we have had no patients with even mild choreoathetosis in more than two years.

Although the limitations of this kind of study caution against premature conclusions, we feel that the data support earlier reparative surgery when children seem less vulnerable to this neurologic complication. We advocate precise preoperative diagnosis and pre- or intraoperative control of collaterals prior to circulatory arrest. We emphasize the importance of further study of pH effects during cardiopulmonary bypass on the development of choreoathetosis, and we encourage clinical trials that examine a less alkaline pH and pCO_2 strategy during cooling on cardiopulmonary bypass.

In our view, the weight of evidence indicates that the lesion causing choreoathetosis is anoxic-ischemic in origin but that no single factor in the management of CPB and DHCA can be held responsible. Multiple factors may play a role, and one or more of these may assume primary importance in a particular patient.

References

1. Bjork VO, Hultquist G. Brain damage in children after deep hypothermia for open-heart surgery. *Thorax* 1960;15:284–291.

2. Bergouignan M, Fontan F, Trarieux M, Julien J. Syndromes choreiformes de l'enfant au d'cours d'interventions cardio-chirurgicales sous hypothermie profonde. *Rev Neurol* 1961;105:48–60.
3. Bjork VO, Hultquist G. Contraindications to profound hypothermia in open-heart surgery. *J Thorac Cardiovasc Surg* 1962;44:1–13.
4. Drew CE. Profound hypothermia in cardiac surgery. *Br Med J* 1961;17:37–42.
5. Brunberg JA, Doty DB, Reilly EL. Choreoathetosis in infants following cardiac surgery with deep hypothermia and circulatory arrest. *J Pediatr* 1974;84:232–235.
6. Brunberg JA, Reilly D, Doty DB. Central nervous system consequences in infants of cardiac surgery using deep hypothermia and circulatory arrest. *Circulation* 1974;49(Suppl II):60–68.
7. Castaneda AR, Lamberti J, Sade RM, Williams RG, Nadas AS. Open-heart surgery during the first three months of life. *J Thorac Cardiovasc Surg* 1974; 68:719–729.
8. Clarkson PM, MacArthur BA, Barratt-Boyes BG, Whitlock RM, Neutze JM. Developmental progress after cardiac surgery in infancy using hypothermia and circulatory arrest. *Circulation* 1980;62:855–861.
9. Robinson RO, Samuels M, Pohl KRE. Choreic syndrome after cardiac surgery. *Arch Dis Child* 1988;63:1466–1469.
10. Wical BS, Tomasi LG. A distinctive neurologic syndrome after induced profound hypothermia. *Pediatr Neurol* 1990;6:202–205.
11. Chaves E, Scaltsas-Persson I. Severe choreoathetosis (CA) following congenital heart disease (CHD) surgery. *Neurology* 1988;38:284. [Abstract]
12. DeLeon S, Ilbawi M, Arcilla R, Cutilletta A, Egel R, Wong A, Quinones J, Husayni T, Obeid M, Sulayman R, Idriss F. Choreoathetosis after deep hypothermia without circulatory arrest. *Ann Thorac Surg* 1990;50:714–719.
13. Kirklin JW, Barratt-Boyes, BG. Hypothermia, circulatory arrest, and cardiopulmonary bypass. In Kirklin JW, Barratt-Boyes BG (eds.), *Cardiac surgery*. New York: Wiley, 1986, pp. 29–82.
14. Almond CH, Jones JC, Snyder HM, Grant SM, Meyer BW. Cooling gradients and brain damage with deep hypothermia. *J Thorac Cardiovasc Surg* 1964; 48:890–897.
15. Ames A III, Wright RL, Kowada M, Thurston AB, Majno G. Cerebral ischemia: the no reflow phenomenon. *Am J Pathol* 1968;52:437–447.
16. Norwood WI, Norwood CR, Castaneda AR. Cerebral anoxia: Effect of deep hypothermia and pH. *Surgery* 1979;86:203–209.
17. Ferry PC. Neurologic sequelae of open-heart surgery in children: An irritating question. *Am J Dis Child* 1990;144:369–378.
18. Wong PC, Barlow CF, Hickey PR, Jonas RA, Castaneda AR, Farrell DM, Lock JE, Wessel DL. Factors associated with choreoathetosis after cardiopulmonary bypass in children with congenital heart disease. *Circulation* 1982;86[suppl II]: 118–126].
19. du Plessis AJ, Treves ST, Hickey PR, O'Tauma L, Barlow CF, Costello J, Castaneda AR, Wessel DL. Abnormalities in regional cerebral blood flow following deep hypothermic cardiac surgery: Tc-99m HMPAO spect in children developing postoperative movement disorders. *J Thoracic Cardiovasc Surg* 1994; 107:1036–1043.
20. Hickey PR, Hansen DD. Temperature and blood gases: The clinical dilemma of acid-base management for hypothermic cardiopulmonary bypass. In Tinker JH

(ed.), *Cardiopulmonary bypass: Current concepts and controversies.* Philadelphia: Saunders & Co., 1989, pp. 1–20.

21. Lane JC, Tennison MB, Lawless SI, Greenwood RS, Zaritsky AL. Movement disorder after withdrawal of fentanyl infusion. *J Pediatrics* 1991;119:649–651.

22. Chugani HT, Phelps ME, Mazziotta JC. Positron emission tomography study of human brain functional development. *Ann Neurol* 1987;22:487–497.

23. Rothman SM, Olney JW. Glutamate and the pathophysiology of hypoxic ischemic brain damage. *Ann Neurol* 1983;19:105–110.

24. Kochhar A, Zivin JA, Lyden PD. Glutamate antagonist therapy reduces neurologic deficits produced by focal central nervous system ischemia. *Arch Neurol* 1988;45:148–153.

25. Greenamyre T, Penney JB, Young AB, Hudson L, Silverstein FS, Johnston MV. Evidence for transient perinatal glutamatergic innervation of globus pallidus. *J Neurosci* 1987;7:1022–1030.

26. Bellinger DC, Wernovsky G, Rappaport LA, Mayer JE, Castaneda AR, Farrell DM, Wessel DL, Lang P, Hickey PR, Jonas RA, Newburger JW. Cognitive development of children following early repair of transposition of the great arteries using deep hypothermic circulatory arrest. *Pediatrics* 1991;87:701–707.

27. Jonas RA, Bellinger DC, Rappaport LA, Wernovsky G, Hickey PR, Farrell DM, Newburger JW. Relation of pH strategy and developmental outcome after hypothermic circulatory arrest. *J Thorac Cardiovasc Surg* 1993;106:362–368.

28. Murkin JM, Farrar JK, Tweed WA, McKenzie FN, Guiraudon G. Cerebral autoregulation and flow/metabolism coupling during cardiopulmonary bypass: The influence of pCO_2. *Anesth Analg* 1987;66:825–832.

29. Kupsky WJ, Drozd MA, Barlow CF. Selective injury of globus pallidus in children with post-cardiac surgery chorea syndrome. *Dev Med Child Neurol* 1995;37:135–144.

30. Dooling EC, Richardson EP. Delayed encephalopathy after strangling. *Arch Neurol* 1976;33:196–199.

31. Ginsberg MD, Hedley-Whyte T, Richardson EP. Hypoxic-ischemic leukoencephalopathy in man. *Arch Neurol* 1976;33:5–14.

32. Plum F, Posner JB, Hain RF. Delayed neurological deterioration after anoxia. *Arch Int Med* 1962;110:56–63.

PART VI

New Strategies for Cerebral Protection

CHAPTER 26

New Strategies for Brain Protection Including NMDA Receptor Antagonists

Michael V. Johnston

Introduction

Glutamate excitotoxicity has been implicated in the pathogenesis of hypoxic brain injury.[1,2] The Boston Circulatory Arrest Study has also suggested that excessive excitation of the brain, as determined by the occurrence of perioperative seizures, may be an indicator of excitotoxic events occurring in relation to hypothermic circulatory arrest.[3] These studies suggest that blockade of excitotoxic mechanisms might be efficacious for preventing brain injury from cardiac surgery.

Potential Receptor-Based Methods of Brain Protection

Figure 26–1 illustrates the cascade of events that can be triggered by overstimulation of excitatory amino acid receptors during and after hypoxia-ischemia. Glutamate in its NMDA (N-methyl-D-aspartate) conformation, together with glycine, operates a channel that passes calcium in large amounts after the magnesium block is removed. Magnesium itself is an effective neuroprotective agent, albeit a short-term one.[4] A number of other potential strategies may be important, only some of which will be mentioned. For example, the glutamate reuptake system is reduced during conditions of hypoxia-ischemia so, potentially, one could reduce dangerous concentrations of glutamate by enhancing the activity of the energy-dependent and sodium-dependent pumps that remove glutamate into

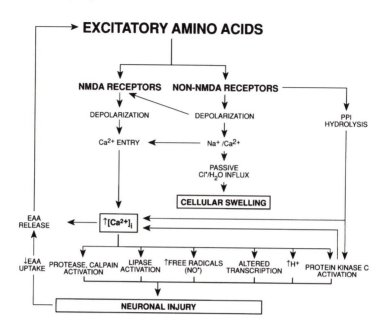

FIGURE 26–1. Overstimulation of excitatory amino acid receptors during hypoxia and ischemia triggers a cascade of events that cause neuronal death. Diminished glutamate uptake is important because it causes an elevation in synaptic concentration of glutamate.

presynaptic terminals and glia.[5] Glutamate receptors other than the NMDA receptor are important in stabilizing the membrane or regulating membrane potential. The so-called AMPA (β-D-aspartylaminomethylphosphoric acid) receptors are also important, and, in fact, antagonists of AMPA receptors have been shown to be effective neuroprotective agents, especially in focal models of stroke.[6] A number of years ago it was shown that hypothermia can reduce glutamate release.[7] Thus, hypothermia may reduce EEG activity and may be protective, in part, by inhibiting the release of glutamate.

NMDA Receptor/Channel Antagonists

The NMDA receptor/channel-blocking drugs are effective agents for shutting down the electrical activity of the brain for a short period of time.[8] The function of the NMDA receptor/channel complex is dependent on the potential of the neuronal membrane as well as receptor occupancy by glutamate and glycine (see Chapter 2). If reduced levels of energy-rich compounds such as ATP lead to a depolarized membrane state, the magnesium block is more easily removed, even though the concentrations of glutamate in the synaptic space are not elevated.[9] This means that a strategy that is simply aimed at blocking the competitive glycine or glutamate receptors may not be as effective as channel blockade during situations such as cardiac surgery, when energy reduction in the cell may allow the channel to open with normal concentrations of glutamate or glycine. At this time, blocking the NMDA channel appears to be the most effective strategy for limiting calcium-mediated neurotoxicity.

The prototypic receptor/channel antagonist is dizocilpine (MK-801), a large molecule that fits inside the channel. Because of the relatively enhanced neurotoxicity mediated by overstimulation of the NMDA receptor in the perinatal period, NMDA antagonists may be particularly effective for salvaging tissue from perinatal hypoxia-ischemia.[2]

Our laboratory has studied the effect of dizocilpine in a perinatal rat model.[2,5] In the model, one carotid artery of a 7-day-old rat is ligated, and the pup is exposed to hypoxia (8% oxygen) for two hours. Over an hour, areas of low flow appear in the periventricular white matter. A 70% reduction in blood flow combined with the hypoxemia leads to a substantial loss of brain tissue in the ipsilateral hemisphere with preservation of the other hemisphere. The fine lamellar organization of the corpus striatum is disrupted in the basal ganglia, and large infarcted areas can often be seen within the smaller hemisphere.[10]

When this rodent model is treated with dizocilpine either before or up to about two hours after the induction of hypoxia-ischemia, infarctions in the basal ganglia and cortex are prevented, and the hemisphere exposed to hypoxia-ischemia is preserved.

Canine Model of Hypothermic Circulatory Arrest and NMDA Receptor Blockade.

Based on the interesting data collected from the rat studies described above, Redmond et al. speculated that the use of an NMDA-receptor antagonist might be effective in a model of hypothermic circulatory arrest.[11] A canine model of hypothermic circulatory arrest had been developed using young male hunting dogs.[12] In these studies, the animals were surface- and core-cooled using closed chest cardiopulmonary bypass to 18°C. The animals then underwent two hours of circulatory arrest after which they were rewarmed on bypass to normal body temperature. After rewarming, the animals were ventilated and monitored for 20 hours. Then they were extubated and neurologically assessed, using a standard scale developed at the University of Pittsburgh.[13] The animals were allowed to survive for 72 hours in an intensive care unit, during which time they underwent regular neurologic assessment. It involved assessment of level of consciousness, ventilation, cranial nerve function, motor and sensory function, and behavior. Using this scale, a high mark indicates a worse outcome, so that 500 is equivalent to brain death while zero represents normality. The animals were then sacrificed for receptor autoradiography studies and brain histopathology.

The neurologic examination scores for animals more than 72 hours after the induction of two hours of hypothermic circulatory arrest showed some improvement over time, but generally the animals had permanently disrupted neurologic function with scores in the range of 300. Two of the animals appeared to have choreoathetosis, or at least what appeared to be a canine equivalent. One dog was bradykinetic and rigid, two signs of Parkinsonism.

The histopathology was performed by a single neuropathologist who was blinded to treatment assignment. Twenty-five brain regions were scored with each region receiving a severity score from 0 to 4. On this scale, similar to the neurologic assessment, a high mark represents severe, multifocal neuropathology; untreated control animals had average scores of 48 ± 9 (± SEM). Generally, the topography of selective necrosis corresponded to the distribution of excitatory amino acid receptors so that it was possible to rationalize the injury based on their distribution. After hypothermic circulatory arrest and 72 hours of recovery, many pyramidal neurons in the hippocampus and Purkinje neurons in the cerebellum were selectively destroyed. Gross infarction was not present, and the area surrounding the pyramidal layer in hippocampus was preserved. The appearance is as though these cells have been selectively scooped out. In the cerebellum, many Purkinje cells appeared to have undergone selective neuronal necrosis.

The hippocampal injury was most prominent in the CA-1 region of the pyramidal layer, which is also vulnerable to other hypoxic-ischemic insults.[14] Receptor autoradiography for excitatory amino acid receptors confirmed that the CA-1 region of the hippocampus in the dog is especially enriched in NMDA-type receptors. There are fewer of the non-NMDA type quisqualate-sensitive receptors and AMPA (β-D-aspartylaminomethylphosphoric acid) receptors. It is the CA-1 region, compared with the regions next to it, that is especially vulnerable to hypoxia-ischemia and is also very enriched in glutamate receptors.

The number of NMDA-type glutamate binding sites was assessed quantitatively using computerized densitometry of glutamate autoradiograms. The number of binding sites in the CA-1 region of the hippocampus was reduced by more than 50% after two hours of hypothermic circulatory arrest.

In the cerebellum, where the Purkinje cells are very vulnerable, autoradiograms suggested that NMDA receptors were especially concentrated on the dendritic candelabra that receives excitatory input onto the Purkinje cells. These Purkinje cells may have been overstimulated by excitatory amino acids, causing the cells to die.

In summary, we showed that two hours of hypothermic circulatory arrest in this canine model produced important functional impairment, with some of the dogs having extra-pyramidal type features. Selective neuronal necrosis was seen in areas of the cortex, basal ganglia, and cerebellum, similar to findings in humans after circulatory arrest.[15-19] Significant reduction in NMDA and AMPA receptor density was found in vulnerable regions. In general, the topography of neuronal injury corresponded to areas of diminished glutamate receptor expression.

We tested the effects of pretreatment with dizocilpine (MK-801), the compound that can block the NMDA channel. In this protocol of MK-801 protection, the details of administration were based on previous experience of our group with this drug.[20,21] A pre-arrest iv bolus of 0.75 mg/kg of dizocilpine was given followed by a continuous infusion until arrest. After arrest, another iv bolus was given. It may also be important to wean this drug over a period of about 24 hours, because in rat experiments it was found that a single dose of MK-801 with rapid withdrawal can actually sensitize the brain to injury.[20] We thought that if the animals were seizing in the period after hypothermic circulatory arrest, the injury might be increased by giving a single bolus alone.

After a single bolus of dizocilpine, the EEG slowed but did not become completely flat, though it is possible to completely flatten the EEG of animals with MK-801. In rats, it is possible to give a dose of dizocilpine that flattens the EEG and yet the animals remain conscious and mobile. The drug has been termed a *dissociative anesthetic* because it is able to disconnect the cortex from the rest of the brain.

The temperature of the dogs undergoing hypothermic circulatory arrest was carefully regulated so that there were no differences between the control and drug study animals (Figure 26–2). This has become an important caveat in experiments such as these because dizocilpine and other glutamate antagonists can themselves lower brain temperature. Because brain temperature was carefully monitored and regulated throughout our study, drug-induced hypothermia is not the explanation for the protective effect.

Results of MK-801 Administration to Dogs
Undergoing Two Hours of Circulatory Arrest

Dizocilpine-treated animals had a neurologic functional score that was considerably better than the untreated hypothermic circulatory arrest-exposed animals (Figure 26–3). On histopathologic scoring, there was quantitative evidence of differences between the two groups in the neocortex, as well as in the hippocampus and basal ganglia (Table 26–1). In the untreated animals, the most severely injured areas were the neocortex and the hippocampus. The basal ganglia in untreated animals also had a fairly high neuropathology injury score, as did the cerebellum. The mean neuropathology score for multifocal neuronal necrosis for saline control animals was 48 versus a score of 7.3 for the study animals treated with dizocilpine.

The powerful protective effect of dizocilpine during hypothermic circulatory arrest can be seen in the cerebellum. In control animals, the Purkinje cell layer is almost totally eliminated so that it is virtually impossible to see

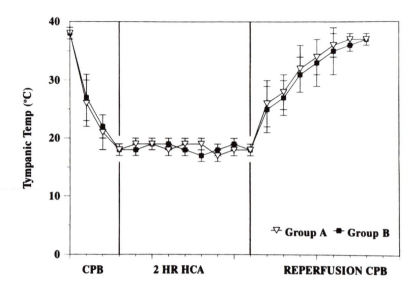

FIGURE 26-2. Tympanic membrane temperatures during cooling, HCA, and rewarming. Group A = Dizocilpine treated; Group B = Saline treated. (Reprinted with permission from Redmond JM, Gillinov AM, Zehr KJ, Blue ME, Troncoso JC, Reitz BA, Cameron DE, Johnston MV, Baumgartner WA. Glutamate excitotoxicity: A mechanism of neurologic injury associated with hypothermic circulatory arrest. *J Thorac Cardiovasc Surg* 1994;107:776–787.)

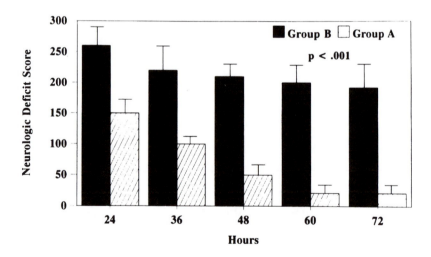

FIGURE 26-3. Neurologic deficit score versus time during neurologic recovery (p <.001 by ANOVA). (Reprinted with permission from Redmond JM, Gillinov AM, Zehr KJ, Blue ME, Troncoso JC, Reitz BA, Cameron DE, Johnston MV, Baumgartner WA. Glutamate excitotoxicity: A mechanism of neurologic injury associated with hypothermic circulatory arrest. *J Thorac Cardiovasc Surg* 1994;107:776–787.)

TABLE 26–1
Histopathologic score after two hours of circulatory arrest in dogs. Animals in group A received dizocilpine. Animals in group B received saline.

	Group A	Group B	p-Value
Neocortex	1.2 ± 1	16 ± 4	<.001
Hippocampus	1	4	<.001
Dentate gyrus	0.3	4	<.001
Entorhinal cortex	0.3	3	<.001
Amygdala	0	2.5 ± 2	<.001
Deep central white matter	0	0	
Basal ganglia	2.4 ± 1	7.7 ± 1	<.001
Brain stem	0	0	
Cerebellum	2.1 ± 1	11.1 ± 1	<.001
Total histopathology score	7.3 ± 3	48.3 ± 9	<.0001

Neocortex includes frontal, parietal, temporal, occipital, insular, and cingulate regions; therefore the most severe cumulative injury score is 24. Basal ganglia includes globus pallidus, putamen, caudate nucleus, and thalamus; the worst score is 16. Brain stem includes midbrain, substantia nigra, periaqueductal gray matter, pons, and medulla; the worst score is 20. Cerebellum includes Purkinje cells and granular and molecular layers; the worst score is 12. Deep central white matter includes the anterior commissure and corpus callosum; the worst score is 12. Total injury score for all 25 brain regions is 100. There were marked differences in scores between groups for each region or related regions, and the total histopathology scores were significantly different (p <.0001).

where it was. In drug-treated animals, these neurons were protected. Autoradiography demonstrated preservation of NMDA receptors in the hippocampus, specifically in the CA-1 region, which were reduced by 50% after hypothermic circulatory arrest. Thus there was a strong correlation between retention of glutamate receptors and histopathologic protection. The loss of AMPA-sensitive receptors, which are usually adjacent but distinct from the NMDA receptors, was also prevented. Interestingly both types of glutamate receptor were protected in the hippocampus.

Summary

Data from our experiments demonstrate that dizocilpine reduces neuropathologic injury following two hours of hypothermic circulatory arrest in the canine model and also promotes functional recovery. Pretreatment and weaning of the drug reduced neuronal injury and preserved both NMDA and non-NMDA glutamate receptor expression in vulnerable regions. The use of NMDA receptor antagonists clearly has promise as a neuroprotective strategy. The fact that dizocilpine and related agents are effective in animal models provides a starting point for the design of clinical protocols. Although dizocilpine may not prove to be the specific drug that is tested clinically, these animal studies provide evidence that excitotoxicity is an important step in the injury that can occur during and after hypothermic circulatory arrest.

References

1. Choi DW, Rothman SW. The role of glutamate neurotoxicity in hypoxic-ischemic neuronal death. *Ann Rev Neurosci* 1990;13:171–178.
2. McDonald JW, Johnston MV. Physiological and pathophysiological roles of excitatory amino acids during central nervous system development. *Brain Res Rev* 1990;15:41–70.
3. Newburger JW, Jonas RA, et al. A comparison of the perioperative neurologic effects of hypothermic circulatory arrest versus low-flow cardiopulmonary bypass in infant heart surgery. *N Eng J Med* 1993;329:1057–1064.
4. McDonald JW, Silverstein FS, Johnston MV. Magnesium reduces NMDA mediated brain injury in perinatal rats. *Neurosci Lett* 1990;109:234–238.
5. Silverstein FS, Buchanan K, Johnston MV. Perinatal hypoxia-ischemia disrupts high affinity [3H]-glutamate uptake into synaptosomes. *J Neurochem* 1986;47: 1614–1619.
6. Li H, Buchan AM. Treatment with an AMPA antagonist 12 hours following severe normothermic forebrain ischemia prevents CA-1 neuronal injury. *J Cereb Blood Flow Metab* 1993;13:933–939.
7. Busto R, Globus MY, Dietrich WD, Martinez E, Valdes I, Ginsberg MD. Effect of mild hypothermia on ischemia-induced release of neurotransmitters and free fatty acids in rat brain. *Stroke* 1989;20:904–910.
8. Meldrum BS. *Excitatory amino acid antagonists.* Oxford, UK: Blackwell Scientific Publication, 1991, pp. 1–350.
9. Novelli A, Reilly JA, Lysko PG, Henneberry RC. Glutamate becomes neurotoxic via the NMDA receptor when intracellular energy stores are reduced. *Brain Res* 1988;451:205–212.
10. Johnston MV. Neurotransmitter alterations in a model of perinatal hypoxia-ischemia brain injury. *Ann of Neurol* 1983;13:511–518.
11. Redmond JM, Gillinov AM, Zehr KJ, Blue ME, Troncoso JC, Reitz BA, Cameron DE, Johnston MV, Baumgartner WA. Glutamate excitotoxicity: A mechanism of neurologic injury associated with hypothermic circulatory arrest. *J Thorac Cardiovasc Surg* 1994;107:776–787.
12. Redmond JM, Gillinov AM, Blue ME, Zehr KJ, Troncoso JC, Cameron DE, Johnston MV, Baumgartner WA. The monosialoganglioside, GMl, reduces neurologic injury associated with hypothermic circulatory arrest. *Surgery* 1993;114: 324–333.
13. Tisherman SA, Safor P, Radovsky A, et al. Profound hypothermia (<10°C) compared with deep hypothermia (15°C) improves neurologic outcome in dogs after two hours circulatory arrest to enable resuscitative surgery. *J Trauma* 1991;31: 1–11.
14. Petito CK, Feldman E, Pulsinelli WA, Plum F. Delayed hippocampal damage in humans following cardiac arrest. In Raichle ME, Powers WJ (eds.), *Cerebrovascular disease.* New York: Raven Press, 1987, pp. 351–355.

15. Tharion J, Johnson DC, Celermajer JM, Hawker RM, Cartmill TB, Overton JH. Profound hypothermia with circulatory arrest. Nine years' clinical experience. *J Thorac Cardiovasc Surg* 1982;84:66–72.

16. Brumberg JA, Doty DB, Reilly EL. Choreoathetosis in infants following cardiac surgery with deep hypothermia and circulatory arrest. *J Pediatr* 1974;84: 232–235.

17. Straussberg R, Shahar E, Gat R, Brand N. Delayed Parkinsonism associated with hypotension in a child undergoing open-heart surgery. *Dev Med Child Neurol* 1993; 35:1011–1014.

18. Huntley DT, Al-Mateen M, Menkes J. Dyskinesia complicating cardio-pulmonary bypass surgery. *Dev Med Child Neurol* 1993;35:631–636.

19. Davis EA, Gillinov AM, Cameron DE, Reitz BA. Hypothermic circulatory arrest as a surgical adjunct: A 5-year experience with 60 adult patients. *Ann Thorac Surg* 1992;53:402–407.

20. McDonald JW, Silverstein FS, Johnston MV. MK-801 pretreatment enhances NMDA mediated brain injury and increases brain NMDA recognition site binding in rats. *Neuroscience* 1990;38:103–113.

21. Williams K, Dichter MA, Molinoff PB. Up-regulation of NMDA receptors on cultured cortical neurons after exposure to antagonists. *Molec Pharmacol* 1992; 42:147–151.

CHAPTER 27

Cerebroplegia and Low Flow

Julie A. Swain

It has become clear over the past several years that circulatory arrest leads to neurological deficits. Wells et al.[1] in 1983 demonstrated that in children the IQ decreased by approximately one point for every three minutes of circulatory arrest with longer arrest times. Other studies have demonstrated neurologic deficits associated with circulatory arrest.[2] Our laboratory embarked on several investigations to try to develop and evaluate methods of cerebral protection during complex cardiac surgery cases. These methods include low-flow cardiopulmonary bypass, cerebroplegia, and intermittent bypass perfusion between periods of circulatory arrest.

Antegrade Cerebroplegia

The increasing use of cardioplegia to protect the heart from ischemia during cardiac surgery led our laboratory to investigate whether cerebroplegia could be useful for the brain. We used phosphorus-31 nuclear magnetic resonance spectroscopy (NMR) to evaluate brain intracellular pH and high-energy phosphates in an adolescent sheep model of circulatory arrest.[3] Animals were placed on cardiopulmonary bypass and cooled to 15°C. Control animals underwent two hours of circulatory arrest and then were reperfused and rewarmed. The cerebroplegia animals had an initial infusion of cold oxygenated crystalloid solution through the carotid arteries and additional boluses every 20 minutes during the arrest period. All animals underwent reperfusion at the end of two hours of circulatory arrest.

Figure 27–1 shows that the control animals had a sudden decrease in ATP that resulted in complete energy depletion by approximately 30 minutes of arrest. The cerebroplegia animals still had measurable amounts of ATP at the end of circulatory arrest, indicating a lessening of ischemia. Reperfusion

% ATP

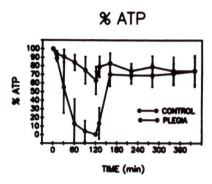

FIGURE 27–1.   Change in adenosine triphosphate (ATP) relative concentration during 2 hours of circulatory arrest at 15°C in the sheep brain and with reperfusion. Control animals had near-total depletion as compared to the preservation in cerebroplegia animals.

resulted in slow resynthesis of high-energy phosphates back to control levels. Intracellular pH was measured in these experiments. The control animals had a marked intracellular acidosis to approximately pH 6.2. Figure 27–2 shows the lessening of intracellular acidosis in the cerebroplegia animals.

In these experiments, the EEG signal in the cerebroplegia animals returned earlier in the reperfusion period. This suggested that there was a functional correlation to the NMR evidence of high-energy phosphate content

pH

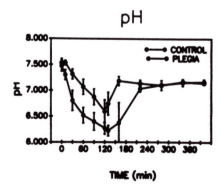

FIGURE 27–2.   The effect of circulatory arrest on the intracellular pH as measured by NMR. Control animals had severe intracellular acidosis; cerebroplegia animals had less acidosis.

and intracellular pH preservation. More quantitative studies correlating functional result with NMR findings were needed.

Correlation of NMR with Functional Studies

This same antegrade cerebroplegia study was then duplicated in a survival situation in the laboratory.[4] Control animals underwent two hours of circulatory arrest followed by reperfusion, another group underwent intermittent perfusion with antegrade cerebroplegia with the oxygenated crystalloid solution, a third group underwent two hours of circulatory arrest with the head packed in ice, and a fourth group underwent retrograde cerebral perfusion intermittently with the cold crystalloid solution. All animals had systemic hypothermia to 15°C. After rewarming and weaning from cardiopulmonary bypass, the animals had sequential neurologic examinations and were observed for seven days.

An ovine coma score was developed and used to assess the neurologic status of the animals. With either antegrade cerebroplegia or simply icing the head combined with systemic hypothermia, all of the animals had enough neurologic function to be extubated and had higher neurologic scores than did the control or retrograde cerebroplegia animals.

Low-Flow and Intermittent Reperfusion

The effect on brain protection of low perfusion flows or intermittent perfusion during systemic hypothermia was examined to determine the minimal hypothermic bypass rate at which cerebral metabolism, as evidenced by NMR, could be preserved.

The experimental protocol consisted of cooling four groups of animals to 15°C. One group of animals underwent two hours of circulatory arrest, another group had two hours of a bypass flow rate of 5 mL/kg/min, and a third group had two hours of flow of 10 mL/kg/min. A fourth group underwent one hour of circulatory arrest, followed by 30 minutes of hypothermic reperfusion, then another hour of circulatory arrest.[5]

Figure 27–3 demonstrates the normal NMR spectrum of the brain during full (100 mL/kg/min) cardiopulmonary bypass and after two hours at 10 mL/kg/min. There was complete preservation of high-energy phosphates with a flow of 10 mL/kg/min. A flow of 5 mL/kg/min resulted in nearly complete depletion of high-energy phosphates after two hours (Figure 27–4). Flows of 10 mL/kg/min resulted in normal intracellular pH, while a flow 5 mL/kg/min resulted in intracellular acidosis nearly as low as that of the circulatory arrest animals. This data is summarized in Figure 27–5.

Intermittent perfusion for 30 minutes between two one-hour periods of circulatory arrest resulted in a moderate amount of resynthesis of high-energy phosphates during reperfusion, and then a rapid decline to nearly complete depletion after two hours of circulatory arrest (Figure 27–6A). The effect on intracellular pH is somewhat different. After 30 minutes of reperfusion, there was only minimal improvement of intracellular pH (Figure 27–6B). Therefore, intracellular acidosis takes far longer to correct than does depletion of high-energy phosphates and brings into question the benefit of shorter periods of reperfusion.

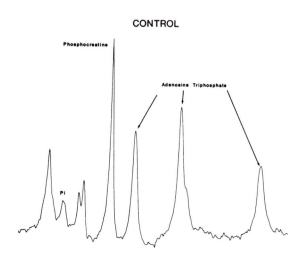

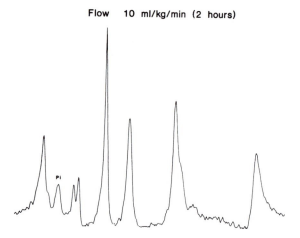

FIGURE 27–3.   Brain phosphorus-31 nuclear magnetic resonance spectra for (*top*) control and (*bottom*) after 2 hours of low-flow cardiopulmonary bypass (10 mL/kg/min). The spectra show no significant changes in metabolite levels. (Reprinted with permission from Swain JA, et al. Low-flow hypothermic cardiopulmonary bypass protects the brain. *J Thorac Cardiovasc Surg* 1991;102:76–84.)

CONTROL

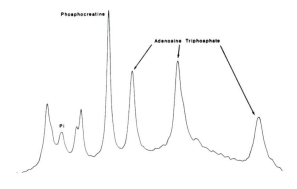

Flow   5 ml/kg/min   (2 hours)

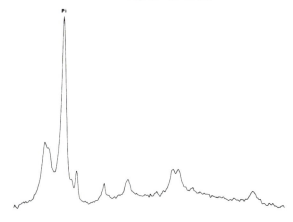

FIGURE 27–4.   Brain phosphorus-31 nuclear magnetic resonance spectra for (*top*) control and (*bottom*) after 2 hours of low-flow cardiopulmonary
bypass (5 mL/kg/min). Note severe depletion of
ATP and PCr. Decrease in signal-to-noise ratio after
2 hours of bypass is due to signal degradation from
coil detuning. (Reprinted with permission from
Swain JA, et al. Low-flow hypothermic cardiopulmonary bypass protects the brain. *J Thorac Cardiovasc Surg* 1991;102:76–84.)

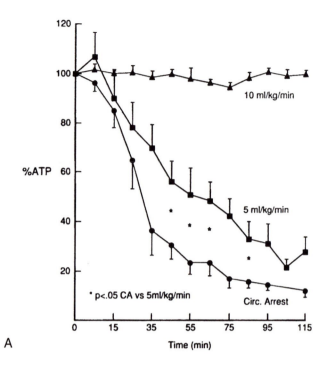

FIGURE 27–5.   High-energy phosphate concentrations (present as percent change from initial concentration) and pH_i changes during 2 hours of either circulatory arrest (CA), cardiopulmonary bypass flow of 10 mL/kg/min, or flow of 5 mL/kg/min. Values are mean ± standard error of the mean. *p <.05, circulatory arrest compared with a flow of 5 mL/kg/min. (A) ATP, (B) PCr, (C) intracellular pH. (Reprinted with permission from Swain JA, et al. Low-flow hypothermic cardiopulmonary bypass protects the brain. *J Thorac Cardiovasc Surg* 1991;102:76–84.)

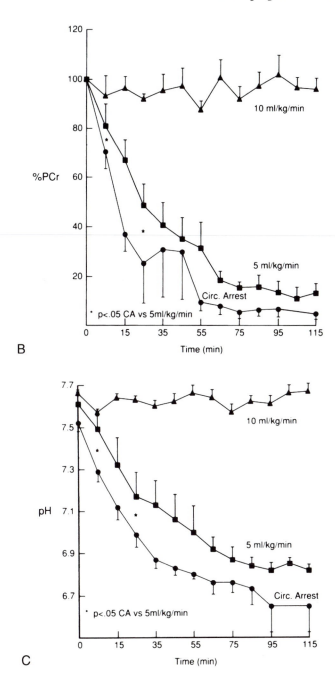

FIGURE 27–5. *(continued)*

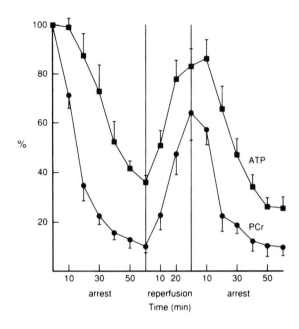

A

FIGURE 27–6. Changes in PCr and ATP (A) and pH (B) during 1 hour of circulatory arrest at 15°C, systemic reperfusion for 30 minutes, followed by a second hour of circulatory arrest. Note that 30 minutes of reperfusion only partially restores PCr and ATP and only incompletely restores pH. (Reprinted with permission from Swain et al. *J Thorac Cardiovasc Surg* 1991;102:76–84.)

Summary

A series of experiments were completed that showed (1) the NMR findings of high-energy phosphate and intracellular pH preservation correlate with neurologic outcome, (2) antegrade cerebroplegia appears to be protective, (3) packing the head in ice during hypothermic circulatory arrest is protective, (4) cardiopulmonary bypass flow as low as 10 mL/kg/min during profound hypothermia maintains normal cerebral metabolism, and (5) intermittent perfusion does not completely restore either high-energy phosphates or intracellular pH.

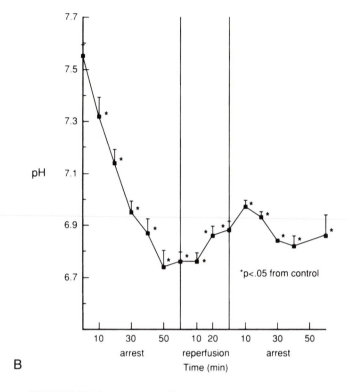

FIGURE 27–6. *(continued)*

References

1. Wells FC, Coghill S, Lincoln C. Psychological development following the use of profound hypothermia and circulatory arrest for the repair of congenital heart defects in infants and young children: A blind controlled study. *J Thor Cardiovasc Surg* 1983;86:823–831.
2. Ferry PC. Neurologic sequelae of open-heart surgery in children: An irritating question. *Am J Dis Child* 1990;144:369–373.
3. Robbins RC, Balaban RS, Swain JA. Asanguinous cerebral perfusion protects the brain during circulatory arrest: A ^{31}P NMR study. *J Thorac and Cardiovasc Surg* 1990;99:878–884.
4. Crittenden MD, Roberts CS, Rosa L, Vatsia SK, Katz D, Clark RE, Swain JA. Brain protection during circulatory arrest. *Ann Thorac Surg* 1991;51:942–947.
5. Swain JA, McDonald TJ, Griffith PK, Balaban RS, Clark RE, Ceckler T. Low-flow hypothermic cardiopulmonary bypass protects the brain. *J Thorac Cardiovasc Surg* 1991;102:76–84.

CHAPTER 28

Pharmacological Modification of a Cerebroplegia Solution

Richard A. Jonas
Mitsuru Aoki

Introduction

Studies such as the Boston Circulatory Arrest Study (see Part V) have demonstrated that deep hypothermic circulatory arrest alone does not provide complete cerebral protection, particularly when the arrest period is extended beyond 30 to 45 minutes. However, this is not adequate time to undertake complex reconstructive procedures for some congenital heart anomalies in children, nor is it adequate for complete replacement of the aortic arch for degenerative disease in adults. For this reason a number of investigators have studied the possibility of adjunctive methods of cerebral protection including the use of cerebral perfusion with cerebroplegia.[1,2] In the previous chapter, Dr. Swain described studies of a cerebroplegia solution which is essentially the same as many cardioplegia solutions. This cold oxygenated crystalloid solution was delivered into the cerebral circulation through the carotid arteries. While control animals demonstrated a complete loss of cerebral ATP, as measured by magnetic resonance spectroscopy after 30 minutes of circulatory arrest (as we have also found in similar studies [see Chapter 20]), the animals that received cerebroplegia had measurable amounts of ATP at the end of the arrest period, showed less intracellular acidosis, and had an earlier return of EEG. In a follow-up survival study, Dr. Swain found that sheep receiving crystalloid cerebroplegia antegrade through the carotid arteries had a greater neurological score than control animals or animals receiving cerebroplegia retrograde through the superior vena cava. Interestingly the animals that had their heads packed in ice during the arrest period did as well as those receiving antegrade cerebroplegia.

Pharmacology of Cerebral Ischemia

In neuroscience circles during the last decade, there has been tremendous interest in the possibility of reducing cerebral ischemic injury by pharmacological means. Much of the incentive for this interest has been driven by the huge population of adults who suffer ischemic strokes every year. In addition there has been an increasing appreciation that the response of the brain to ischemia is extremely complex (see Part III).

Focal Versus Global Cerebral Ischemia

It is important to distinguish focal from global ischemia. In cases of *focal* ischemia the area of central necrosis is surrounded by a penumbra of potentially salvageable tissue with borderline adequate blood flow to maintain cellular viability. Generally there is no reperfusion of the area of central necrosis. *Global* ischemia, in contrast, is often transient and is followed by a period of reperfusion, which introduces numerous potentially deleterious effects such as oxygen free radicals. Even though perfusion is reduced to the entire brain during global ischemia, there is usually non-uniform distribution of cellular injury. This is in part determined by vascular factors; for example, the watershed areas of periventricular white matter and the optic cortex are notoriously vulnerable to ischemia related to their tenuous vascular supply. However, in addition certain cells in the brain are more susceptible than others to ischemia.

Selective Neuronal Vulnerability

One factor that determines a specific neuron's susceptibility to a given ischemic insult is the concentration of specific receptors which are sensitive to neurotransmitters such as glutamate on the surface membrane of the cell. This results from the large increase in extracellular levels of glutamate which are seen after an ischemic insult. Stimulation of NMDA receptors, for example, by glutamate results in calcium influx, which probably further threatens the viability of the cell by promoting intraneuronal synthesis of nitric oxide, which is potentially neurotoxic.[3] This excitotoxic hypothesis of brain injury[4] offers multiple potential sites for pharmacological intervention directed against ischemia including inhibiting glutamate release, using NMDA receptor antagonists, inhibiting nitric oxide synthase, and increasing calcium buffering proteins within cells, for example by transfecting appropriate DNA within neurons. In fact, all of these methods have already been demonstrated in various animal models to reduce cerebral ischemic injury.[5] Other areas of intense interest include the potential application of free radical scavengers, the study of the interaction of glial cells and neurons in responding to ischemia, the role of growth factors and cytokines, the possible role of programmed cell death, as well as the inhibition of gene transduction to reduce the production of protein second messengers that exacerbate brain injury. The significance of seizures following ischemia, as both a marker of injury as well as a possible secondary mechanism of injury, remains unclear. However the results of the Boston Circulatory Arrest Study (see Part V) strongly implicate seizures as either a marker or mechanism of delayed injury, or perhaps both, in young infants undergoing hypothermic circulatory arrest.

Pharmacologically Modified Cerebroplegia

In light of the promising results described by Swain et al., and with a view to applying one or more of the pharmacological methods of cerebral protection described above, we embarked on a study of pharmacologically modified cerebroplegia.

Preliminary Study of Systemic Administration of Glutamate Antagonists

We applied our immature piglet model of deep hypothermic circulatory arrest to study the potential use of agents that had been demonstrated in rodent models to reduce excitotoxic brain injury.[6]

MK-801

MK-801 is a noncompetitive N-methyl-D-aspartate (NMDA) receptor antagonist which blocks calcium influx triggered by excitatory transmitters. Ment et al.[7] administered 10 mg/kg of MK-801 to newborn dogs 15 minutes before an hypoxic insult. Treated animals had improved recovery of cerebral phosphocreatine, determined by magnetic resonance spectroscopy, as well as less accumulation of cerebral lactate and less intracellular acidosis. Haraldseth et al.[8] studied acute recovery of cerebral high-energy phosphates using magnetic spectroscopy in rats subjected to 10 minutes of normothermic global ischemia. They also found improved early recovery with MK-801. Redmond et al.[4] subjected 18 dogs to 2 hours of hypothermic circulatory arrest with core cooling and rewarming. Animals that received MK-801 before arrest, as well as continuous infusion, had significantly better neurological function over the next 3 days and less histological evidence of neuronal injury. Receptor autoradiography revealed preservation of NMDA receptor expression only in animals that received MK-801. Careful control of temperature is necessary in studies using MK-801 because this compound may have a direct central action on temperature control.[9]

NBQX

NBQX is a non-NMDA, or AMPA (a-amino-3-hydroxy-5-methyl-4-isoxazole) receptor antagonist. AMPA receptor activation results in depolarization of the cell membrane and an increase in sodium and potassium flux, and it can produce excitotoxic neuronal injury in the immature brain. In studies using mature rodents, NBQX has been demonstrated to reduce ischemic neuronal injury.[10] However these studies were performed at normothermia and did not include the added insults of cardiopulmonary bypass, anticoagulation, and hemodilution.

MK-801 and NBQX in a Piglet Model of Deep Hypothermic Circulatory Arrest[6]

We evaluated the effects of MK-801 and NBQX on recovery of brain cellular energy state and metabolic rates in 34 4-week-old piglets undergoing cardiopulmonary bypass and hypothermic circulatory arrest at 15°C (nasopharyngeal temperature) for one hour. MK-801 or NBQX was given intravenously before bypass. Equivalent doses were placed in the cardiopulmonary bypass prime and continuous infusions after reperfusion were given. Changes in high-energy phosphate concentrations and pH were analyzed by magnetic resonance spectroscopy in 17 animals until 225 minutes after reperfusion. Cerebral blood flow (determined by radioactive microspheres) as well as cerebral oxygen and glucose consumption were studied in 17 other animals. Cerebral blood flow and oxygen consumption were depressed relative to control by both MK-801 and NBQX at baseline. Recovery of phosphocreatine (p = .01), ATP (p = .03), and intracellular pH (p = .004) was accelerated by MK-801 and was retarded by NBQX over the first 45 minutes of rewarming/reperfusion and the first hour of normothermic reperfusion (Figure 28–1). The final recovery of ATP at 225 minutes of reperfusion was significantly reduced by NBQX versus control and MK-801. Cerebral oxygen consumption recovered to 105% baseline in the animals receiving MK-801 and to 61% baseline in those receiving NBQX. Cerebral blood flow stayed significantly lower in the animals receiving NBQX relative to control animals. Cerebral edema was exacerbated by NBQX although it was reduced by MK-801. Systemic lactate acidemia was decreased by MK-801 and was unaffected by NBQX. Neither drug affected the systemic hypertension observed in control animals following 225 minutes of reperfusion after hypothermic circulatory arrest.

Laboratory Study of Pharmacologically Modified Cerebroplegia

In this study,[11] we used our juvenile piglet model to explore the effects of pharmacologic manipulation of cerebroplegic solutions on recovery of cerebral blood flow and metabolism using University of Wisconsin (UW) solution as a delivery solvent and the excitatory neurotransmitter antagonist, MK-801. We chose to study asanguineous solutions because our previous studies had shown that activation of blood protease cascades[12] and leukocytes[13] play important roles in the pathogenesis of brain injury after

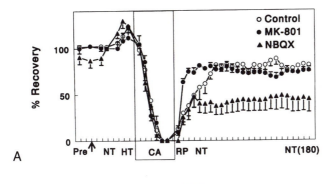

ATP

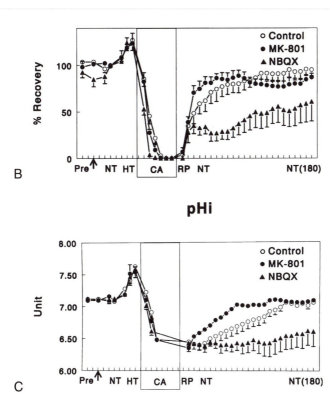

PCr

pHi

FIGURE 28–1. Cerebral high-energy phosphates and intracellular pH determined by NMR spectroscopy in young piglets before, during, and after 1 hour of hypothermic circulatory arrest at 15°C nasopharyngeal temperature. (A) Percent recovery of cerebral ATP (adenosine trisphosphate). Baseline (100%) is following 20 min of normothermic CPB (NT). Pre, before

hypothermic cardiopulmonary bypass and circulatory arrest. Furthermore, partial oxygen or substrate supply during cerebral ischemia can exacerbate accumulation of toxic metabolites.

Experimental preparation

Forty-six Yucatan miniature piglets (mean age 29.5 ± 0.3 [standard error] days, mean weight 3.9 ± 0.3 kg) were studied. The animals were obtained 1 to 2 days before the study and fasted for 12 hours prior to surgery.

In 24 piglets, cerebral blood flow and oxygen and glucose consumption were studied. Animals were anesthetized with intraperitoneal injection of methohexital (40 mg/kg) and were ventilated with 100% O_2 to achieve arterial pCO_2 levels of 35 to 45 mmHg. After a bolus intravenous injection of 20 μg/kg of fentanyl and 0.3 mg/kg of pancuronium, anesthesia was maintained with continuous infusion of fentanyl (25 μg/kg/h) and pancuronium (0.1 mg/kg/h). The animal's temperature was monitored throughout the study by rectal and nasopharyngeal temperature probes (Yellow Springs Instruments, Yellow Springs, OH). Temperatures were maintained above 35°C except for the induced hypothermic period. A 30-gauge needle temperature probe (Model HYP-1, Omega Engineering, Inc., Stamford, CT) with styrofoam for support was inserted 15 mm deep into the right occipital region of the brain through a 1 mm burr hole in the skull for continuous monitoring of brain temperature.

The heart was exposed through a median sternotomy incision. The brachiocephalic trunk, which divides into the right and left common carotid artery beyond the takeoff of the right subclavian artery, was exposed. The right subclavian artery was dissected and a 6 French (Fr) catheter was inserted retrograde into the artery to the point of vertebral artery takeoff for infusion of cerebroplegia solutions and pressure monitoring in the carotid artery system. All branches of the subclavian artery except the vertebral artery were ligated. A snare with a tourniquet was passed around the common carotid trunk for occlusion during circulatory arrest. A 4-mm diameter electromagnetic flow probe (FB-040, Nihon Kohden, Irvine, CA) was placed on the now single common carotid trunk to assess the carotid arterial blood flow by a flowmeter (MFV-3 100, Nihon Kohden). A 5 Fr sampling catheter was inserted through the right internal jugular vein retrograde to the level of the jugular bulb. Position of the catheter tip was determined by measure-

FIGURE 28–1 continued.   initiation of CPB; arrow indicates drug infusion; HT, hypothermic CPB; CA, total circulatory arrest; NT (180), after 180 min of reperfusion at normothermia. (B) Percent recovery of cerebral phosphocreatine (PCr). (C) Recovery of cerebral intracellular pH (pH_i).

ment in all animals as well as dissection at the end of the study in preliminary experiments. The piglet was fully heparinized (300 IU/kg), and a 10 Fr arterial cannula and a 20 to 24 Fr venous cannula were inserted through purse-string sutures in the ascending aorta and into the right atrial appendage, respectively, for institution of CPB. The pump-oxygenator system consisted of a roller pump and a Bio-2 infant bubble oxygenator (Bentley Laboratories Inc, Irvine, CA). The venous drainage was accomplished by gravity. No arterial filter was used. After systemic heparinization, shed blood in the operating field was returned to the system through a 20-micron transfusion filter. An electromagnetic flow probe (FF-060T, Nihon Kohden) was placed on the arterial perfusion tubing to verify the pump flow rate. The pump-oxygenator system was primed with 400 mL of heparinized homologous blood collected 2 days prior to the study and 350 mL of Normosol R pH 7.4 to achieve a hematocrit of 20 to 25%. To mimic our clinical application of hypothermic circulatory arrest, methylprednisolone 30 mg/kg, cephazolin sodium 25 mg/kg, and sodium bicarbonate to achieve a pH of 7.4 were added to the prime. Normosol R pH 7.4 heparinized with 2500 IU/L was used when there was a decrease in reservoir volume during bypass. Temperature of the perfusate was controlled by the heat exchanger within the oxygenator and a water bath system warmed by a thermostat-controlled heater-circulator. During the cooling phase, ice water was circulated.

Perfusion protocol

Bypass flow was set at 150 mL/kg/min calibrated at a perfusate temperature of 37°C. The alpha-stat strategy of acid-base management during hypothermia was accomplished by adjusting the flow of 100% oxygen to the oxygenator. The piglet was initially perfused for 20 minutes at normothermia (37°C arterial temperature) to stabilize body temperature and metabolism. The baseline measurements were made at the end of this period. Then the perfusate was cooled to an arterial temperature of 13°C maintaining a gradient of less than 10°C between blood and nasopharyngeal temperatures. Ice packs were placed around the head throughout the cooling and hypothermic circulatory arrest periods. After 30 minutes of perfusion cooling, when nasopharyngeal temperature was 14.0° to 15.0°C, the second measurements were made. The carotid trunk snare was tightened (complete occlusion was confirmed by a drop of pressure monitored from the right subclavian artery line). The perfusion was stopped for 2 hours. The animal was exsanguinated through the venous drainage line for two minutes, and then arterial and venous lines were clamped. No cardioplegic solution was given. Reperfusion was begun at 150 mL/kg/min with the perfusate at room temperature (20° to 25°C), and then rewarmed to 37°C by circulating warm water (40°C) to the oxygenator. Boluses of phentolamine (0.2 mg/kg) were given at the beginning of both the cooling and rewarming periods as is done in our clinical practice. Sodium bicarbonate (8.4%, 10 mL) was given after five minutes of reperfusion to correct metabolic acidosis. Additional bicarbonate was given when blood pH was less than 7.30, but not immediately before measurements. Measurements were made at five minutes after reperfusion and at 45 minutes, by which time normothermia was achieved. When the animal was normothermic, ventilation was restarted, and the pump-perfusion was continued for three hours with the blood temperature at 37°C to ensure adequate perfusion without inotropic support as well as stable body and brain temperature. During the last three hours of normothermic perfusion, pulsatile assistance from the heart was achieved by raising central venous pressure minimally (<5 mmHg).

Another set of 22 animals, which underwent the same surgical procedure and cardiopulmonary bypass as described above, were studied with ^{31}P magnetic resonance spectroscopy (MRS) using an Oxford horizontal-bore superconducting 4.7 Tesla magnet, as described elsewhere in detail.[14] A 3.0-cm diameter surface coil was sutured on the scalp overlying the cerebral hemispheres. After placement, the surface coil was matched and tuned to the phosphorous frequency. Arterial and venous lines were inserted for blood gas measurement and drug infusion, but no instrumentation for metabolic or blood flow measurements was applied. All ferromagnetic surgical instruments were removed or substituted with plastic equivalents before placing in the magnet.

Data Collection

Blood Flow Measurement.   Cerebral blood flow was measured by radioactive microspheres at 20 minutes after the initiation of CPB; at 30 minutes into cooling; and at 15 minutes, 45 minutes, and 225 minutes after reperfusion. Fifteen-micron diameter microspheres were labeled with one of the following radioactive nuclides: [141]Ce, [113]Sn, [85]Sr, [95]Nb, [46]Sc and were suspended in 0.5 mL of 10% dextran (approximately 2.5×10^6 microspheres). The suspension was injected into a side port on the arterial tubing 50 cm from the tip of the cannula to ensure complete mixing. A measured quantity of blood (approximately 7 mL) as reference was withdrawn at a constant rate by a syringe pump (Dye dilution pump model 2603, Harvard Apparatus, South Natick, MA) from the thoracic aorta catheter throughout the duration of, and until 30 seconds after completion of, the microsphere injection. At the end of the experiment, the brain was removed and weighed for measurement of water content. It was divided into the right and the left cerebral hemispheres, basal ganglia, midbrain, cerebellum, and lower brainstem (pons and medulla oblongata). After desiccation and measurement of dry weight, the brain parts were dissolved in 2N KOH-methanol solution, and the radioactivity was counted (Compugamma 1282, LKB Int., Wallac, Finland) with a spillover correction between the nuclides. The regional blood flow was calculated from the rate of withdrawal of the reference blood and the ratio of the radioactivity of the brain parts to the reference blood.

Metabolic Measurements. Blood gas tensions, and pH, hemoglobin, plasma glucose, and lactate concentrations were measured in arterial and jugular venous blood before cardiopulmonary bypass and after each microsphere injection. Blood gas and hemoglobin were measured with a blood-gas analyzer. Plasma glucose and lactate levels were determined by the glucose oxidase method and the enzymatic fluorometric micromethod, respectively. Cerebral oxygen and glucose consumption were calculated from the difference between the arterial and internal jugular venous oxygen contents and glucose concentrations and total cerebral blood flow. The oxygen content was calculated by the following formula:

$$O_2 \text{ content} = 1.34 \times \text{hemoglobin(g/dL)} \times O_2 \text{ saturation} + 0.003 \times pO_2$$

Lactate concentrations in the return effluent of cerebroplegia solutions also were analyzed.

Magnetic Resonance Spectroscopy. ^{31}P magnetic resonance spectra were acquired in the Fourier transform mode on a custom-built spectrometer using the Oxford horizontal-bore 4.7 Tesla magnet and surface coil. The field homogeneity was optimized with the brain water signal. Spectra were acquired using a 90-degree excitation pulse of 60 microseconds. Each spectrum was the average of 128 acquisitions (nine minutes). Peak areas of inorganic phosphate (Pi), creatine phosphate (PCr), and beta nucleoside triphosphate were determined by Lorentzian curve fitting and peak integration (NMRI Software, New Methods Research, East Syracuse, NY). Changes in ATP concentration were assessed from the beta nucleoside triphosphate peak area. The inorganic phosphate, creatine phosphate, and ATP data are reported as percentage of the baseline data obtained during the last nine minutes of the initial full-flow normothermic bypass period. The intracellular pH in the brain (pH_i) was calculated from the chemical shift of the inorganic phosphate peak relative to the creatine phosphate peak.

Vascular Reactivity to Vasodilators. To assess preservation of endothelial function, vascular reactivity to the endothelium-dependent vasodilator, acetylcholine, and the endothelium-independent vasodilator, nitroglycerin, was evaluated in the carotid circulation by calculating vascular resistance change during drug infusion. The concentration of acetylcholine solution was calculated to give a concentration of 10^{-7} M/L in the arterial blood at a certain infusion rate assuming that the solution mixed thoroughly with the perfusate in the arterial tubing during infusion. The concentration of nitroglycerin solution was calculated to give an arterial concentration of 10^{-5} M/L. These concentrations were selected after preliminary experiments determined a dose-response relationship for cerebral vascular resistance. A near linear dose-response relationship was observed in the range of concentrations used. The solutions were infused into the side port on the arterial tubing used for microsphere injection for a period of 60 seconds by an infusion pump (Model 975, Harvard Apparatus, South Natick, MA). Vascular resistance response was defined as percent change in vascular resistance, calculated from baseline and maximum change in blood pressure, and carotid blood flow, measured by the electromagnetic flowmeter during the infusion, assuming a venous pressure of zero. The evaluation was made at 10 minutes after initiation of cardiopulmonary bypass (pre-hypothermic circulatory arrest baseline), and at 60 and 230 minutes after reperfusion.

Brain water content.   The whole brain was weighed immediately after the experiment (wet weight) and after desiccation for 72 hours at 60°C (dry weight). The brain water content was calculated as (wet weight − dry weight)/ (wet weight).

Experimental Groups

Twelve piglets (n = 7 for blood flow and metabolic study; n = 5 for MRS study) had 50 mL/kg of saline infused in the carotid artery system through the catheter in the subclavian artery at the initiation of hypothermic circulatory arrest. Doses of 10 mL/kg were repeated every 30 minutes during the hypothermic circulatory arrest (Group CPS). Eleven (n = 5 for blood flow and metabolic study; n = 6 for MRS study) received the same volumes of UW solution (Viaspan, Dupont Pharmaecuticals, Wilmington, DE) (Group CPU). Ten piglets (n = 5 for blood flow and metabolic study; n = 5 for MRS study) received the UW solution with 7.5 mg/L of MK-801 (Biochemical Research Laboratories, Natick, MA) (Group CPM). The dose of MK-801 was determined from calculated blood concentration in our previous study (see above) which explored systemic administration of MK-801 in a similar piglet model of hypothermic circulatory arrest. All solutions were infused at 4°C. Glutathione (3 mM/L reduced form, Sigma Chemical, St. Louis, MO) was added to the UW solution immediately prior to usage. The pH of the solutions was 6.30 ± 0.01(saline), 7.10 ± 0.02(UW), 7.00 ± 0.02(UW ± MK801). pO$_2$ of the solutions ranged from 200 to 290 mmHg as measured at 37°C. The return effluent of the infused solution was drained and collected from a side arm from the venous cannula. Thirteen piglets (n = 7 for blood flow and metabolic study; n = 6 for MRS study) received no solution and served as controls.

Statistics

All values are reported as mean ± standard error of the mean (SEM). Analyses were conducted with a statistical analysis system (SPSS, SPSS Inc., Chicago, IL). Data were analyzed with two-way repeated measures analysis of variance(ANOVA). The paired t-test was used to detect differences within a group, and one-way ANOVA and Student-Newman Keuls test were used to detect differences between groups.

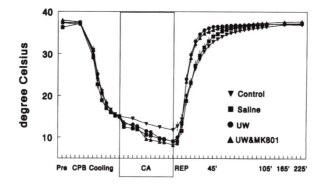

FIGURE 28–2. Brain temperature of young piglets before, during, and after 2 hours of hypothermic circulatory arrest. All animals had ice packed around the head. Cerebroplegia solution consisting of either saline, UW solution, or UW solution with MK-801 (UW & MK801) was infused every 30 minutes throughout the circulatory arrest period.

Results

Experimental Conditions.   Arterial pO_2 levels were above 200 mmHg and arterial pCO_2 levels were controlled within a range of 25 to 55 (40.1 ± 0.3) mmHg in all animals throughout the experiments. All groups had a metabolic acidosis (pH = 7.27 ± 0.01) five minutes after beginning reperfusion (before bicarbonate injection), but pH was 7.34 ± 0.01 at 15 minutes reperfusion and 7.35 ± 0.01 at 45 minutes reperfusion. There were no significant differences (ANOVA p > .13) among the four groups in arterial pH, pO_2 and pCO_2, and rectal temperatures at all measurements. Nasopharyngeal temperature during hypothermic circulatory arrest was significantly lower in the cerebroplegia-treated groups compared with the control group (CNT: 20.8 ± 0.8°C; CPS: 17.2 ± 0.7°C; CPU: 17.7 ± 0.5°C; CPM: 16.6 ± 0.5°C, at the end of hypothermic circulatory arrest). Brain temperature at the onset of hypothermic circulatory arrest was 15.0 ± 0.11°C and dropped to 13.0 ± 0.29°C after cerebroplegia infusion and stayed lower than control throughout hypothermic circulatory arrest (Figure 28–2). The nasopharyngeal and brain temperatures warmed faster in the CPU group during reperfusion relative to the other groups. Brain temperature returned to normothermic baseline levels within two hours of reperfusion in all groups.

Cerebral High-Energy Phosphates and Intracellular pH.   In all animals, except for one in the group CPM, the phosphocreatine and nucleoside triphosphate concentrations became unmeasurable within 90 minutes of the onset of hypothermic circulatory arrest (Figure 28–3A,B). The intracellular brain

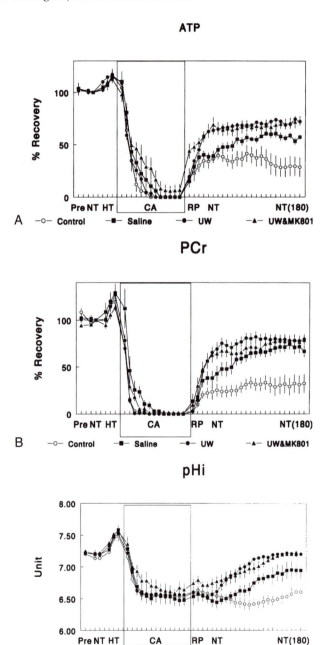

FIGURE 28–3. Cerebral high-energy phosphates and intracellular pH determined by magnetic resonance spectroscopy before, during, and after 2 hours of hypothermic circulatory arrest either with or without

pH became acidotic during circulatory arrest with a tendency for group CPM to have slower decline than other groups (Figure 28–3C). Recovery of ATP (p = .004) and PCr (p = .002) was significantly greater during the first 45 minutes of reperfusion in the groups CPU and CPM relative to the control, but not relative to group CPS. The final recovery of ATP (p < .001), and PCr (p < .001) was significantly better in all the cerebroplegia-treated groups relative to the control group, and the recovery of ATP was further improved by UW solution and UW solution with MK-801 relative to saline (ATP: 28.5 ± 9.3% and PCr:32.4 ± 9.9%, respectively, in group CNT; ATP:53.7 ± 2.6% and PCr:66.7 ± 6.1%, respectively, in group CPS; ATP:72.2 ± 3.0% and PCr:79.8 ± 11.4%, respectively, in group CPU; ATP:72.9 ± 4.6% and PCr:78.9 ± 5.3%, respectively, in group CPM). Intracellular brain pH showed slower recovery than the high-energy phosphates. There was a period of further progression of the intracellular acidosis during early reperfusion, which tended to be longer in groups CNT and CPS. The final recovery of intracellular brain pH was significantly better (p < .001) in all the cerebroplegia groups compared with the control group (6.57 ± 0.11 in group CNT, 6.90 ± 0.14 in group CPS, 7.14±0.02 in group CPU, 7.15 ± 0.01 in group CPM). It returned to the baseline levels within the observation period only in groups CPU and CPM, with the control animals showing a final intracellular brain pH that was profoundly acidotic.

Cerebral Blood Flow. The mean values for all groups for cerebral blood flow was 55.5 ± 1.6 mL/min/100g tissue at the normothermic cardiopulmonary bypass baseline. There were no intergroup differences. Recovery of cerebral blood flow was significantly greater in group CPU relative to the control and saline-treated groups and was also greater than group CPM (Figure 28–4). UW solution significantly improved the recovery of regional blood flow to the cerebral hemispheres, basal ganglia, midbrain, and cerebellum but not to the lower brainstem.

Vascular Response to Vasodilators. There were no significant intergroup differences in cerebral vascular resistance response at the normothermic cardiopulmonary baseline. Groups CPS and CPU showed greater vascular resistance response to acetylcholine (p = .008) and nitroglycerin (p = .048) at 60 minutes of reperfusion relative to groups CNT and CPM. The same

---

FIGURE 28–3 continued. cerebroplegia infusion. (A) ATP (B) Phosphocreatine (C) Intracellular pH. Pre, before initiation of cardio-pulmonary bypass; NT, normothermic cardiopulmonary bypass; HT, hypothermic cardiopulmonary bypass; CA, total circulatory arrest; RP, reperfusion and rewarming; NT(180), after 180 minutes of reperfusion at normothermia.

trend was seen at 230 minutes of reperfusion but did not attain statistical significance (p = .069 for acetylcholine and p = .133 for nitroglycerin).

Cerebral Oxygen and Glucose Consumption.   The mean values for all groups for cerebral oxygen consumption and cerebral glucose consumption were 2.49 ± 0.13 mL/min/100 g tissue, and 6.83 ± 0.58 mg/min/100 g tissue at the normothermic cardiopulmonary bypass baseline. There were no intergroup differences. Recovery of cerebral oxygen consumption was more complete and occurred earlier in the piglets receiving UW solution than in either the control or saline-treated piglets (Figure 28–5). In contrast, there were no differences between the groups in the recovery of glucose consumption, with the values remaining around 50% of the pre-cooling value after three hours of normothermic reperfusion.

Lactate Levels.   The lactate levels in the cerebroplegia effluent were 2.42 ± 0.20 mM/L in group CPS, 2.69 ± 0.20 mM/L in group CPU, and 2.89 ± 0.09 mM/L in group CPM (p = .215). The systemic lactate levels were 2.69 ± 0.19 mM/L at baseline, increased to 8.48 ± 0.39 mM/L at 15 minutes of reperfusion, and stayed high until the end of reperfusion (7.07 ± 0.60 mM/L). There were no significant intergroup differences at any time.

Brain Water Content.   The brain water content at the end of experiment was significantly lower in the cerebroplegia-treated groups (80.7 ± 0.3% in group CPS, 80.5 ± 0.4% in group CPU, and 80.6 ± 0.3% in group CPM) than in the control group (82.1 ± 0.2%).

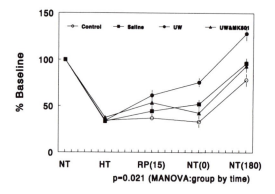

Cerebral Blood Flow

FIGURE 28–4.   Recovery of cerebral blood flow after two hours of hypothermic circulatory arrest in piglets receiving cerebroplegia solution.

CMRO2

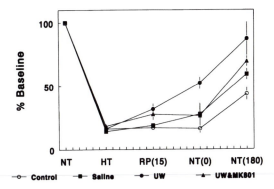

FIGURE 28–5. Recovery of cerebral oxygen consumption following two hours of hypothermic circulatory arrest in piglets receiving cerebroplegia solution.

Comment

This study demonstrated that simple saline infusion at 4°C improves the acute recovery of cerebral blood flow and metabolism after two hours of hypothermic circulatory arrest. Modification of the solution with UW solution further improved the recovery. The excitatory neurotransmitter antagonist MK-801 did not augment the protective effects of UW solution and reduced the recovery of cerebral blood flow.

The UW solution was developed for cold storage of organs for transplantation.[15] Improved organ preservation has been reported in the liver, kidney, pancreas, and heart. The UW solution does not contain glucose or any other substrates for energy production, and therefore does not preserve cellular high-energy phosphate levels during ischemia, as was observed in the present study and in studies of other organs. The beneficial effects of UW solution appear to be due to other cellular protective mechanisms during hypothermic ischemia and reperfusion. Adenosine, glutathione, allopurinol, and lactobionate seem to be particularly important components for the improved preservation.

Adenosine is an endogenous neuroprotective agent.[16,17] High levels of endogenous intracellular adenosine, which result from a breakdown of ATP during ischemia, depress cellular metabolic rate. Adenosine also blocks the release of the neurotransmitter glutamate (A1 receptor). Adenosine thereby may reduce the severity of excitotoxic injury. In addition, adenosine is a potent vasodilator (A2 receptor) and also blocks neutrophil activation (A2 receptor). We observed a hyperemic response in animals receiving UW solution alone; this response was not seen in the other groups. This hyperemia may have contributed to the more rapid warming of the brain during the reperfusion period as well as to the more rapid recovery of intracellular pH and ATP. Detrimental effects of blocking adenosine receptors by antagonists and protective effects of exogenous adenosine agonists on ischemic brain injury have been reported previously.

Glutathione is an intracellular compound that is essential for the reduction of cytotoxic agents, including hydrogen peroxide, lipid peroxides, and free radicals. These agents are thought to have important roles in reperfusion injury. Cellular glutathione is depleted during ischemia.[18] It has been demonstrated in liver and kidney preservation that the reduced form of glutathione plays an important role in the efficacy of UW solution. *Allopurinol* acts as both an inhibitor of xanthine oxidase and is also a scavenger of free radicals. Xanthine oxidase can produce superoxide radicals by catalyzing oxidation of hypoxanthine during reperfusion. The role of xanthine oxidase in cerebral ischemia/reperfusion injury seems limited. However, beneficial effects of allopurinol in reducing cerebral ischemic injury have been reported. *Lactobionate* is an impermeant anion and has been demonstrated to have important effects on suppressing cell swelling during cold storage of the liver.[19] Other components of UW solution include raffinose, an impermeant trisaccharide that may play a role in prevention of cellular swelling, and hydroxyethyl starch, which acts as a colloid to prevent interstitial edema. However, since brain water was the same in all the cerebroplegia groups, the role of these latter two compounds in the cerebroplegia may be less important.

In our study of systemic administration of MK-801 we demonstrated beneficial effects of MK-801 on postischemic recovery of high-energy phosphates after hypothermic circulatory arrest in our piglet model. However, when delivered as a cerebroplegia solution, MK-801 failed to add to the beneficial effects of UW solution on the postischemic recovery. The inhibitory effects of adenosine on excitatory amino acid release may partly explain the lack of an additional effect of MK-801 in the presence of UW solution. Another possibility is that the reduced cerebral blood flow recovery seen with MK-801, relative to UW solution alone, might have offset the protective effects of MK-801.

The effects of MK-801 on cerebral blood flow have not been well-studied. MK-801 could reduce cerebral blood flow by NMDA receptor blockade. Stimulation of NMDA receptors has been shown to increase nitric oxide (intraneuronal) production. Both neuronal as well as endothelial cell production of nitric oxide have a role in cerebral blood flow regulation. However, our finding that cerebral vascular reactivity to acetylcholine (i.e., endogenous nitric oxide production by endothelial cells) and to nitroglycerin (i.e., exogenously derived nitroglycerin) were both reduced by MK-801 relative to UW solution alone suggests a direct vasoconstrictive action of MK-801. Torregrosa and colleagues[20] have also reported a direct vasoconstrictive effect of MK-801.

The final ATP recovery of 73% at the end of 225 minutes reperfusion in the UW groups, while better than the other groups, is nevertheless less satisfactory in comparison with the recovery of 90% after one hour of hypothermic circulatory arrest observed in our previous study using the same model. Furthermore, in contrast to the previous study by Robbins et al.[1] using a simple crystalloid cerebroplegia solution, we continued to see complete loss of measurable high-energy phosphates as we had in previous studies in which cerebroplegia was not used. Perhaps use of the pH-stat strategy rather than alpha-stat may have improved recovery. We chose to use alpha-stat in the cerebroplegia study despite our previous findings suggesting improved recovery with pH-stat[21a] because alpha-stat continues to be widely used clinically and we wished to observe a maximal effect from the cerebroplegia solution. Perhaps further modification of the cerebroplegia solution may improve recovery. The high potassium concentration (140 mEq/L) in the standard UW solution raises a concern. High potassium concentrations depolarize the neuronal membrane and activate voltage-dependent ion channels including the calcium ion channel. Although UW solution contains no calcium, calcium ions in the interstitial space may not be washed out completely. Calcium ion influx plays an important role in ischemic neuronal injury . It has been reported that reversing the sodium/potassium concentration ratio does not alter the protective effects of UW solution in the liver or kidney.[21b] However, just as with cardioplegic solutions, the protective effects of UW solution may be improved by reversing the sodium/potassium ratio in an excitable tissue such as the brain. Further studies are needed for determination of optimal composition of the cerebroplegia solution.

The acute nature of this cerebroplegia study, i.e., the lack of correlation with neurological outcome or histopathology, was one of the important limitations of the study. This led us to undertake a survival study in which piglets were allowed to survive for five days following hypothermic circulatory arrest.[22] Ten Yorkshire pigs, age 5 weeks, were placed on cardiopulmonary bypass, cooled to 15°C, and subjected to 90 minutes deep hypothermic circulatory arrest. Group UW (n = 5) received one dose of 50 mL/kg 4°C UW solution delivered antegrade to the cerebral circulation. Group CON (n = 5) received no intervention other than circulatory arrest. Animals were reperfused, rewarmed to 35°C, and weaned from CPB. Neurologic assessments using neurologic deficit scoring (NDS, 0 = normal, 500 = brain death) and overall performance categories (OPC, 1 = normal, 5 = brain death) were performed at 24-hour intervals for five days. On the fifth postoperative day, brains were perfusion fixed and examined for histologic evidence of neuronal injury (0 = normal, 5 = severe injury).

UW solution delivered as antegrade cerebroplegia did not improve neurologic recovery at any time following deep hypothermic circulatory arrest. Three of the UW animals, but none of the control animals, experienced generalized seizures. Histologic examination revealed more damage in UW brains, primarily in the cerebral cortex. Unlike control animals, UW animals demonstrated extracortical injury in the cerebellum and hippocampus.

It is interesting to speculate why there should have been contradictory results between the short-term study and the survival study. The most likely explanation is that the very high potassium concentration in the UW solution, which resulted in an increase in the serum potassium to greater than 12 mM/L (despite attempts to discard the effluent from the cerebroplegia), significantly compromised the cardiac performance of these animals postoperatively. Previous studies have demonstrated that cerebral autoregulation is compromised after circulatory arrest. Therefore, a marginal cardiac output postoperatively may have compromised the cerebral outcome. An important methodological difference between the two studies may also help to explain the different results. In the short-term study the cerebroplegia was administered every 30 minutes during the total arrest time of two hours. In preliminary studies of the survival study, this protocol resulted in an unacceptably high serum potassium concentration. Therefore only a single dose was administered at the beginning of the 90-minute arrest period.

Retrograde Cerebral Perfusion

An alternative to antegrade delivery of a cerebroplegia solution to extend the safe duration of circulatory arrest is retrograde cerebral perfusion. This method has become popular in recent years and is now being widely applied for clinical surgery of the aortic arch in adults, even though there is relatively little information regarding the efficacy of this method in humans.[23,24]. The only study that has looked at any solution (other than the blood perfusate from the cardiopulmonary bypass circuit) delivered in a retrograde fashion is the study by Crittenden et al.[2] published in 1991 and described above (see Introduction). The animals employed in those studies were juvenile sheep. The methods of cerebral protection that were compared were systemic hypothermia alone, systemic hypothermia with external cooling of the head, retrograde cerebroplegia, and antegrade cerebroplegia. The solution used for cerebroplegia was a simple crystalloid solution. The only group that did not demonstrate a progressive improvement in neurological score following two hours of circulatory arrest was the group receiving retrograde cerebroplegia.

In a study by Mohri et al.[25] using dogs, histopathology, including examination for carbon black infused retrograde, suggested nonhomogeneous distribution of perfusate when delivered in this fashion, analogous to the heterogeneous distribution of retrograde cardioplegia to the myocardium. The authors cautioned against clinical use of this method until it has been more carefully examined. Midulla et al.[26] studied retrograde cerebral perfusion in the Yorkshire piglet. They were unable to use their usual model, the beagle puppy, because they found that venous valves prevented adequate cerebral perfusion. This problem has also been recognized in humans, leading to the recommendation of inserting the perfusion cannula into the internal jugular vein rather than relying on retrograde perfusion from the superior vena cava. Midulla et al. compared retrograde cerebral perfusion, antegrade perfusion, circulatory arrest alone, and circulatory arrest with the head packed in ice. In each group systemic hypothermia to an esophageal temperature of 20°C was employed within 90 minutes of the intervention. During a seven-day recovery period the behavioral score was lower in the animals with circulatory arrest alone than the other three groups. Recovery of quantitative EEG was better in the antegrade perfusion group than all other groups. Histological examination revealed ischemic injury in the circulatory arrest animals whether or not they had the head packed in ice, while only 1 of 6 animals with retrograde perfusion and none of those with antegrade perfusion had histopatholgic evidence of injury. Interestingly they found that only 5% of the perfusate delivered retrograde into the venous system returned to the aortic cannula, with the remainder finding its way to the inferior vena caval system. They also found that in some animals it was necessary to use very high pressure (70 mmHg) in the SVC to achieve an adequate superior saggital sinus perfusion pressure. They attributed this to the presence of venous valves.

Usui et al.[27] and a number of other Japanese groups have published extensively regarding retrograde cerebral perfusion. Usui et al. measured cerebral blood flow, oxygen consumption, and CSF pressure in dogs during retrograde cerebral perfusion. They found that CSF pressure remained lower than 25 mmHg so long as external jugular pressure remained lower than 25 mmHg. High external jugular pressure was associated with high intracranial pressure, which restricts cerebral blood flow and may cause brain edema. Usui et al. concluded that a venous pressure of 25 mmHg is the optimum pressure for retrograde cerebral perfusion. Nojima et al.[28] found in a similar study that a perfusion pressure of 20 mmHg resulted in satisfactory oxygen consumption and carbon dioxide production with no excess lactate. ATP and energy charge were significantly higher than with circulatory arrest alone. Perfusion at a pressure of 32 mmHg resulted in a significant increase in brain tissue water. It should be noted that it was necessary to cannulate both the right and left maxillary veins in these dogs because there is no internal jugular vein draining the brain as in the human. In addition there are many competent venous valves in the maxillary/external jugular venous system.

There have been a small number of clinical reports of the use of retrograde cerebral perfusion. Ueda et al. described 33 patients.[24] They used mean 40 minutes of retrograde cerebral perfusion in 33 patients at mean nasopharyngeal temperature 17°C. Two patients had strokes and four patients died. The remaining patients were said to have had no complications related to the use of retrograde cerebral perfusion, though there is no information regarding careful prospective neurological and behavioral analyses of this new technique of cerebral protection. The same is true of the paper by Safi et al.[23] in which 11 patients underwent retrograde cerebral perfusion for mean 35 minutes at a mean nasopharyngeal temperature of 15°C. One patient suffered a stroke and no patients died. It is hoped that in future clinical studies there will be appropriately careful neuropsychometric analysis. Until such studies are available it would be prudent for surgeons considering using this method not to exceed the limits considered acceptable for hypothermic circulatory arrest alone.

References

1. Robbins RC, Balaban RS, Swain JA. Intermittent hypothermic asanguineous cerebral perfusion (cerebroplegia) protects the brain during prolonged circulatory arrest: A phosphorous 31 nuclear magnetic resonance study. *J Thorac Cardiovasc Surg* 1990;99:878–884.
2. Crittenden MD, Roberts CS, Rosa L, et al. Brain protection during circulatory arrest. *Ann Thorac Surg* 1991;51:942–947.
3. Dawson VL, Dawson T, London E, Bredt D, Snyder S. Nitric oxide mediates glutamate neurotoxicity in primary cortical cultures. *Proc Natl Acad Sci USA* 1991;88:6368–6371.
4. Redmond JM, Gillinov AM, Zehr JK, et al. Glutamate excitotoxicity: A mechanism of neurologic injury associated with hypothermic circulatory arrest. *J Thorac Cardiovasc Surg* 1994;107:776–787.
5. Kriegelstein J, Oberpichler-Schwenk H. *Pharmacology of cerebral ischemia.* Stuttgart: Wissenschaftliche Verlagsgesellschaft mbH, 1994.
6. Aoki M, Nomura F, Stromski ME, Tsuji MK, Fackler JC, Hickey PR, Holtzman D, Jonas RA. Effects of MK-801 and NBQX on acute recovery of piglet cerebral metabolism after hypothermic circulatory arrest. *J Cereb Blood Flow Metab* 1994;14:156–165.
7. Ment LR, Stewart WB, Petroff OA, Duncan CC, Montoya D. Beagle puppy model of perinatal asphyxia: Blockade of excitatory neurotransmitters. *Pediatr Neurol* 1989;5:281–286.
8. Haraldseth O, Gronas T, Southon TE, Jynge P, Gisvole SE, Unsgard G. The NMDA antagonist MK-801 improved metabolic recovery after 10 minutes global cerebral ischemia in rats measured with ^{31}P magnetic resonance spectroscopy. *Acta Neurochir* (Wien) 1990;106:32–36.
9. Corbett D, Evans S, Thomas C, Wang D, Jonas RA. MK-801 reduces cerebral ischemic injury by inducing hypothermia. *Brain Res* 1990;514:300–304.
10. Sheardown MJ, Nielson EO, Hansen AJ, Jacobsen P, Honore T. 2,3-Dihydroxy-6-nitro-7-sulfamoyl-benzo(F)quinoxaline: A neuroprotectant for cerebral ischemia. *Science* 1990;247:571–574.
11. Aoki M, Jonas RA, Nomura F, Stromski ME, Tsuji MK, Hickey PR, Holtzman D. Effects of cerebroplegic solutions during hypothermic circulatory arrest and short-term recovery. *J Thorac Cardiovasc Surg* 1994;108:291–301.
12. Aoki M, Jonas RA, Nomura F, Stromski ME, Tsuji MK, Hickey PR, Holtzman DH. Effects of aprotinin on acute recovery of cerebral metabolism in piglets after hypothermic circulatory arrest. *Ann Thorac Surg* 1994;58:146–153.
13. Aoki M, Jonas RA, Nomura F, Kawata H, Hickey PR. Impact of monoclonal antibody to leukocyte adhesion molecule CD18 on deleterious effects of cardio-

pulmonary bypass and hypothermic circulatory arrest in immature piglets. *J Card Surg*, in press.

14. Kawata H, Fackler JC, Aoki M, Tsuji MK, Sawatari K, Offutt M, Hickey PR, Holtzman D, Jonas RA. Recovery of cerebral blood flow and energy state after hypothermic circulatory arrest versus low-flow bypass in piglets. *J Thorac Cardiovasc Surg* 1993;106:671–685.

15. Belzer FO, Southard JH. Principles of solid-organ preservation by cold storage. *Transplantation* 1988;45:673–676.

16. Marangos PJ, Boulenger JP. Basic and clinical aspects of adenosinergic neuro-modulation. *Neurosci Biobehav Rev* 1985;9:421–430.

17. Dragunow M, Faull RL. Neuroprotective effects of adenosine. *Trends Pharmacol Sci* 1988;9:193–194.

18. Fuller BJ, Lunec J, Healing G, Simpkin S, Green CJ. Reduction of suscepti-bility to lipid perooxidation by deferoxamine in rabbit kidneys subjected to 24-hour cold ischemia and preservation. *Transplantation* 1987;43:604–606.

19. Jamieson NV, Lindell S, Sundberg R, Southard JH, Belzer FO. An analysis of the components in UW solution using the isolated perfused rabbit liver. *Transplantation* 1988;46:512–516.

20. Torregrosa G, Salom JB, Miranda FJ, Alabadi JA, Alvarez JA, Alborch E. In vivo and in vitro effects of the NMDA receptor antagonist dizocilpine (MK-801) on the cerebrovascular bed of the goat. *J Cereb Blood Flow Metab* 1991;11 (suppl 2):S287.

21a. Aoki M, Nomura F, Stromski ME, Tsuji MK, Fackler JC, Hickey PR, Holtzman D, Jonas RA. Effects of pH on brain energetics after hypothermic circulatory arrest. *Ann Thorac Surg* 1993;55:1093–2103.

21b. Jamieson NV, Lindell S, Sundberg R, Southard JH, Belzer FO. An analysis of the components in UW solution using the isolated perfused rabbit liver. *Transplanation* 1988;46:512–516.

22. Forbess JM, Ibla JC, Lidov H, Cioffi M, Hiramatsu T, Laussen P, Miura T, Jonas RA. Survival of immature swine after cardiopulmonary bypass and hypo-thermic circulatory arrest: The delivery of University of Wisconsin solution. *Ann Thorac Surg*, in press.

23. Safi HJ, Brien HW, Winter JN, Thomas AC, Maulsby RL, Doerr HK, Svensson GL. Brain protection via cerebral retrograde perfusion during aortic arch aneurysm repair. *Ann Thorac Surg* 1993;56:270–276.

24. Ueda Y, Miki S, Okita Y, Tahata T, Ogino H, Sakai T, Morioka K, Matsuyama K. Protective effect of continuous retrograde cerebral perfusion on the brain dur-ing deep hypothermic systemic circulatory arrest. *J Card Surg* 1994;9:584–595.

25. Mohri H, Sadahiro M, Akimoto H, Haneda K, Tabayashi K, Ohmi M. Protection of the brain during hypothermic perfusion. *Ann Thorac Surg* 1993;56:1493–1496.

26. Midulla PS, Gandsas A, Sadeghi AM, Mezrow CK, Yerlioglu ME, Wang W, Wolfe D, Ergin MA, Griepp RB. Comparison of retrograde cerebral perfusion to antegrade cerebral perfusion and hypothermic circulatory arrest in a chronic porcine model. *J Card Surg* 1994;9:560–575.

27. Usui A, Oohara K, Liu TL, Murase M, Tanaka M, Takeuchi E, Abe T. Deter-mination of optimum retrograde cerebral perfusion conditions. *J Thorac Car-diovasc Surg* 1994;107:300–308.

28. Nojima T, Magara T, Nakajima Y, Waterida S, Onoe M, Sugita T, Mori A. Optimal perfusion pressure for experimental cerebral perfusion. *J Card Surg* 1994;9:548–559.

Index

Illustrations appear on pages that are set in **boldface** type. Tables appear on pages that are set in *italic* type.